Edited by
GRAHAM THORNIC
CHRIS R. BREWIN
JOHN WING

Measuring Mental Health Needs

GASKELL

Gaskell is an imprint of the Royal College of Psychiatrists,
17 Belgrave Square, London SW1

British Library Cataloguing-in-Publication Data
  Measuring Mental Health Needs
    I. Thornicroft, G. J.
    362.2

ISBN 0-902241-51-6

Distributed in North America
by American Psychiatric Press, Inc.
ISBN 0-880486-17-1

Phototypeset by Dobbie Typesetting Ltd., Tavistock, Devon
Printed in Great Britain by Henry Ling Ltd., Dorchester, Dorset

Contents

Contributors

Paul Bebbington, Reader, MRC Social and Community Psychiatry Unit, Institute of Psychiatry, De Crespigny Park, London SE5 8AF

Jeni Beecham, Personal Social Services Research Unit, Cornwallis Building, University of Kent, Canterbury, Kent CT2 7NF

Sir Douglas Black, The Old Forge, Duchess Close, Whitchurch on Thames, Berkshire RG8 7EN

William R. Breakey, Department of Psychiatry and Behavioral Sciences, The Johns Hopkins University School of Medicine, 600 N. Wolfe Street, Baltimore, MD 21287 USA

Chris Brewin, Professor, Department of Psychology, Royal Holloway, University of London, Egham Hill, Egham, Surrey TW20 0EX

Tom Fryers, District Offices, Priors Lea, Abbey Road, Barrow-in-Furness, Cumbria LA13 9JU

Howard Goldman, Director, Mental Health Policy Studies, Department of Psychiatry, University of Maryland School of Medicine, 645 West Redwood Street, Baltimore, MD 21201 USA

Ian Greatorex, Department of Community Medicine, Manchester University, Swinton Road, Manchester M13

Steven Hirsch, Professor of Psychiatry, Department of Psychiatry, Charing Cross Hospital, Fulham Palace Road, London W6 8RF

Brian Jarman, Professor, Department of General Practice, Lisson Grove Health Centre, Gateforth Street, London NW8 8EG

Rachel Jenkins, Mental Health Division, Department of Health, Wellington House, 133–135 Waterloo Road, London SE1 8UG

Martin Knapp, Personal Social Services Research Unit, Cornwallis Building, University of Kent, Canterbury, Kent CT2 7NF

Liz Kuipers, DSC, The Maudsley Hospital, Denmark Hill, London SE5 8AZ; Department of Psychology, Institute of Psychiatry, London SE5 8AF

Joseph P. Morrissey, Sheps Center for Health Services Research, University of North Carolina, Chapel Hill, NC 27599 USA

Elaine Murphy, Section of Psychogeriatrics, United Medical and Dental Schools, Guy's Hospital, St Thomas' Street, London SE1 9RT

James Raftery, Department of Public Health, St George's Hospital Medical School, Blackshaw Road, Tooting, London SW19

M. Susan Ridgely, Mental Health Policy Studies, Department of Psychiatry, University of Maryland School of Medicine, 645 West Redwood Street, Baltimore, MD 21201 USA

Peter Rohde, Emeritus Consultant, Riverside Health Authority, 53 Harley Street, London W1N 1DD

Philip Seager, Director, Health Advisory Service, Sutherland House, 29–37 Brighton Road, Sutton, Surrey SM2 5AN (retired)

Andrew Stevens, Wessex Institute of Public Health Medicine, Down House, Highcroft, Romsey Road, Winchester SO22 5DH

Geraldine Strathdee, Consultant Psychiatrist, Maudsley Hospital, Denmark Hill, London SE5 8AZ

Ezra Susser, Box 24, New York State Psychiatric Institute, 722 W. 168th Street, New York, NY 10032 USA

Jason Taylor, Locum Consultant Psychiatrist, Whittington Hospital, Highgate Hill, London N19 5NF

Graham Thornicroft, Senior Lecturer, PRiSM Director, Institute of Psychiatry, and Consultant Psychiatrist, Maudsley Hospital, Denmark Hill, London SE5 8AF

Philip Timms, Registrar, Department of Psychiatry, Guy's and St Thomas' UMDS, Guy's Hospital, St Thomas' Street, London SE1 9RT

John Wing, Director, Research Unit, Royal College of Psychiatrists, 17 Belgrave Square, London SW1X 8PG

Foreword

SIR DOUGLAS BLACK

In an ideal world, demands for health care would accurately reflect health needs, and would themselves in turn be satisfied by adequate and appropriate provision of services. In the world in which we actually live, there are health needs which fail to arouse demand, being either accepted as part of life's burden, or unappreciated through simple failure to detect them or to recognise that anything can be done about them. However, demands are voiced from time to time for which it is difficult to detect or define any corresponding needs – unless perhaps the very making of a health-related demand itself constitutes a health need. This discrepancy between need and demand is important in relation to service provision, perhaps particularly because choices between alternative provisions are commonly made not as a sequel to a dispassionate appraisal and comparison of conflicting needs, but in response to the demands of pressure groups or to simple political expediency.

Such considerations make it particularly important for those qualified to do so to undertake an objective study of the constellation of needs in the field in which they are expert. Only after such an analysis is it possible to argue for what would seem to be a desirable transition, from a 'demand-led' service to a 'needs-led' service. Of course, in relation to provision of services, the weighting given to a defined need has to be modulated by considering whether in the present state of the art it can be 'cured', 'relieved', 'palliated', or in the last resort 'accepted'. The recognition and quantification of those needs which can be met is obviously of immediate importance; less obviously there is also value in the recognition and definition of needs for which there is at present no available remedy. That value consists not only in stimulating research towards a future remedy, but also in laying down the base of information for planning support services for what cannot yet be cured.

The task implicit in the title of this book is thus important; it is also distinctly difficult. Assessment of need in relation to physical illness is hard enough; when I was involved in studying the relationship between deprivation and ill health we had very largely to wield the Occam's razor of analysing the bills of mortality. Such draconian measures have fortunately little relevance to analysing needs in mental impairment and illness. However, in relation to both bodily and mental disorder, there has in the past decade been considerable interest and advance in the analysis of the effects of illness on various aspects of well-being. Such analysis has to be multidimensional, comprising measures of physical and mental performance, subjective perception of well-being, fitness for work, social adaptation, and ability to participate in leisure activities. Such studies of what has been grouped under the term 'quality of life' are a necessary complement to older approaches based on diagnostic categories which may be less than clear-cut.

The editors of this book deserve warm commendation, first for tackling a difficult and important range of problems; then for assembling a group of experts capable of discussing the various aspects of a complicated and still evolving field of study; and finally for producing a work which is both scholarly and practical. As with physical disease, the provision of services for mental health is far too important to be left to the uninstructed play of market forces. I am confident that this book makes an important, and indeed necessary, contribution to the logical development of mental health services in this and other countries.

1 Defining mental health needs

JOHN WING, CHRIS R. BREWIN and GRAHAM THORNICROFT

This chapter sets the agenda for the book by listing and defining the terms used in needs assessment. The topics covered include both clinical audit, i.e. analysis of face-to-face assessment of need followed by intervention and reassessment of outcome, and the epidemiologically-based equivalents required to plan and manage a geographical area rationally.

The chapter is divided into individual needs and those of an 'average' Health District. The limitations of the restriction to NHS services are obvious and will become more so as the book proceeds and the all-pervading overlap with other social and private services is documented. The principles of definition, however, remain constant as these boundaries are crossed, and will be highly relevant when joint commissioning becomes mandatory. A further limitation is imposed by the omission of primary prevention. This requires a book to itself.

Most of the following chapters deal in a practical way with specific aspects of needs assessment. The many problems raised are reconsidered in the final chapter, using the issues raised somewhat theoretically in this one to systematise the discussion.

The needs of individuals

Mental health and mental illness

Mental health is a social concept, which varies from one society or culture to another. It is therefore dangerous to define mental illness in terms of a deviation from health. However, personal concepts of illness and the recognition of need for help are affected by prevailing social expectations. Such concepts cannot be ignored now that 'mental health budgets' are in competition with the budgets of all other health specialities and, within the speciality, limited funds must be divided between common but less severe and rarer but more persistently disabling disorders.

Mental illness is based on concepts of symptoms and signs of 'dysfunction', resulting from deviation from normal psychological and physiological systems of functioning. Links between the two kinds of system are firmer and less controversial at two ends of the spectrum of severity – cognitive and autonomic disorders. In the case of psychotic, particularly schizophrenic, disorders, the argument is based on the absence of social content from the definition of basic psychological symptoms, which are technically recognisable irrespective of social or cultural context. The affective disorders come somewhere in between.

Symptoms and signs can now be recognised fairly reliably by trained practitioners in most parts of the world. The application of standardised sets of rules then results in reasonably reliable diagnoses. But diagnosis, in itself, does not lead directly to the formulation of needs; other factors must be taken into account. A consideration of concepts of disability and handicap illustrates some of these.

Concepts of disability

The World Health Organization's Illness, Disability, and Handicap (IDH) classification of the consequences of disease and injury works well for many straightforward medical problems (World Health Organization, 1980). The first level of the classification is concerned with a concept of 'impairment', which involves loss or abnormality of function. This concept is appropriate for the psychological impairments or dysfunctions that underlie the basic psychiatric symptoms.

At a second level lie 'disabilities', which involve restrictions on personal activities that may be directly caused by impairments.

At a third level, impairments and disabilities usually lead to 'handicaps', which involve disadvantages in interacting with or adapting to the individual's environment. A simple example is a violinist who develops arthritis of a finger joint (disease), which results in some loss of movement (impairment), little personal restriction (disability), but a serious occupational block (handicap).

There are two kinds of problem in adapting the IDH system for use with psychiatric disorders. Firstly, the distinction between impairment and disability is difficult (although not impossible) to draw when the impairment is psychological. Secondly, the direction of cause and effect is drawn firmly from left to right. Although there is some discussion in the IDH text as to how social factors might influence disorder, impairment, and disability (right to left), no criteria are suggested and the classification, in effect, ignores these possibilities.

In addition there is a semantic problem. The terms 'disability' and 'handicap' are used interchangeably in common speech and it is very difficult to allocate separate meanings to them. For present purposes, we need to begin, rather than end, with a concept of social disablement that includes any substantial inability to perform up to personal expectation, or to the expectations of important others, and is associated with psychiatric disorder or impairment. Someone who *can* perform to expectation, but chooses not to, would be excluded by definition.

Severity of disablement

The severity of disablement, therefore, results (a) from the severity and duration of impairment, that is, psychological and physiological dysfunctions, (b) from adverse circumstances and disadvantages both past and present that can affect social functioning independently, and (c) from personal reactions to the first two factors, including loss of self-esteem and motivation. For convenience, (a) is measured in terms of the presence and severity of symptoms and behaviour of various kinds, (b) in terms of environmental adversity, and (c) in terms of self-attitudes.

Each component should be assessed separately so that a profile of problems is available, on which judgements of need can be made. The clinical severity of symptoms, for example, can be measured in terms of intensity and persistence. Intensity tends to be equivalent to intrusiveness, which affects more general mental functioning and, in turn, affects behaviour and lowers social functioning. This is true across the whole range of symptoms, from anxiety to auditory hallucinations. Psychotic symptoms are more likely to be intrusive and persistent, and to affect behaviour more severely, than neurotic or non-specific symptoms, but both groups of disorders can be manifested throughout the whole range of severity.

Specific features of behaviour are often determined by symptoms. For example, overactivity associated with mania has features that differentiate it from overactivity associated with delirium, schizophrenia, agitated depression, or panic. However, there are also features in common that require a similar pattern of treatment or management. People with many different disorders, or none, may harm themselves or be violent to others. Socially embarrassing behaviour can occur across all diagnoses.

Social disablement is therefore associated with an amalgam of factors that produce a pattern, level, and persistence of malfunctioning that is not diagnosis-specific. It is this pattern, level, and duration that principally determine need for care and services. Both in the general population (Hurry & Sturt, 1981) and in cross-sections of people in contact with specialist services (Clifford & Webb, personal communication), the greater the number and severity of symptoms, the more severe social disablement tends to be.

Duration carries further implications, since the other two components may be amplified if impairment persists. For example, persisting impairment may itself lead to stigma, a low standard of living, and demoralisation. These, in turn, can amplify clinical manifestations such as depression and anxiety.

Diagnosis-related groups (DRGs) cannot, therefore, be used in isolation to determine needs. One DRG, such as 'psychosis' can account for a substantial proportion of all admissions, allowing no discrimination between real needs. A multifactorial, or 'casemix', approach is essential (Taube *et al*, 1984). Casemix allows the assignment of patients to recognisable groups, which reflect the problems that give rise to a need for some form of care and the cost of that care.

Targets: health gain and the prevention of disability

Thus the target for interventions by the health and social services, in practice, should be two-fold. One aim is to reduce the severity of social disablement associated with mental disorder. Any such reduction can be called a 'health gain'. The other aim is to prevent the amplification of any disablement that cannot be further reduced. Both aims require disentanglement of the three components of disablement, despite the difficulty of doing so, because each may require its own forms of intervention.

An analysis of this kind leads to setting specific targets for the provision of treatment and care, professional staff (agents) to provide it, and settings for staff and user to work in. These targets must be realistic and defined in such a way that it is possible to measure the extent to which they are being met, i.e. measurable outcomes. Detailed examples of mental health targets are given in Chapter 2.

Care and services: terminology

Care will be defined in terms of the medical, psychological, and social interventions that are used as 'state of the art' by well trained mental health practitioners. It includes treatment, rehabilitation, counselling, training, supervision, resettlement, and welfare. Since the term comprises reduction and further prevention of social disablement (not only the care required for symptoms and behavioural problems), it automatically includes the provision of special enabling opportunities to individuals who cannot use ordinary amenities because of temporary or persisting impairments, and therefore also includes attention to quality of life. By the same token, care also involves attention to the environment of sheltered or protected settings or activities, in order to preserve and enhance social functioning. Interventions of these kinds which are designed to prevent disablement becoming worse, rather than to reduce its severity, are included in the same way.

The term *services* includes several components. Three need to be separately specified – the agents, settings, and the organisation necessary to deliver care.

Care is provided by formal *care agents* or staff, specifically trained for their functions, or by non-specific formal agents whose work often brings them into contact with mentally ill people – for example, police, firefighters and, ambulance staff. Informal agents include relatives, friends, befrienders, and voluntary workers.

Care agents require *settings* to work in, including every kind from a domiciliary visit (or even a visit 'on the street') to a high security ward.

Case management is a term with unduly patronising, if not authoritarian, overtones but it is intended to connote a process to ensure continuity of needs-led services. *Care co-ordination* is perhaps a more accurate term. There are National Health Service (NHS) and social service department (SSD) versions. Whatever the term used, the intention is that the case manager should be a care worker, such as nurse or a social worker, who assesses needs and who coordinates the delivery of a 'package of care' to the service user (Thornicroft, 1991*a*). However, it appears from Social Service Inspectorate guidance documents, that this concept is being superseded by a narrower one, that of a 'care manager' who is seen as a purchaser and coordinator of care, using a brokerage model, and without any necessary direct care responsibilities (see Chapter 16).

Needs for care and service

Economical definitions of terms used in needs assessment were provided by Matthew (1971). Suitably adapted and broadened (Wing, 1972; Brewin & Wing, 1989), they will be used throughout the rest of this chapter. More specifically, needs are defined in terms of problems for which 'state of the art' solutions exist. The following definitions are based upon a needs-assessment system intended to promote comparisons between different populations, whether for clinical, research, or planning purposes (Brewin *et al*, 1987; Brewin & Wing, 1989). The principles are derived from a model of day-to-day clinical practice but they are not intended to be prescriptive.

Need

Need can be defined either in terms of the type of impairment or other factor causing social disablement or of the model of treatment or other intervention required to meet it, for example, hip replacement, insulin regime for diabetes, medication for auditory hallucinations.

If an individual is socially disabled, in association with a mental disorder for which an effective and acceptable form or model of care exists, either for amelioration or prevention, the individual is in need of that intervention. There will usually be a hierarchy of methods, at the top of which may be one that produces a complete and rapid recovery with no extra ill-effects. At the bottom there will usually be methods of amelioration, or prevention of relapse or amplification of disablement.

The fact that needs are defined does not mean that they will be met. Some may remain unmet for the immediate future because other problems must be dealt with first, or because the more effective method is not available locally, or because availability is limited by rationing, or because the person in need objects, or because there are other reasons why the intervention should not be made. There are also 'potential' needs for forms of care that do not at the moment exist but which research may eventually provide. Moreover, voluntary organisations may develop services for needs that are not at present recognised or understood by most professionals.

Two further points should be clearly understood. Firstly, the definition does not exclude interventions that, for whatever reason, are locally unavailable. If a method of help is known, a need for it exists. Secondly, the acquiescence of an individual in a situation that precludes the needed intervention does not overrule the need. Thus many people in mental hospitals in the 1960s had grown used to their situation and a needs assessment would not have revealed problems requiring such a setting. Some who wished to stay were helped to move to less occupationally and residentially restrictive settings and, in retrospect, were pleased to have done so (Wing & Brown, 1970). A similar problem arose when a new long-stay hostel-ward was introduced as an alternative to remaining on busy acute wards (Wykes, 1982). A needs assessment is not intended to endorse the status quo. It is important not to define need in terms of the care, agent or setting already in place, thus automatically perpetuating the present allocation and priorities. It is not intended either to lead to the imposition of an official set of priorities on unwilling people. A professionally defined need may remain unmet, and have to be replaced by one lower in the hierarchy, simply because the user disagrees that there is such a need.

The specification of an intervention, if available, and accepted by the user following 'negotiation', leads to the choice of an agent to provide the care and a setting in which user and carer can interact (Mangen & Brewin, 1991).

Demand

A demand for care exists when individuals express a wish to receive it. Some demands are expressed in an unsophisticated form, for example, 'something needs to be done'. The user should be involved in a negotiation as to what interventions should be provided for what problems. This includes an explanation of the options. The process should not be purely top-down.

Provision

Provision includes interventions, agents, and settings, whether or not used. Care coordination entails providing such a pattern of service after initial assessment and then updating the assessment regularly in order to check outcomes and to modify the pattern if needs remain unmet or change.

Overprovision is provision without need. Underprovision is need without provision (unmet need).

Utilisation

Utilisation occurs when an individual actually receives care, for example, bed occupancy.

Need may not be expressed as demand; demand is not necessarily followed by provision or, if it is, by utilisation; and there can be demand, provision and utilisation without real underlying need for the particular service used.

The clinical audit cycle

The definition of audit provided by the Department of Health (1989) has frequently been quoted and widely accepted:

> "Medical audit can be defined as the systematic, critical analysis of the quality of medical care, including the procedures used for diagnosis and treatment, the use of resources, and the resulting outcome and quality of life for the patient."

This definition can be complemented by the description of quality of care by the Institute of Medicine of the National Academy of Medicine, Washington (Lohr, 1990).

> "The degree to which health services for individuals and populations increase the likelihood of desired health outcomes and are consistent with current professional knowledge."

Psychiatry is necessarily practised in a multidisciplinary environment because the problems presented by patients usually have a substantially larger psychosocial component than in most other medical specialities. With the exception of some who have accumulated from the past in long-stay wards, nearly all patients are treated in community settings most of the time. The switch from large single-speciality hospitals to small psychiatric day and in-patient departments in District General Hospitals, backing up (at least by intention) a broad range of community services, will continue to cause changes in clinical practice for a decade to come. Part of this responsibility is shared with clinical psychologists, general practitioners, community psychiatric nurses, social workers and other professionals involved in day and residential care and domiciliary visiting, and a significant portion of the work involves settings that are not part of the hospital services.

It is not appropriate to apply the term 'medical' audit to such a broad range of activities, particularly since the integrated team approach to patient care has gained acceptance throughout medicine. 'Clinical audit' covers both the strictly medical and the more psychosocial aspects of psychiatric practice, whatever the setting. The multidisciplinary context means that the role of the consultant psychiatrist can be central for audit, in terms of influence, guidance, coordination, training and, above all, continuity. Most consultants stay in post in their districts for years and are in a position to acquire a deep and comprehensive knowledge of all the local services, their management and their personnel. In particular, psychiatrists must be aware of the social as well as the health aspects of their practice and that it will often be impractical to audit one without the other.

These considerations are underlined by the proposals in the National Health Service and Community Care Act 1990 (House of Commons, 1990), which require health, social and non-statutory services to cooperate closely in the provision of care for people with chronic or frequently recurring mental disorders of all kinds. The interdependence of health and social care for such people cannot be overemphasised. Health Authorities are charged with the responsibility for providing 'health care' to people for whom social services departments are providing 'social care', and vice versa. The specific grant for provision of social-care services for people with a mental illness is intended precisely to promote this collaboration. Questions of assessment and care coordination have also been addressed.

The classical audit cycle, with its three central components – the measurement of structure (staff and settings), process (care activities), and outcome – is usually discussed in the context of peer review, 'a frank discussion between doctors, on a regular basis and without fear of criticism, of the quality of care provided as judged against agreed standards'. The aims of audit are to identify and act on opportunities to improve the quality of face-to-face clinical care, and to enlarge the scope of clinical education. And 'where deficiencies in care can be attributed to lack of resources it necessarily impinges on resource provision and financial audit'. These aims go beyond single-case audits and merge into those of clinical and services research, which are dealt with later. An example, auditing the reasons for admission to a psychiatric hospital, is given in Chapter 12.

Needs-assessment techniques

Methods of needs assessment can be used to extend, systematise and generalise from the principles of clinical audit, by measuring structure, process and outcome against standard guidelines, which are specified in advance. Chapter 13 describes one technique in particular. The guidelines suggested can be challenged, but use of the system allows comparisons to be made, and the construction and publication of alternatives.

Quality of care and quality of life

Decreasing disablement does not automatically lead to an increase in the quality of life but it will usually increase the options available to the individual to make use of the amenities available to the generality of local people although, clearly, the richness and variety of the social and economic opportunities available will vary. Some impairments, however, affect motivation and drive, or impose a pattern of behaviour or thought that makes it difficult for the person afflicted to use 'open' amenities. Access to public facilities may be denied or unwise. Enabling measures are then necessary in order to find other ways of realising unused potentialities.

Quality of life is therefore measurable in terms of physical necessities such as heat, light, shelter, food, security, and so on, which must be provided for people who cannot procure them otherwise. A second measure should be concerned with the quality of such provisions themselves – in particular, in terms of the quality of the environment and the choice available. Finally, there is the quality of personal life, the extent to which a disabled individual can maintain self-respect and autonomy, keep up interests, make a recognised contribution to society and increase in self-knowledge.

In serving these ends, quality of care and quality of life are two sides of the same coin. Fig. 1.1 shows the inter-relationships between the factors involved in decreasing social disablement, and in enabling quality assurance.

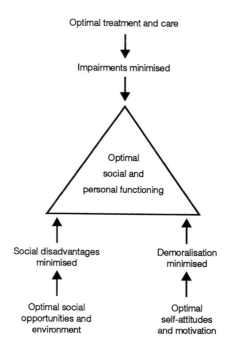

Fig. 1.1. Three components of quality assurance

The needs of groups

The epidemiology of need

The model for ordinary clinical practice has been outlined above. It is to assess an individual in order to construct a partial or complete care plan, implement it, and then follow-up for reassessment. The single-case audit cycle follows the same model. This contrasts with assessment of the needs of a diagnostic group, or of people with a particular type of clinical problem (for example, parasuicide, or admission under the Mental Health Act), or of those requiring a particular form of treatment, or agent, or setting. In such cases, the same assessment model can be used to measure the needs of each member of the relevant group, in order to obtain a summary profile of group needs.

The needs of a defined population, such as the one for which a district health authority (DHA) is responsible, can most thoroughly be assessed in the same bottom-up way (see Chapter 6). The top-down information requirements of management and planning (based on national, regional, and local targets and guidelines) involve the collection of administrative and financial data as well.

Mental health information systems

A comprehensive mental health information system, therefore, would cover both kinds of collection and use, and the output would be available, within the limits of confidentiality, to all. Such a system would include both statistical and non-numerical information concerning:

(a) local history, topography, and communications
(b) sociodemographic indices and epidemiology
(c) local services (agents and settings), their functioning and efficiency
(d) clinical data about the needs of people in contact with services and how far they are being met
(e) opinions of local users and informal carers.

Such systems would provide a database for national and regional returns, local resource allocation and target setting, district needs and outcome assessment, casemix, care plans, clinical records, and the audit of clinical care. In order to create and maintain the system, high quality clinical information is needed that can only be obtained with the consistent collaboration of clinical teams, who have to be convinced of the practical value to them and to the people they are caring for.

The Körner Committee (Department of Health and Social Security, 1982) recommended a 'minimum data set' that should be collected across the whole of the hospital services. It was not principally concerned with the needs of people with mental disorders or with services that were community-based. The Mental Health Enquiry (MHE), which had provided a more or less continuous series of mental health statistics for decades, required only that a relatively simple manually-produced set of data should be collected and sent for central processing. It was abandoned in 1986, together with the Hospital Activity Analysis.

A new set of indicators, based on the Körner data set, was issued in 1989, but it was chiefly concerned with the needs of acute medicine and surgery. The needs of psychiatry were not well represented; the gap being particularly obvious for psychiatric services not based in hospital wards. This was not so important in the days of the MHE, when the budget for mental-illness services was relatively non-competitive – in effect, 'ring-fenced', as Griffiths (1988) later recommended. However, the increasing specificity of management requirements backed by financial budgeting has changed the situation.

It therefore becomes very important to judge the quality of the data collected for health service indicators (HSIs) such as CP35 (% total number of mental-illness nurses employed in community), or DC41 (% discharges to NHS hospitals outside the district). Cooper (1989) pointed out that a system of local psychiatric case registers had existed for which quality of data-collection had been a high priority. He recommended that the experience be utilised when setting up any alternative system to the MHE. In particular, the staff who oversee the data collection should also be concerned with the final output, and since sequences of data about individuals have to be collected, a series of checks should be introduced to make sure that new data are consistent with the old. Such psychiatric case registers are described in Chapter 5.

A further problem arises from the multi-agency nature of psychiatric services, in which people follow complex paths from unit to unit, only some of which come under the aegis of the Health Authority. Domiciliary visiting has now taken a broader meaning. Some CPNs work directly with general practitioners (GPs), without being part of a specialist mental health team. A Mental Health Information System must be capable of coping with such forms of service, and provide data of value to clinical teams, purchasers, and providers.

In particular, the setting of clinical, as well as financial and administrative targets, demands the continuous collection of data that would serve to determine the outcome of interventions for problems, as in the classic audit and needs-assessment cycles. It is as important for members of clinical teams to take part in such a monitoring process and to learn how to utilise the knowledge that it can provide, as it is for administrators to understand the central requirement for planning of good quality bottom-up information.

Further changes in information requirements are being made as a result of the White Paper *Working for Patients* (NHS Management Executive, 1991).

These are set out, in draft, in a series of massive volumes called *The Data Manual*. A substantial increase in coverage, both of in-patient services (Module 1) and of day units, community teams, and other forms of non-hospital services, is suggested (Module 2). Clinical psychology and private mental nursing homes are included in Module 3, devoted to 'paramedical' services. The fourth module is concerned with estates and the others are technical. Whether all this information can, in fact, be collected, accurately and on time, depends on the collectors, not the designers.

A substantial change arises from the new distinction between purchaser (DHA) and provider functions, which entails a requirement to identify each party to the contract separately, for all spells of care.

> "Each DHA is required to monitor the health needs of its resident population and place contracts to cover its anticipated health needs. Data on past and current utilisation of services are essential for planning health care." (House of Commons, 1990)

This purchasing responsibility, however, can only be carried out by obtaining data from the providers under contract. A 'hospital provider spell' replaces the concept of a 'district spell'. Homelessness also makes for difficulty (see Chapter 16), as does the definition of who is a district resident. Thus, there may be problems in collecting data with an epidemiological base (Wing, 1992). The more general needs of purchasers are discussed in Chapter 3.

A long-term aim, strongly to be welcomed, is the proposal to establish patient-based information systems, 'so that contacts with individual clients can be built into person-identified episodes of care, each with an agreed provider minimum data set'. This principle of record linkage allows counts based on individuals as well as on events. It is most economically implemented, as demonstrated by the Psychiatric Case Registers (Wing, 1989), by relating information to dates of contact. Rohde & Taylor describe two recently developed computerised case-record systems in Chapter 14, while further discussion of the present and future scope for computerised clinical assessments is provided by Thornicroft in Chapter 15.

Sociodemographic indices of need

The classic epidemiological studies of the early post-war years provided strong evidence that people who developed schizophrenia and people who committed suicide had often moved away from their usual area of residence before (sometimes long before) the time of clinical onset or fatality (Ödegård, 1932; Sainsbury, 1955; Hare, 1956; Dunham, 1965). The areas to which they moved were characterised by social isolation or 'anomie'. Indices of social isolation tend to be correlated with others that measure poverty although, when there are exceptions, social isolation appears more important (Stein, 1957). The inclusion, for example, of marital status in the Resource Allocation Working Party (RAWP) formula for allocations to psychiatric services recognised the significance of isolation, practical as well as theoretical, for the prediction of morbidity.

More recently, administrative indices such as first admission and readmission rates, and rates of accumulation beyond a year's residence in hospital, have been found empirically to be associated with a composite measure of 'deprivation', which includes marital status as one component (Thornicroft, 1991b, 1992). A recent example of such an index is presented by Jarman & Hirsch in Chapter 4. The question of how to allocate a budget to regions and thence to districts, when sociodemographic proxies for need vary so widely is considered in the final chapter.

Setting priorities

Setting targets raises the issue of priorities in several ways. Firstly, the targets themselves must be chosen from a wide range of possibilities. Secondly, once measured and found unmet, they force further selection, even when only those with roughly equivalent and affordable costs are considered. Thirdly, the priority given to targets that are being met can be reappraised.

The problem of priorities can be illustrated quite starkly by a consideration of the common problems of mental disorder treated in general practice (a large proportion of which are minor disorders that are not referred on) compared with those of the far fewer people with more severe disorders who are admitted to hospital. From the Mental Health Enquiry for 1986 it can be estimated that there were 22 002 200 'in-patient days'. At £44.05 per day this comes to £5 122 619 for an average-sized district (250 000 people) for that year. Croft-Jefferys & Wilkinson (1989) estimated that there were 5.79 m consultations with GPs for neurosis in 1985. The average cost per visit, including home visits, medication and referrals, was £19.44, omitting indirect costs. This totals £594 913 per 250 000 population per year.

Taking such figures at face value, and without examining the clinical evidence for the effectiveness and efficiency of current treatments, staff and settings, it might appear that some of the money spent on in-patients could be spared to help the much larger numbers in general practice. Indeed, there already appears to be a diversion of CPN activity in this direction in some areas (Wooff et al, 1986, 1988). But without a proper mental health information system it is impossible to have a clear idea of what such shifts might mean in terms of priorities, targets and outcomes for the two groups.

A second illustration of problems because of the allocation of priorities arises from the rule enunciated earlier in this chapter – that preventing the amplification of social disablement is as important as demonstrating a diminution. Targets have to be set in such a way that the effects of preventive care can be measured positively, even though the degree of impairment is no longer expected to be much reduced. One way to do this is to ensure, as part of the regular needs assessments, that interventions previously not found successful may be offered again from time to time, without pressure.

These considerations raise the issue of priority starkly, and illustrate why it is necessary for Mental Health Information Systems (MHIS) to generate data that accurately reflect the needs for caring, enabling, and prophylactic services, based on the clinical and social characteristics of all those known to all the responsible authorities. The Audit Commission (1992) has calculated that public expenditure on community-based care in England (including that provided by primary-care services) now costs more than in-hospital care, whereas 10 years ago, at equivalent prices, the expenditures were more or less equal. The report points out:

> "no authority visited had any information systems that could tell managers in either authority the range of services deployed to a particular individual from health and social services – let alone from the independent sector or from relatives and friends. There was very little available on unit costs of services, and there was only occasional systematic information available to managers (let alone users and carers) on the range of services available throughout an area. Such information systems as exist are nearly always service orientated. There is a particular need to strengthen the information available to users and carers outlining their entitlement and services available to them."

A more detailed account of ways of determining priorities for mental health care within districts is given by Murphy in Chapter 7, and within sectors by Strathdee & Thornicroft in Chapter 8, while the closely related issues of costing care and services are considered by Beecham & Knapp in Chapter 9.

The way in which a MHIS, based on a combination for good quality bottom-up clinical information and top-down administrative data can underpin both clinical care and resource management is summarised in Fig. 1.2.

Conclusions and plan of the book

Until now, the assessment of needs for mental health care and services has proceeded in a relatively haphazard and informal way, particularly in areas not served by a psychiatric case register. Little attention has been paid to basic questions about what needs are and how to measure them. Assessment of individual needs has relied on the expertise and implicit models of care held by individual clinicians, on informal audit procedures and, in cases where patients have been compulsorily detained, on the Mental Health Act Commissioners. Routine assessment of clinical services has been mainly the province of the Hospital Advisory Service (described in Chapter 10 by

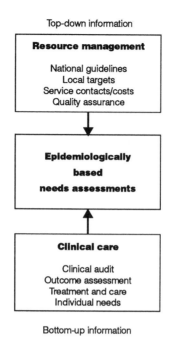

Top-down information

Resource management

National guidelines
Local targets
Service contacts/costs
Quality assurance

**Epidemiologically
based
needs assessments**

Clinical care

Clinical audit
Outcome assessment
Treatment and care
Individual needs

Bottom-up information

Fig. 1.2. Use of a mental health information system for high-quality local planning

Seager), which has relied on the judgements of small groups of highly experienced practitioners rather than creating generally applicable standards.

The trend is now clearly evident for the evaluation of clinical practice to become more systematic and routine. At the individual level, models of good practice are being specified, along with increased recognition of the needs of others in patients' social networks, such as relatives (see Chapter 17 by Kuipers). The technical challenge of computerising information collection and deployment in such a way that it can aid routine decision-making is being addressed. Assessment tools are now available for comparing patients' needs across time and across settings. At the service level, comprehensive assessments are now being developed that examine not only patient outcomes but aspects of organisation, funding, and structure (see for example Chapter 11 by Ridgely *et al*).

In attempting to cover the many disparate topics that are relevant to needs assessment, we have organised the book in an approximate sequence, beginning with the most general considerations and ending with the most specific techniques and issues. Part I deals with basic definitions of need as they can be applied to mental health, differentiating them from associated concepts such as demand, utilisation and quality of life. Needs assessments are put into a general context of audit, evaluation and planning. The setting of general targets for the assessment of need is discussed from a national perspective.

In Part II the focus is on the needs of populations and the information requirements of districts. Sources of information, both local and national, are discussed, with the aims of purchasing authorities and provider units in mind. Part III deals with the issues involved in choosing between the competing needs of a population, that is, setting priorities and costing services.

The emphasis then shifts in Part IV to evaluating the ability of services to meet needs, starting with central monitoring as practised by the Hospital Advisory Service, continuing with an example of a heavily researched and coordinated evaluation of new arrangements for the delivery of community-care services, and concluding with an example of a local audit of admissions to a particular hospital-provider unit.

Part V, by contrast, deals with the needs of individuals. The first chapter gives an account of the methods that have been used to assess the needs of individual patients, and of the differing levels of detail required for community surveys, the long-term mentally ill, and so on. The next chapter is concerned with how the collection of data required for assessing individual needs can be incorporated into routines and describes a number of patient-information systems. This is followed by a description of the advantages and disadvantages of new techniques for computerising patient assessment.

Becoming yet more specific, Part VI describes the needs of special groups such as the homeless and relatives of the mentally ill. The final part gives an overview of the material presented in the book, concluding with a critical look at the problems of and prospects for needs assessment in mental health.

References

AUDIT COMMISSION (1992) *Community Care: Managing the Cascade of Change.* London: HMSO.
BREWIN, C. R., WING, J. K., MANGEN, S., *et al* (1987) Principles and practice of measuring needs in the long term mentally ill. The MRC Needs for Care Assessment. *Psychological Medicine*, **17**, 971–981.
—— & —— (1989) *The MRC Needs for Care Assessment: Manual for version Two/2.* London: Institute of Psychiatry (unpublished manuscript).
COOPER, J. (1989) Information for planning. Case registers and Körner. In *Health Services Planning and Research. Contributions from Psychiatric Case Registers* (ed. J. K. Wing), pp. 115–120. London: Gaskell.
CROFT-JEFFERYS, C. & WILKINSON, G. (1989) Estimated costs of neurotic disorder in UK general practice. *Psychological Medicine*, **19**, 549–558.
DEPARTMENT OF HEALTH (1989) *Working for Patients, Cm 555. Working Paper 6, Medical Audit.* London: HMSO.
DEPARTMENT OF HEALTH AND SOCIAL SECURITY (1982) *A Report on the Collection and Use of Information about Hospital Clinical Activity in the NHS.* London: HMSO.
DUNHAM, H. W. (1965) *Community and Schizophrenia. An Epidemiological Analysis.* Detroit: Wayne State University Press.
GRIFFITHS, R. (1988) *Community Care. Agenda for Action.* London: HMSO.

HARE E. H. (1956) Mental illness and social conditions in Bristol. *Journal of Mental Science*, **102**, 349–357.

HOUSE OF COMMONS (1990) *National Health Service and Community Care Act*. London: HMSO.

HURRY, J. & STURT, E. (1981) Social performance in a population sample. Relation to psychiatric symptoms. In *What is a Case? The Problem of Definition in Psychiatric Community Surveys* (eds J. K. Wing, P. Bebbington & L. N. Robins), pp. 202–213. London: Grant McIntyre.

LOHR, K. N. (ed) (1990) *Medicare: A Strategy for Quality Assurance*. Washington DC: National Academy Press.

MANGEN, S. & BREWIN, C. R. (1991) The measurement of need. In *Social Psychiatry. Theory, Methodology and Practice* (ed. P. E. Bebbington), pp. 162–182. London: Transaction Publishers.

MATTHEW, G. K. (1971) Measuring need and evaluating services. In *Problems and Progress in Medical Care. Sixth Series* (ed. G. McLachlan). London: Oxford University Press.

NHS MANAGEMENT EXECUTIVE (1991) *Health Service Indicators. New Perspectives. Consultation Draft*. London: Department of Health.

ÖDEGÅRD, Ö. (1932) Emigration and insanity. A study of mental diseases among Norwegian-born populations in Minnesota. *Acta Psychiatrica et Neurologica Scandinavica* (suppl. 4).

SAINSBURY, P. (1955) *Suicide in London*. London: Chapman and Hall.

STEIN, L. (1957) Social class gradient in schizophrenia. *British Journal of Preventive and Social Medicine*, **11**, 181.

TAUBE, C., LEE, E. S. & FORTHOFER, R. N. (1984) Diagnosis-related groups for mental disorders, alcoholism and drug abuse. Evaluation and alternatives. *Hospital and Community Psychiatry*, **35**, 452–455.

THORNICROFT, G. (1991*a*) The concept of case management for long-term mental illness. *International Review of Psychiatry*, **3**, 125–132.

—— (1991*b*) Social deprivation and rates of treated mental disorder: developing statistical models to predict psychiatric service utilisation. *British Journal of Psychiatry*, **158**, 475–484.

—— (1992) The TAPS Project (6): new long stay psychiatric patients and social deprivation. *British Journal of Psychiatry*, (in press).

WING J. K. (1972) Principles of evaluation. In *Evaluating a Community Psychiatric Service. The Camberwell Register, 1964–71* (eds J. K. Wing & A. H. Hailey), pp. 11–40. London: Oxford University Press.

—— (Ed) (1989) *Health Services Planning and Research. Contributions from Psychiatric Case Registers*. London: Gaskell.

—— (1992) *Epidemiologically-Based-Needs Assessments. Review of Research on Psychiatric Disorders*. London: Department of Health.

—— & BROWN, G. W. (1970) *Institutionalism and Schizophrenia*. Cambridge: Cambridge University Press.

—— & HAILEY, A. M. (Eds) *Evaluating a Community Psychiatric Service. The Camberwell Register, 1964–1971*. London: Oxford University Press.

WORLD HEALTH ORGANIZATION (1980) *International Classification of Impairments, Disabilities and Handicaps*. Geneva: WHO.

WOOFF, K., GOLDBERG, D. & FRYERS, T. (1986) Patients in receipt of community psychiatric nursing care in Salford 1976–82. *Psychological Medicine*, **16**, 407–414.

——, —— & —— (1988) The practice of community psychiatric nursing and mental health social work in Salford: some implications for community care. *British Journal of Psychiatry*, **152**, 783–792.

WYKES, T. (1982) A hostel-ward for 'new' long-stay patients. An evaluative study of 'a ward in a house'. In *Long-term community care. Experience in a London borough* (ed. J. K. Wing). *Psychological Medicine Monograph Supplement No 2*, pp. 57–97. Cambridge: Cambridge University Press.

2 Health targets

RACHEL JENKINS

The reason for having a national health service is to improve the health of the nation. At its most fundamental, the purpose of health services is to achieve some overall health gain: specifically, to improve the overall health of the nation, to prevent the onset of illnesses, to increase detection and improve the management of existing illness, to slow down the rate of deterioration of incurable diseases and to minimise the accompanying social disability, and to improve the quality of life of those who are ill. As in all organisations, we need to know how far we are achieving our primary goal.

How do we know if we are improving the health of the nation?

We cannot know unless we measure it. The simple fact of doing one's clinics faithfully over a working life time does not translate automatically into having improved the health of one's patients, or of the overall population one is serving. In other words, efficiency is not the same as effectiveness and there is no point in considering efficiency without reference to effectiveness (Butt & Palmer, 1985). For example, it is pointless for a consultant to see 20 patients in an afternoon if few are improved by that contact. It is better for him or her to see six patients and deliver effective treatment to each. We must look at how effective we are in our work, and we cannot do this without measuring health, social functioning, and quality of life. While health has been measured in research studies for several decades now, it has not been measured routinely or used in routine statistics. Mortality statistics in the health services have of course been collected routinely since the 18th Century.

However, mortality, while interesting and important in its own right, is not remotely a good proxy indicator of health or morbidity, except for illnesses which are almost invariably and rapidly fatal, for example, lung cancer. For other diseases such as asthma, diabetes, hypertension, heart disease, and mental illness, mortality is a small part of the overall task of the health services, and the mortality that does occur does not in any way measure the size and severity of the remaining morbidity in the population at large.

How can we measure health?

We measure health and health care using indicators. An 'indicator' is a measure which summarises information relevant to a particular phenomenon, or a seasonable proxy for such a measure. Ideally, indicators should actually measure what they are supposed to measure (validity), and they should provide the same answer if measured by different people in similar circumstances (reliability) (Cook & Campbell, 1976). They should be able to measure change (sensitivity), and they should reflect changes only in the situation concerned (specificity) (World Health Organization, 1981). Of course, in real life these criteria are hard to achieve, and indicators at best are indirect or partial measures of a complex situation. A health indicator, therefore, is a variable, susceptible to direct measurement, that reflects aspects of the state of health of a community, while a health-care indicator is a variable that reflects aspects of the state of health care in a community (World Health Organization, 1981). Health-care indicators can be categorised, using a general systems approach, into input, process, and outcome. The resources put into the health-care system in terms of finance, personnel, building, etc., are the input, the activity of the personnel form the process, and the changes in functioning, morbidity and mortality are the outcome. (Thus, in general, outcome indicators in health care will be health indicators.) Outcome may of course be influenced not only by the health-care system, but also by other aspects of public policy, social change, and environment factors (Smith, 1992).

The measurement of input is relatively straightforward – a simple accounting procedure – and the measurement of process has been tackled for some time, in the shape of 'performance' or 'activity' indicators, although this has sometimes tended to follow the approach of establishing what is collectable first and seeing what it can tell us, rather than specifying the key aspects of performance and devising appropriate indicators.

The measurement of outcome is a more complex task, and the fact that outcome information is hard to obtain has led to health-service inputs and processes being used as proxy measures for outcomes, which of course they are not (Bergner *et al*, 1979). It was also argued that because chronic health problems, morbidity, and mortality are insensitive variables, and are seemingly unrelated to health-care changes in the short term, the use of input and process indicators as proxy measures for outcome was justified. The initial assumption was that use is cure, and amount of use equates with severity of condition, but it is now well recognised that use is not necessarily cure, and that use of services varies not only with sociodemographic factors, independent of the severity of symptoms and disability, but also with characteristics of the service, including factors relating to the doctors themselves (see for example Goldberg & Huxley, 1980). This variation greatly compromises the use of services as a proxy for outcome measures of health and leaves us no nearer our goal of measuring the impact of health care on the health of the population.

It is generally helpful for all organisations to have a goal to work towards. In the private sector, it is usually profitability. In the public sector, it is the service outputs which are the goal, and so in the case of the NHS, it is the health outcomes which matter. Likewise, for education, it is the actual educational achievements and skills of the children which matter.

What indicators are available to us to measure health outcomes?

The official mortality statistics are a very good indicator of actual mortality, and relatively good indicators of the treatment of life-threatening diseases; however, they do not indicate health, but rather lack of survival. This may seem self-evident, but it is extraordinary how widespread the use of mortality is as an indicator of health. Mortality data do not adequately reflect changes in health status within populations (Patrick & Erickson, 1987). Decreased mortality may not signal a healthier population. On the contrary, it may reflect the longer life of chronically ill and seriously disabled people (Wilson, 1981).

In people with mental illness, there are two major classes of avoidable mortality: suicide and death from physical illness. The mortality statistics are very helpful indicators of both of these (Sainsbury, 1983; Fox & Goldblatt, 1982) and as such, are extremely useful in monitoring progress towards the objective of reducing these classes of avoidable mortality. However, such mortality in mental illness is not in any way a measure of the overall morbidity from mental illness in the population.

Direct measures of health and social functioning have by far the strongest conceptual basis as relevant indicators of health outcome. Many measures have separate physical, psychological and social axes, while there are also combined measures, including measures of quality of life. Good reviews are available (e.g. McDowell & Newell, 1987; Thompson, 1989), and some of the best scales are listed in the Appendix.

Subjective health indicators are measures that focus on experiential aspects of illness, distress, and discomfort, instead of the more objective evaluation of health status by a professional. They are important to consider because of the research evidence that self-perceived health correlates with mortality and rate of recovery, even after controlling for objective measures of health.

Furthermore, subjective measures of health correlate more closely with the use of health services than do the medical conditions themselves (Hunt, 1988). There is often a disparity between judgements of professionals and lay people on whether a particular treatment has been successful, and it is crucial to take the lay view as well as the medical view.

'Unmet needs' have been defined as the differences between those services judged necessary to deal appropriately with defined health problems and those services actually being received. Changes in unmet need are measures of the outcome of health services, but they are not in themselves measures of health status (Carr & Wolfe, 1979). They do not measure the level of health of an individual or a population, but the capacity of the health and social-care system to care for the sick. There is a strong tradition of measuring unmet need in the US, reviewed by Carr & Wolfe (1979), and more recently Brewin *et al* (1987, 1988) have developed measures of unmet need applicable to chronic mental illness. Indicators of unmet needs and health-care outcomes, although not the same, are related. Indicators of unmet needs relate to the services and resources necessary to maintain and improve health status. Carr & Wolfe (1979) suggested that the provision of appropriate health services according to need is an intermediate outcome of a health system whose ultimate goal may be to improve the health status of a population.

Disability days, bed days, and restricted activity are indicators which may reflect many conditions other than health, such as provision for paid sick leave, the number and age of children in a family, and the division of responsibilities within families, as well as psychosocial factors such as the tendency to assume a sick role or to express problems through somatic symptoms. Disability days are more properly regarded as a measure of social disability (Wilson, 1981). However, they are also useful as a measure of self-care during illnesses. (It is worth remembering that in a prospective investigation of 6928 adults, a pattern of greater mortality was found among persons with no disability days in comparison with those who reported one to three sick days during a year (Berkman, 1975); the greater mortality of people with no sick days was independent of age, sex, objective and subjective health status, and health habits.)

Bed usage and hospital admission/discharge figures are not in themselves outcome indicators because they are affected not only by the availability of beds, but also by:

(a) inflow factors, such as the availability of alternative services (e.g. day hospitals or community psychiatric nurses could reduce the need for admission)
(b) factors influencing length of treatment, such as the admission of heavily dependent patients when alternative arrangements in the community take a long time to set up, or the special interests of the team (e.g. a brief-admission policy, the admission of forensic cases under a court order, in-patient psychotherapy)

(c) outflow factors, which influence the transfer of patients back to the community or to other appropriate units.

If these factors are explored and understood, then admission figures can become helpful to us in monitoring interventions to rationalise inflow, length of stay, and outflow. However, psychiatric in-patients represent only 1–2% of the total of psychiatric morbidity. In mental illness, as with other medical conditions of varying severity such as asthma or hypertension, not all cases reach hospital or even come to medical attention. It is therefore important for us to develop health indicators that apply not only to hospital in-patients, but also to the rest of the iceberg of morbidity in the community. Similarly, we need input and activity indicators not only for hospital services, but also for the primary-care services.

How do we set the targets?

A target is a specified goal, set within the framework of an overall objective. In order to set the target there are a number of preliminary steps:

(a) deciding on the overall objective in the light of evidence from preva-
    lence studies, evaluation of preventive, treatment, and rehabilitative
    strategies, and views from health-service professionals, users and carers
(b) establishing the strategy to achieve the objective
(c) choosing an indicator which can measure progress towards the
    objective, and for which there is research evidence on its validity and
    reliability
(d) setting the precise target to a precise timetable
(e) monitoring the strategy to see when it is achieved.

The overall objectives should be clear, compelling, visionary and easy to communicate, not only to health professionals but also to the general public. Furthermore, they should be implementable by being subsequently developed down into action plans which are well balanced between people, the organisational systems, and the techniques used for prevention, treatment, and rehabilitation. The objectives must gain the commitment of the organisation as a whole, and they must be feasible in terms of what people are asked to do, and over what time period.

What targets might be set for mental illness?

The range of mental disorders is very wide, but in public-health terms, the three most important areas are severe psychotic illness (because of its severity, social disability, and mortality); chronic non-psychotic illness (mostly depression and anxiety) because of its consequences for physical health, consumption of health services, and consequences for family relationships, cognitive and emotional development of children, sickness, absences, labour turnover, and accidents etc.; and dementia. This chapter concentrates on the first two.

The overall goal is to reduce morbidity and mortality caused by mental illness by an appropriate balance of prevention, treatment, and rehabilitation. There is considerable research evidence that it is possible for service interventions to achieve an impact on incidence, relapse and readmission rates, total disability, and mortality.

The major objectives for severe mental illness are to improve health and social functioning, and to reduce mortality from suicide and physical illness. The intermediate stages to achieve these objectives in health or reduced mortality include the development of adequate and appropriate community-care services for treatment and rehabilitation of the severely mentally ill.

The major objectives for non-psychotic illness are to improve health and social functioning, and to reduce mortality from suicide and physical illness. The intermediate steps to be taken to achieve these objectives in health and reduced mortality include the development of adequate and appropriate primary-care services for mental illness.

The relative importance of different risk factors varies between the different categories of mental illness, as do the relative benefits from prevention, treatment and rehabilitation. However, for all categories, to a greater or lesser degree, the causes, treatment and outcome are influenced by social as well as health factors. Therefore, the hoped-for improvements in health will be slow to occur unless social care and health care are truly integrated.

Through prevention, treatment and rehabilitation, it is possible that the incidence of schizophrenia, affective psychosis and depression can be reduced.

(a) *Schizophrenia*. The aetiology of schizophrenia may be at least half genetic (Rosenthal, 1971), probably due to a polygenic rather than a single-gene mechanism (Cutting, 1985). Rainier (1982) quotes the life-time risk of developing the disorder as 10–15% for a child with one schizophrenic parent. Therefore, adequate access to simple genetic counselling (by ensuring the education of primary-care and secondary-care teams to provide this on request) and the availability of contraceptive services may help a little in the long term (Reveley, 1985).

(b) *Affective psychosis*. The aetiology of affective psychosis is at least partially genetic (Reich *et al*, 1982). Morbid risk in relatives varies with unipolar and bipolar illness, age of onset, and responsiveness to treatment.

(c) *Depression*. The causes of non-psychotic depression are environmental rather than genetic (Torgensen, 1983; Jenkins, 1985). Some depression is secondary to physical disease, pain, and disability (particularly loss of mobility and sensory function) for which specific treatment and prevention measures are available (e.g. Cooper, 1976). Some cases of depression are precipitated by acute life events and can be prevented by crisis intervention, and other systems of support (Newton, 1988). Some are precipitated by lack of social support and can be prevented by setting up systems for at-risk groups (e.g. isolated mothers of pre-school children). Organisations such as CRUSE and NEWPIN, as well as adequate child and family psychiatric services may all help.

It may also be possible to reduce relapse rates and readmission rates, as outlined below.

(a) *Schizophrenia*. Research has demonstrated that the delivery of family interventions (which reduce those family stresses and conflicts that precipitate relapse and readmission), and direct education of sufferers about the management of their own illness, can significantly reduce rates of relapse and readmission (Falloon *et al*, 1982, 1985; Birchwood *et al*, 1989). Intensive home treatment can significantly reduce the requirement for admission to hospital (e.g. Dean & Gadd, 1990).

(b) *Affective psychoses*. These can be reduced by prophylactic drug therapy, and by adequate early-warning communication between family, primary-care and secondary-care teams and by the provision of adequate social support (Bennett, 1982). Intensive home treatment for acute psychiatric illness can dramatically reduce the need for hospital admission (Dean & Gadd, 1990).

(c) *Depression*. The prognosis can be improved by improving the detection and treatment of depression in general practice. Research has shown that depression detected by the general practitioner (GP) has a better prognosis than 'hidden' morbidity (Johnstone & Goldberg, 1976; Ormel *et al*, 1990). At present GPs only identify about half of the total morbidity presenting in their surgeries (Goldberg & Huxley, 1980).

Reduction in total disability may be achieved for some patients in the following ways.

(a) *Schizophrenia*. Research has demonstrated that the provision of adequate rehabilitative services can have a major impact on total disability (Wing, 1982). There are perhaps 100 research reports on the benefits of transferring patients from long-stay hospital care to treatment in the community, and none that demonstrates that hospital treatment is better than equally competent community treatment for any psychiatric disorder (Andrews, 1990). The accretion of severely dependent patients is much lower in the presence of such services (Hyde *et al*, 1987; James & Margolius, 1989; Shepherd, 1990; Thornicroft, 1992).

(b) *Affective psychosis*. The disability is generally far less than for schizophrenia, as deterioration of personality does not occur to the same extent and multiple handicaps are less likely to accumulate. Adequate occupational opportunities are crucial after recovery (Bennett, 1982).

The question of whether there is an avoidable mortality is discussed below.

(a) *Schizophrenia.* The standardised mortality ratios of people with schizophrenia are grossly elevated, at approximately 2.5. This is partly due to cardiovascular, malignancy, and respiratory disease (Fox & Goldblatt, 1982), presumably contributed to by smoking, poor nutrition, poor environmental conditions, and lack of medical and social care; and partly due to suicide – 10% of schizophrenia patients commit suicide (Hawton, 1987).

(b) *Affective psychosis.* Of those with affective psychosis, 15% commit suicide (Miles, 1977). Continuing education of primary-care and secondary-care teams in how to assess suicidal risk is vital if the rates are to be reduced.

(c) *Depression.* A small proportion of depressed people commit suicide, and the risk of death from all causes including accidents is twice the norm in severe neurotic depression (Sims & Prior, 1978).

We can now establish the major objectives within the central goal, which are listed below.

The major objectives for severe mental illness are:
    1A Improve health and social functioning
    2B Reduce mortality from suicide and physical illness
Strategic interventions to achieve objectives in health and mortality:
    1S Develop adequate and appropriate community-care services for treatment and rehabilitation.
The major objectives for depression and anxiety are:
    2A Improve health and social functioning
    2B Reduce overall suicide rate
Strategic interventions to achieve objectives in health and mortality:
    2S Develop adequate and appropriate primary-care services for prevention and treatment.

Improvements in health and social functioning of severe mental illness

National baseline data on prevention of severe mental illness

Taking our first objective, improvement in health and social functioning of people with severe mental illness, the first and most fundamental problem we encounter is that we do not have national baseline data on prevalence of severe mental illness, and therefore find it difficult both to set informed targets to reduce the prevalence rates of mental illness, and to know if we are reaching them. Other countries, such as the USA and New Zealand are able to set detailed targets of prevalence relating to different categories of mental illness, informed by national surveys, for example, in the US, the Epidemiological Catchment Area Survey. The Department of Health is currently commissioning the Office of Population Censuses and Surveys (OPCS) to do initial development work on a national mental illness survey in England. Therefore our first target is to achieve a national survey of prevalence rates of severe mental illness.

Target 1Ai A national survey of prevalence rates of severe mental illness.

Improved health and social functioning

Once we have good baseline data, the next step is to set targets for improving health and social functioning of severe mental illness, and these targets will be informed by current research on health outcomes of mental illness. The Department of Health is commissioning a few detailed research projects to evaluate outcome indicators of improved mental health and social functioning in good community-care settings, which can be routinely collected by health and social-care professionals.

Target 1Aii for improving health and social functioning of SMI to be set, informed by current research on health outcomes of mental illness. (Possible target date: 1998.)

Standardised assessments of health, social functioning and social disability, and quality of life

The next obvious requirement is that, in order to monitor improvements in health and social functioning, every multidisciplinary team will need a standardised assessment procedure, which takes account of symptom state, social functioning and social disability, and quality of life, and which is used routinely, for example at admission, discharge and at regular specified follow-up intervals. (Examples of such assessment procedures are in the Appendix.)

Target 1Aiii All districts should use standardised assessment procedures for assessing symptom state, social functioning and social disability, and quality of life at specified intervals to develop a health-status profile of the population in contact with their local services, and track it over time. Drs Strathdee and Thornicroft at the Maudsley and others elsewhere are starting to do this. (Possible target date: 1994.)

Our second objective – a reduction in mortality from severe mental illness – has two strands to it: firstly, suicide, and secondly, mortality from physical illness.

Suicide (both recorded and open verdicts)

Patients with SMI have a large avoidable mortality from suicide. In total, 15% of patients with affective psychosis and 10%–15% of patients with schizophrenia kill themselves despite most, if not all, being in contact with services. To reduce this mortality, lessons must be learnt from the audit of suicide, and national and local targets to reduce the suicide rate must be set.

> Target 1Bi All suicides of SMI should be audited at district level, and targets for reducing rates should be set. (Possible target date: all suicides audited 1993, targets set 1994, if realistic at district level, if not, at regional and national levels only.)

Mortality from physical illness

Patients with SMI also have a significant avoidable mortality from general medical illness including cardiovascular and respiratory diseases, and malignancy. In order to reduce this mortality, it is necessary to monitor and audit all deaths of SMI under age 65, and then to set targets to reduce this avoidable mortality.

> Target 1Bii All deaths under the age of 65 of people with SMI should be monitored at district level, and targets for reducing standardised mortality ratios (SMRs) should be set. (Possible target date: monitoring introduced 1993, targets set 1994.)

People with SMI have more physical illness than the general population, and their physical health is often sadly neglected while health-care staff focus rather exclusively on their mental states. Positive efforts are needed to redress this balance, and every patient with SMI should have a general practitioner (GP) who provides regular physical health checks, and health promotion information (e.g. diet, exercise, smoking, contraception) such as is generally given to the rest of the population. (Each GP has, on average, about seven such patients (Kendrick *et al*, 1991).)

> Target 1Biii All patients with SMI should be registered with a GP and receive annual physical health checks, and health-promotion information. (Possible target date: 1993.)

In order to expedite this, it is important to develop a system of flagging patients with SMI on computerised general-practice registers, so that the GP can ensure they receive annual physical health checks and health-promotion information.

> Target 1Biv Each GP surgery should have a practice case register of patients with SMI. (Possible target date: 1995.)

It seems only reasonable that if we are to set health targets for SMI, then adequate resources must be in place for these targets to be achieved. What are the resources required? Research has demonstrated that the provision of adequate rehabilitative services has a major impact on total disability (Wing, 1982). Such rehabilitative services have three essential components: supported housing, therapy, and occupational activities. When these three components are delivered in the community, as opposed to within an old-style large psychiatric institution, this is preferred by the patients and their families and furthermore is of health and social benefit (TAPS, 1990) and it is this research that underpins the policy of community care. However, the ultimate success of this policy will depend on the adequacy and balance of the three essential components of the community services, and the extent to which they meet the needs of the local population.

In order to achieve the best community services, it is essential to continue the process of running down and closing the old, large, out-of-district psychiatric institutions, in order to release the heavy capital and revenue expenditure currently tied up in them, and this should be carried out in the context of a planned and phased implementation programme. However, it is essential that some long-term 24-hour residential nursing care and 12-hour nursing care is provided, albeit locally, rather than in the traditional large institutional settings (Clifford *et al*, 1991).

Target 1Si By 1994, every region should have agreed with its districts a strategic plan which covers the planned closure of all large old-style psychiatric institutions over a realistic timetable. (Possible target date: 2000.)

Joint purchasing mechanisms

Mental illness services are the joint responsibility of both the health authority (HA) and the local authority (LA), and there is considerable variability in the relative proportion of provision by HAs, LAs, and the voluntary and private sector. Clearly, the amount of LA provision for the SMI directly affects the amount of HA provision required. For instance, an LA with a good range of residential accommodation together with a good supply of domiciliary support by both health and social services, for example nurses working in residential care would reduce the HA requirement for in-patient beds. Less provision on one side leads to a requirement for more provision on the other side. The aim is to provide a 'seamless service', and the most cost-effective method to achieve this is for district health authorities (DHAs) and LAs jointly to purchase mental health services, and for central government to consider ring-fencing mental health budgets, including the Social Services Department (SSD), DHA and current Social Security income support for residential-care components.

Target 1Sii All HAs and LAs establish joint purchasing mechanisms for the full range of mental health services. (Possible target date: 1995.)

The three essential components of the rehabilitative services, namely supported housing, therapy, and structured occupational activities, make it vital to develop close interagency collaboration between health services, social services, and housing and voluntary bodies.

Target 1Siii Each HA and SSD to publish a jointly agreed 'purchasing' strategy for mental health services for the period to 2000, agreed with Regional Health Authorities and SSI. (Possible target date: 1995.)

Computerised record of service contacts

In order to monitor the care of SMI, and to assess morbidity and mortality, it is essential for every district to have computerised records of everyone subject to the Care Programme Approach in order to supply the population denominator. In addition, it should be used as a proactive administrative aid to help ensure that patients are in fact receiving the agreed package of care, and to prevent people being missed out. A properly established information system would not only underpin the administrative process, but would also demonstrate outcomes in terms of key indicators such as symptoms and social functioning.

Target 1Siv All districts to establish a computerised record of service contacts. (Possible target date: 1993.)

Requisite service infrastructure and facilities

Every person with SMI should have a care programme coordinated by a case manager, and which is regularly reviewed at a clinical meeting with the identified key worker present. As from 1 April 1991, health authorities in conjunction with local authorities are required to draw up care-programme plans for all patients being considered for discharge and all new patients accepted by the specialist psychiatric services. All regional health authorities have confirmed that care programmes are in place in their regions, but there is strong circumstantial evidence to indicate that this is not the case. A key worker should be nominated to keep in close contact with the patient and monitor that the agreed care programme is effected by the multidisciplinary team.

Target 1Sv All HAs and Local Authority Social Services Departments (LASSDs) to establish a specified qualitative range of facilities and personnel, appropriate to local circumstances. (Possible target date: establish range by 1995 and complete implementation by 2000.)

Proportion of SMI in appropriately supported housing, and in appropriate day time activity

Every person with SMI should have housing at the appropriately supported level, and structured day-time activity at the appropriate level (e.g. employment, sheltered work placement, occupational therapy). While there is now a general consensus about the range of provision required, numbers of places and personnel will be determined on the basis, appropriately assessed, of the needs of the individual district.

Target 1Svi HAs and LASSDs and local housing authorities to secure adequate provision of suitable supported housing for people with SMI. (Possible target date: 75% by 1995, 95% by 2000.)

Multidisciplinary training in community care for secondary-care teams

Training for the multidisciplinary team in community care is essential for the effective delivery of services. Staff have both vocational and continuing training needs.

Target 1Svii An integrated and multi-professional staff training and development programme geared to the achievement of the other targets. (Possible target date: jointly agreed HA/LASSD plan by 1995.)

Proportion of districts with multidisciplinary training programmes for primary-care teams

Furthermore, primary-care teams also need to be trained in the management of mental illness crises, and in the use of the Mental Health Act.

Target 1Sviii An integrated training programme jointly organised by Health and Social Services for primary care teams in the management of crisis and use of the Mental Health Act. (Possible target date: 1993.)

Research on effects of service interventions for SMI

There is a need for specific research devoted to establishing baseline data on the long-term effects of service interventions on health, social, and economic outcomes.

Target 1Six Specific research commissioned by the Department of Health to clarify further the long-term effects of service interventions for the SMI on health, social, and economic outcomes. (Possible target date: 1997.)

Improvements in health and social functioning of chronic non-psychotic disorders

The prevalence during any year of non-psychotic disorders is 10–25% of the adult population, and between one-third and a half of these last over six months, and may lead to chronic alcohol abuse, tranquilliser dependency, excessive use of general medical services, and loss of economic activity.

National baseline data on prevalence of non-psychotic disorders

As with psychotic illness, we do not have a national baseline, and therefore find it difficult to set an informed target. Other countries, for example, the USA, have set detailed targets relating to non-psychotic disorders, informed by the Epidemiological Catchment Area Survey. The Department of Health is currently commissioning the OPCS to do initial development work on a national mental illness survey in England.

> Target 2Ai A national survey of prevalence rates of non-psychotic illness, to run simultaneously with a survey of psychosis. (Possible target date: 1993/4.)

Improved health and social functioning

The Department of Health requires research to evaluate outcome indicators of improved health and social functioning of chronic non-psychotic disorders in primary-care settings.

> Target 2Aii Targets for improved health and social functioning of chronic non-psychotic disorders to be set by 1998, informed by current research. (Possible target date: 1998.)

Objective 2B – reduction in overall suicide rate of people with depression

Suicide (defined as E950–959 plus 'open verdicts' E980–989) was responsible for 5594 deaths in England in 1990, a rate of 11.7 per 100 000 population. In England, suicide kills about 1000 more people per year than die in motor-vehicle traffic accidents. While there has been a general downwards trend over recent decades for suicide rates in both sexes over the complete age range, in young men the suicide rate is rising (Monk, 1987; Department of Health, 1990, 1991). The UK is not unique in this respect as there is a similar trend in the USA and the rest of Europe.

Key variables in the aetiology of suicide include mental disorder (Barraclough, 1974), alcohol and drug misuse (Raj & Linnoila, 1986), age (Trovato, 1986), employment variables (Pritchard, 1988), imprisonment (Dooley, 1990), migration (Kushmer, 1984), marital breakdown, AIDS (Marzuk *et al*, 1988), and post-traumatic stress disorders (including combat neuroses). In addition, the availability of easy methods of suicide is known to be an important factor in influencing suicide rates, as shown by the fall in suicide rates in the early 1960s following the reduction of the proportion of carbon monoxide in coal gas (Murphy *et al*, 1986). In contrast, inhalation of car exhaust fumes has increased dramatically in recent years, and parallels the increased availability of the motor car, and the hatchback in particular (Bulusu *et al*, 1984), probably because it is easier to run a tube from the exhaust pipe into the car. While self-poisoning as a method of suicide has declined in recent years, in parallel with reduced prescriptions for barbiturates, suicide by hanging and other violent means is rising, with no obvious explanation.

Target 2Bi National, regional and district targets for reduction in suicide rates to be set. (Possible target date: 1992.)

Strategic intervention 2S – develop adequate primary-care services for prevention and treatment of depression and anxiety

Primary-care services are crucial for the prevention and treatment of depression and anxiety because it is at the primary-care level that recognition of patient risk factors and detection of illness usually occurs. Primary preventive strategies include identification and support of those at high risk of depression, for example, the elderly, bereaved, socially isolated, physically disabled, the blind and the deaf, those who have been exposed to disasters, and children who have suffered sexual and physical abuse.

Secondary preventive strategies include the prompt treatment of those who are depressed and anxious. Depression, which is frequently unrecognised and untreated, has a better prognosis if it is identified by the GP. It is, therefore, crucial to improve detection and management in order to avoid the consequences of untreated depression, which include an increased risk of physical illness and hence increased mortality, increased risk of suicide and parasuicide, marital breakdown, and considerable occupational problems such as sickness absence, labour turnover, problems with colleagues, poor performance, and accidents. There are also problems for the children of depressed parents; they are more vulnerable to emotional and cognitive impairment, which in turn can predispose to adult mental illness on maturity as well as having an adverse effect on the children's ultimate intellectual attainment. Chronic non-psychotic illness such as chronic depression, persistent unresolved grief states, chronic phobias, and tranquilliser dependency leads not only to considerable distress, and a low quality of life, but also may act as a trigger for alcohol and drug abuse, excessive burden on health services, and a loss of productive economic activity.

Proportion of general practices with a written mental health policy

Policies within primary care and those to run between primary and secondary care are becoming more common. Research into practice policies, and the outcomes on which these policies should be based, is one of the Department's priorities for research in primary care. However, the use of policies is not specified in the GP contract. The incentive to use policies comes from a realisation that they can make life easier, particularly when running health clinics. They become essential when other members of the primary health-care team assist. GP fundholders have found that they can contract at cheaper rates if they follow an agreed policy. One mechanism for encouraging the use of policies is the requirement for GPs to supply an annual report to family health services authorities (FHSAs) that include total numbers of referrals within the major clinical specialities, including psychiatry. It will be easier to defend a particular referral rate if an agreed policy of care has been followed.

> Target 2Si Each general practice to develop a written mental health policy for detecting and managing mental illness in the practice, both depression and anxiety (and for ensuring the physical health care of people with chronic psychotic illnesses, see Target 1A) which clearly identifies at least one member of the team who takes special responsibility/interest in the area, and who goes on regular training courses, and also organises training for the other members of the team. (Possible target date: 1994.)

Proportion of FHSAs with a written mental health policy

At present, FHSA operational plans could include a mental health policy which covered staffing. The present GP contract may limit how far FHSA operational plans could cover training and audit, but nonetheless FHSAs could act as a local liaison point.

> Target 2Sii Each FHSA to have a written mental health policy which covers training, staffing and audit. (Possible target date: 1994.)

Proportion of general practices auditing mental health

FHSAs in their management role may be able to direct medical audit to local need, for example, of mental health via the Medical Audit Advisory Group. However, it is unclear whether the requirement for GPs to take part in medical audit will be made a contractual matter.

> Target 2Siii General practice audit to include mental health, particularly the identification and management of illness lasting more than 12 months, such as chronic phobias, tranquilliser dependency, and persistent unresolved grief states to ensure they are receiving optimal management, and not being missed. (Possible target date: 1994.)

Proportion of general practices screening the over-75s for depression

The current GP contract specifies that the mental state of the over-75s should be screened annually.

> Target 2Siv Each GP surgery to screen the over-75s for depression. (Possible target date: 1994 although this could be interpreted as already being within the existing GP contract.)

Proportion of GPs and other primary-care staff taking courses on depression and suicide

Postgraduate education of GPs: the 1990 contract emphasises postgraduate education more than ever before. GPs can qualify for a substantial allowance if they do enough accredited courses over a period of five years. A balanced number of courses under three topics – health promotion and prevention, disease management, services management – has to be followed.

That is as far as the specification goes. There is a role here for postgraduate deans to encourage education in particular fields. FHSAs, in their management role, may care to 'bend the ears' of the postgraduate deans.

> Target 2Sv Vocational training and continuing education of GPs and other primary-care staff in risk factors for depression, and assessment of depression (see also target on suicide). (Possible target date: 1994.)

Proportion of DHAs with training courses in cognitive and behaviour therapy

The appropriate management of anxiety includes cognitive and behaviour therapies, and training courses are required for this.

> Target 2Svi Training opportunities in cognitive and behaviour therapies should be expanded for mental health care staff and GPs so that 50% of the former have completed introductory courses. (Possible target date: 1995.)

Prescriptions for benzodiazepines for anxiolytic and hypnotic purposes

> Target 2Svii A reduction in prescriptions for tranquillisers by x%. (Possible target date: 1994.)

Mental health content of the core curriculum of qualifying courses for the Diploma in Social Work

In the same way that GPs encounter substantial amounts of morbidity (some chronic psychotic but mostly serious depression), so social workers in all settings encounter the same types of morbidity. Several studies (Corney, 1984; Huxley *et al*, 1987; Cohen & Fisher, 1988) have all shown that psychiatric morbidity (defined using the PSE in Huxley *et al*, 1987) runs at a minimum of 50% of all cases on social-workers caseloads. These studies and others (Isaac *et al*, 1986) show that this morbidity is present whether cases are 'classified' by social services as mental health, elderly, child, etc.

Therefore, all social workers need basic education in the recognition of mental health problems and in taking appropriate steps to help clients, including referral for specialist opinion and treatment. This knowledge should be included as part of the core curriculum of the new Diploma in Social Work (DipSW) qualifying courses. For specialist psychiatric social work in community-, primary-, or secondary-care settings, social workers should undertake practice in psychiatric social work as part of the special emphasis in the DipSW, and they should also have the opportunity to undertake further studies after qualifying. These recommendations are all consistent with Social Services Inspectorate (SSI) and Central Council for the Education and Training of Social Workers (CCETSW) policy, although, in practice, the policy is not working out very well.

A number of studies (e.g. Chiu, 1991) have argued that there needs to be a better system of joint work between social workers and GPs so that this morbidity, which is often social in origin, can be treated by clinical *and* social interventions concurrently.

> Target 2Sviii The core curriculum of the new DipSW qualifying courses should include basic education in the recognition of mental health problems and in taking appropriate action to help clients, including referral to appropriate health care. (Possible target date: 1994.)

Proportion of districts with jointly prepared FHSA/SSD/DHA good practice protocols for local management of common conditions

> Target 2Six All local secondary- and primary-care teams to develop good practice protocols for the local management of common psychiatric conditions. (Possible target date: 1993.)

GPs are independent practitioners operating under a contract who have their obligations specified with a high level of precision. Inevitably, there will be contractual changes over the years, and if GPs are to be encouraged to make important contributions in this field, consideration should be given to reviewing their contractual commitments with this in mind.

Conclusions

I have attempted in this chapter to give examples of how far strategic targets can be set in order to stimulate and monitor progress towards achieving our health objectives, in relation to severe mental illness, and to non-psychotic disorders (mostly depression and anxiety). These targets could be simplified to a set of seven key targets, as outlined below.

(a) To establish a national picture of prevalence and composition, and progress over time, by a national survey of the prevalence of mental illness, which is repeated at intervals.
(b) All districts should use standardised assessment procedures for assessing symptom state, social functioning and social disability, and quality of life, at specified intervals to develop a health-status profile of the population in contact with local services, and track over time.
(c) To reduce mortality from MI, by auditing suicide rates of SMI and overall suicides, and to set targets for reduction.
(d) To develop and implement joint HA/LA plans for locally based services.
(e) To establish joint purchasing strategies for providing local services including supported housing.
(f) All provider units should establish computerised records of service contacts with SMI.
(g) All local secondary- and primary-care teams should develop good practice protocols for local management of common psychiatric conditions.

Acknowledgements

The targets suggested in this chapter have been developed in discussion with a number of expert colleagues both within and outside the Department of Health, and I would like to express my thanks to the following: Mr Robert Anderson, Mr Peter Gant, Dr Richard Gater, Professor David Goldberg, Dr Keith Hawton, Professor Peter Huxley, Dr David Kingdon, Professor Anthony Mann, Dr Gethin Morgan, Mrs Elizabeth Parker, Dr John Reed, Dr Geoff Shepherd, Dr Geraldine Strathdee, Dr Graham Thornicroft, and Mr Clive Wilson.

Appendix

Brief scales to measure symptoms in the chronic mentally ill

(a) Manchester or K-G-V Scale (Krawiecka *et al*, 1977): nine ratings based on interview and observation, including positive psychotic symptoms and negative symptoms. Appropriate for chronic psychotics, sensitive to change, video training tapes available. Items correspond to areas thought important in clinical assessment. Developed in UK. (10–15 minutes.)

(b) Brief Psychiatric Rating Scale (Overall & Gorham, 1962): 16 ratings based on observation and interview, includes conceptual disorganisation, hallucinatory behaviour, unusual thought content, emotional withdrawal, motor retardation and blunted affect, suspiciousness, grandiosity, and mannerisms and posturing. Criticism: overlap of symptoms, questionable inter-rater reliability and inconsistent guidelines. Some items do not correspond well with clinically relevant areas. (15–30 minutes.)

(c) Schizophrenia Change Scale (Montgomery *et al*, 1978): 12 items selected from Comprehensive Psychopathological Rating Scale to detect change in response to antipsychotic drugs. Includes positive psychotic symptoms but lacks hallucinations (except commenting voices) and no rating of negative symptoms. Developed in UK and Sweden. (10–15 minutes.)

(d) Global Assessment Scale (Endicott *et al*, 1976): Single global severity measure on continuum from sickness to health. Does not distinguish positive and negative symptoms, nor other symptoms/syndromes (e.g. depression, delusions, hallucinations, flattened affect, etc.). Developed in US. (5 minutes.)

(e) Global Assessment of Functioning Scale, 1987 (American Psychiatric Association, 1987).

Another option would be to select items from a longer, more comprehensive scale such as the Present State Examination (Wing *et al*, 1974), the Comprehensive Psychopathological Rating (Asberg *et al*, 1978) or the Structured Clinical Inverview for DSM–III–R (Spitzer & Endicott, 1987).

Brief scales to measure social disability in the chronic mentally ill

(a) Social Behaviour Schedule (Wykes & Sturt, 1986): 21 specific behaviours relevant to patients with long-term impairments in community or in hospital. Developed in UK.

(b) Social Role Performance Schedule (Stevens, 1973): Alternative approach to measure social disability in which performance in socially accepted roles rather than behaviour is measured. Developed in UK.

An alternative is to select a single dimension (e.g. occupation) from one of the more comprehensive interviews such as the Social Behaviour Assessment Schedule (Platt *et al*, 1980) the Groningen Social Disability Schedule (Wiersma *et al*, 1990), or the Psychiatric Disability Assessment Schedule (World Health Organization, 1988).

Brief scales to measure quality of life

Generic measures of quality of life can be applied to individuals suffering from different diseases. There are several generic measures of quality of life which can be applied to individuals suffering from diseases, for example,

Rosser Classification of Health States (Rosser & Kind, 1978), Health Measurement Questionnaire (Gudex & King, 1988), Nottingham Health Profile (McEwan, 1983), and Ewoqot Questionnaire (Brooks *et al*, 1991). However, they do not have specific relevance to severe mental illness and include components such as physical mobility and pain. They can therefore be applied across disciplines of medicine in evaluating health care services, but include a lot of 'noise' if applied to a specific group. They are untested in the chronic mentally ill.

The Lancashire Quality of Life Profile has been specifically developed for use with the chronic mentally ill, the first application takes 25 minutes and subsequent applications an average of 15 minutes. At present it also contains the affect balance scale and Rosenberg's self concept scale so without these it would be even shorter. It has been designed for and used in operational settings.

American instruments include the Sickness Impact Profile (Bergner *et al*, 1976), Quality of Well Being Scale (Patrick *et al*, 1973), Q-L Index (Spitzer *et al*, 1985), and the Karnofsky Performance Status Index (Karnofsky *et al*, 1948).

Quality of Life Schedules (Lehman *et al*, 1982, 1986).

References

AMERICAN PSYCHIATRIC ASSOCIATION (1987) *Diagnostic and Statistical Manual of Mental Disorders* (3rd edn, revised) (DSM–III–R). Washington, DC: APA.

ANDREWS, G. (1990) *The Tolkein Report: A Description of a Model Mental Health Service*. Sydney: University of New South Wales.

ÅSBERG, M., MONTGOMERY, S. A., PERRIS, C., *et al* (1978) The comprehensive psychopathological rating scale. *Acta Psychiatrica Scandanavica* (suppl. 271), 5–27

BARRACLOUGH, B., BIRCH, J., NELSON, B., *et al* (1974) A hundred cases of suicide: clinical aspects. *British Journal of Psychiatry*, **125**, 355–373.

BENNETT, D. H. (1982) Management and rehabilitation of affective psychoses. In *Handbook of Psychiatry, Vol 3, Psychoses of Uncertain Aetiology* (eds J. K. Wing & L. Wing). Cambridge: Cambridge University Press.

BERGNER, M., BOBBIT, R. A., KRESSEL, S., *et al* (1979) The sickness impact profile: conceptual formulation and methodology for the development of a health status measure. In *Sociomedical Health Indicators* (eds J. Elinson & A. Siegmann). New York: Baywood.

——, ——, POLLARD, W. E., *et al* (1976) The sickness impact profile: validation of a health status measure. *Medical Care*, **14**, 157.

BERKMAN, P. (1975) Survival and a modicum of indulgence in the sick role. *Medical Care*, **13**, 85.

BIRCHWOOD, M., SMITH, J., MACMILLAN, S., *et al* (1989) Predicting relapse in schizophrenia: the development and implementation of an early signs monitoring system using patients and families as observers. *Psychological Medicine*, **19**, 649–656.

BREWIN, C. R., WING, J. K., MANGEN, S. P., *et al* (1987) Principles and practice of measuring needs in the longterm mentally ill; the MRC Needs for Care Assessment. *Psychological Medicine*, **17**, 971–981.

——, ——, ——, *et al* (1988) Needs for care in the longterm mentally ill: a report from the Camberwell High Contact Survey. *Psychological Medicine*, **18**, 457–468.

BROOKS, R. G., JENDTEG, S., LINDGREN, B., *et al* (1991) EuroQol: health related quality of life measurement. Results of the Swedish questionnaire exercise. *Health Policy*, **18**, 37–48.

BULUSU, L. & ALDERSON, M. (1984) Suicides 1950–1980. *Population Trends*, **35**, 11–17.

BUTT, H. & PALMER, B. (1985) *Value for Money in the Public Sector*. Oxford: Blackwell.

CARR, W. & WOLFE, S. (1979) Unmet needs as social indicators. In *Sociomedical Health Indicators* (eds J. Elinson & A. E. Siegmann). New York: Baywood.

CHIU, M. (1991) *A Comparison of two Community Based Mental Health Social Work Services*. Unpublished MSc thesis. Manchester: University of Manchester.

CLIFFORD, P., CHARMON, A., WEBB, Y., *et al* (1991) Planning for community care. Long stay populations of hospitals scheduled for rundown or closure. *British Journal of Psychiatry*, **158**, 190–196.

COHEN, J. A. & FISHER, M. (1988) *The Tip of the Iceberg*. Bradford: Department of Applied Social Studies University of Bradford North Yorkshire SSD and the Joseph Memorial Trust.

COOK, T. D. & CAMPBELL, D. T. (1976) The design and conduct of quasi experiments and true experiments in field settings. In *Handbook of Industrial and Organisational Psychology* (ed. M. D. Dunnette). Chicago: Rand McNally.

COOPER, A. F. (1976) Deafness and psychiatric illness. *British Journal of Psychiatry*, **129**, 216–226.

CORNEY, R. H. (1984) The mental and physical health of clients referred to social workers in a local authority department and a general practice attachment scheme. *Psychological Medicine*, **14**, 137–144.

CUTTING, J. (1985) *The Psychology of Schizophrenia*. Edinburgh: Churchill Livingstone.

DAVIES, L. & DRUMMOND, M. (1990) The economic burden of schizophrenia. *Psychiatric Bulletin*, **14**, 522–525.

DEPARTMENT OF HEALTH (1991) *On the State of the Public Health – The Annual Report of the Chief Medical Officer of the Department of Health for the Year 1990*. London: HMSO.

DOOLEY, E. (1990) Prison suicide in England and Wales 1972–87. *British Journal of Psychiatry*, **156**, 40–45.

ENDICOTT, J., SPITZER, R. L., FLEISS, J. L. *et al* (1976) The global assessment scale, a procedure for measuring overall severity of psychiatric disturbance. *Archives of General Psychiatry*, **33**, 766–771.

FALLOON, I. R. H., BOYD, J. L., McGILL, C. W., *et al* (1982) Family management in the prevention of exacerbations of schizophrenia. *New England Journal of Medicine*, **306**, 1437–1440.

—— , —— , —— , *et al* (1985) Family management in the prevention of morbidity of schizophrenia: clinical outcome of a two year longitudinal study. *Archives of General Psychiatry*, **42**, 887–896.

FOX, A. J. & GOLDBLATT, P. O. (1982) *Longitudinal Study – Sociodemographic Mortality Differential, LS No 1, 1971–1975*. London: HMSO.

GOLDBERG, D. & HUXLEY, P. (1980) *Mental Illness in the Community: The Pathway to Psychiatric Care*. London: Tavistock.

GUDEX, C. & KING, P. (1988) *The QALY Toolkit*. York: University of York Centre for Health Economics Discussion Paper 38.

HAWTON, K. (1987) Assessment of suicide risk. *British Journal of Psychiatry*, **150**, 145–153.

HUNT, S. M. (1988) Subjective health indicators and health promotion. *Health Promotion*, **3**, 23–24.

HUXLEY, P. J., KORER, J. & TOLLEY, S. (1987) The psychiatric 'caseness' of clients referred to an urban social services department. *British Journal of Social Work*, **17**, 507–520.

HYDE C., BRIDGES, K., GOLDBERG, D., *et al* (1987) Evaluation of a hostel ward. A controlled study using modified cost-benefit analysis. *British Journal of Psychiatry*, **151**, 805–812.

ISAAC, B., MINTY, E. B. & MORRISON, R. M. (1986) Children in care – the association with mental disorder in the parents. *British Journal of Social Work*, **16**, 325–329.

JACKSON, H. J., BURGESS, P. M., MINAS, I. H., *et al* (1990) Psychometric properties of the Manchester Scale. *Acta Psychiatrica Scandinavica*, **81**, 108–113.

JAMES, D. & MARGOLIUS, O. (1989) The accumulation of 'new long stay' patients at Claybury and Friern Hospitals. In *Team for the Assessment of Psychiatric Services 4th Annual Conference Report*. London: North East Thames Regional Health Authority.

JENKINS, R. (1985) Sex differences in minor psychiatric morbidity. *Psychological Medicine* (monograph suppl. 7).

JOHNSTONE, A. & GOLDBERG, D. (1976) Psychiatric screening in general practice. *Lancet, i*, 605-608.

KARNOFSKY, D. A., ABELMANN, W. H., *et al* (1948) The use of nitrogen mustards in the palliative treatment of carcinoma. *Cancer*, November 1948, 635-656.

KENDRICK, A., SIBBALD, B., BURNS, T., *et al* (1991) Role of general practitioners in care of long term mentally ill patients. *British Medical Journal*, **302**, 508-511.

KRAWIECKA, M., GOLDBERG, D. P. & VAUGHAN, M. (1977) A standardised psychiatric assessment scale for rating chronic psychotic patients. *Acta Psychiatrica Scandanavica*, **55**, 299-308.

KUSHMER, H. I. (1984) Immigrant suicide in the United States: toward a psychosocial history. *Journal of Social History*, **18**, 3-24.

LEHMAN, A., REED, S. & POSSIDENTE, S. (1982) Priorities for longterm care: comments from board and care residents. *Psychiatric Quarterly*, **54**, 181-189.

——, POSSIDENTE, S. & HAWKER, F. (1986) The quality of life of chronic patients in a state hospital and in community residences. *Hospital and Community Psychiatry*, **37**, 901-907.

MCDOWELL, I. & NEWELL, C. (1987) *Measuring Health: A Guide to Rating Scales and Questionnaires*. Oxford: Oxford University Press.

MCEWAN, J. (1983) The Nottingham Health Profile: a measure of perceived health. In *Measuring the Social Benefits of Medicine* (ed. G. T. Smith), pp. 75-83. London: Office of Health Economics.

MARK, M. (1987) Epidemiology of suicide. *Epidemiology Review*, **9**, 51-57.

MARZUK, P. M., TIERNEY, H., TARDIFF, K., *et al* (1988) Increased risk of suicide in persons with AIDS. *Journal of the American Medical Association*, **159**, 1333-1337.

MILES, C. P. (1977) Conditions predisposing to suicide: a review. *Journal of Nervous and Mental Disease*, **164**, 231-246.

MONTGOMERY, S. A., TAYLOR, P. & MONTGOMERY, D. (1978) Development of a schizophrenia scale sensitive to change. *Neuropharmacology*, **17**, 1061-1063.

MURPHY, E., LINDESAY, J. & GRUNDY, E. (1986) 60 years of suicide in England and Wales. *Archives of General Psychiatry*, **43**, 969-976.

NEWTON, J. (1988) *Preventing Mental Illness*. London: Routledge and Kegan Paul.

ORMEL, J., KOETER, M. W. J., VAN DEN BRINK, W., *et al* (1990) The extent of non-recognition of mental health problems in primary care and its effects on management and outcome. In *The Public Health Impact of Mental Disorder* (eds David Goldberg & Digby Tantam), pp. 154-165. Toronto: Hogrefe and Huber.

OVERALL, J. E. & GORHAM, D. R. (1962) The Brief Psychiatric Rating Scale. *Psychological Reports*, **10**, 799-812.

PATRICK, D. & ERICKSON, P. (1987) *Assessing Health Related Quality of Life in General Population Surveys: Issues and Recommendations*. Washington DC: National Center for Health Statistics.

PATRICK, D. L., BUSH, J. W. & CHEN, M. (1973) Methods of measuring levels of well-being for a health status index. *Health Services Research*, **8**, 228.

PLATT, S., WEYMANN, A., HIRSCH, S., *et al* (1980) The Social Behaviour Assessment Schedule (SBAS): Rationale, contents, scoring and reliability of a new interview schedule. *Social Psychiatry*, **15**, 455.

PRITCHARD, C. (1988) Suicide, gender and unemployment in the British Isles and EEC 1974-1985. *Social Psychiatry and Psychiatric Epidemiology*, **23**, 85-89.

RAINIER, J. D. (1982) Genetics of schizophrenia. In *Handbook of Psychiatry, vol 3. Psychoses of Uncertain Aetiology* (eds J. K. Wing & L. Wing). Cambridge: Cambridge University Press.

RAJ, A. & LINNOILA, M. (1986) Alcoholism and suicide. *Suicide and Life Threatening Behaviour*, **16**, 244-273.

REICH, T., CLANINGER, C. R., SUZREZ, B., *et al* (1982) Genetics of the affective psychoses. In *Handbook of Psychiatry, vol 3. Psychoses of Uncertain Aetiology* (eds J. K. Wing & L. Wing). Cambridge: Cambridge University Press.

REVELY, A. (1985) Genetic counselling for schizophrenia. *British Journal of Psychiatry*, **147**, 107-112.

ROSENTHAL, D. (1971) *Genetics of Psychopathology*. New York: McGraw Hill.

ROSSER, R. & KIND, P. (1987) A scale of valuations of states of illness: is there a social consensus? *International Journal of Epidemiology*, **7**, 347-358.

SAINSBURY, P. (1983) Validity and reliability of trends in suicide statistics. *World Health Statistics Quarterly*, **36**, 339–348.

SHEPHERD, G. (1990) Need in the community. In *Community Care* (eds Sheila Sharkey & Sara Barna), pp. 181–188. London: Routledge.

SIMS, A. & PRIOR, P. (1978) The pattern of mortality in severe neuroses. *British Journal of Psychiatry*, **133**, 299–305.

SMITH, A. (1992) Setting a strategy for health. *British Medical Journal*, **304**, 376–378.

SPITZER, R. L. & ENDICOTT, J. (1987) *Structured Clinical Interview for DSM–III–R Personality Disorders*. Biometrics Research Department, New York State Psychiatric Institute, 722 West 168th Street, New York, NY 10032.

SPITZER, W. O., DOBSON, A. J., *et al* (1985) Measuring the quality of life of cancer patients. *Journal of Chronic Diseases*, **34**, 585–597.

STEVENS, B. (1973) The role of fluphenazine decanoate in lessening the burden of chronic schizophrenics on the community. *Psychological Medicine*, **3**, 141–158.

STURT, E. & WYKES, T. (1986) The measurement of social behaviour in psychiatric patients: an assessment of the reliability and validity of the SBS schedule. *British Journal of Psychiatry*, **148**, 1–11.

TAPS (Team for the Assessment of Psychiatric Services) (1990) *Better Out than In?* London: North East Thames Regional Health Authority.

THOMPSON, C. (ed) (1989) *The Instruments of Psychiatric Research*. Chichester: Wiley.

THORNICROFT, G. (1991) Social deprivation and rates of treated mental disorder: developing statistical models to predict psychiatric service utilisation. *British Journal of Psychiatry*, **158**, 465–484.

THORNICROFT, G., MARGOLIUS, O. & JONES, D. (1992) The TAPS Project (6): New long-stay psychiatric patients and social deprivation. *British Journal of Psychiatry*, **161**, 621–624.

TORGENSEN, S. (1983) Genetics of neuroses: the effects of sampling variation upon the twin concordance ratio. *British Journal of Psychiatry*, **142**, 126–132.

TROVATO, F. (1986) A time series analysis of international immigration and suicide mortality in Canada. *International Journal of the Society of Psychiatry*, **32**, 38–46.

WIERSMA, D., DE JONG, A., KRAAIJKAMP, H. J. M., *et al* (1990) *GSDS-II The Groningen Social Disabilities Schedule, 2nd Version*. Groningen: University of Groningen, Department of Social Psychiatry.

WILSON, R. (1981) Do health indicators indicate health? *American Journal of Public Health*, **71**, 461.

WING, J. (1982) Rehabilitation and management of schizophrenia. In *Handbook of Psychiatry, vol 3. Psychoses of Uncertain Aetiology* (eds J. K. Wing & L. Wing). Cambridge: Cambridge University Press.

WING, J. K., COOPER, J. E. & SARTORIUS, N. (1974) *The Measurement and Classification of Psychiatric Symptoms*. London: Cambridge University Press.

WORLD HEALTH ORGANIZATION (1981) *Development Indicators for Monitoring Progress Towards Health for All by the Year 2000*. Geneva: WHO.

WORLD HEALTH ORGANIZATION (1988) *Psychiatric Disability Schedule (WHO/DAS)*. Geneva: WHO.

WYKES, T. & STURT, E. (1986) The measurement of social behaviour in psychiatric patients: an assessment of the reliability and validity of the SBS schedule. *British Journal of Psychiatry*, **148**, 1–11.

3 The purchasers' information requirements on mental health needs and contracting for mental health services

ANDREW STEVENS and JAMES RAFTERY

In England and Wales since April 1991 a new factor has been injected into the planning of health (including mental health) services – that of the purchasers. Traditionally, planning has been dominated by providers, defined here to include psychiatrists, general practitioners (GPs) and other practising health professionals. Providers made decisions on the ways that patients should be managed with little overt reference to the costs incurred, but within a system which rationed the overall level of services. The new purchasing agencies comprise mainly the District Health Authorities (DHAs), which are now responsible for spending the resources available, to improve the health of their resident population. Although the overall level of resources available will be set nationally, the purchasers will be responsible for the pattern of spending between different services, and are obliged to determine this pattern on the basis of an assessment of the needs of the population so as to maximise health gain.

Because of the blurred border between primary and secondary care, and the necessity for health-care provision to reflect GP referral preferences, DHA purchasing takes place in consultation with both the local family health services authority (FHSA) and the local GPs.

Local authorities also have an interest in 'needs assessment' – specifically of the social-care requirement for individuals with mental health problems which is a formal requirement from April 1993 (Department of Health, 1990). The ill-defined boundary between health care and social care in the mental health field necessitates close working arrangements between local authorities and health authorities. The overlap of responsibilities, the possible tightening of local-authority finance, the different geographical boundaries of different authorities, and the differing nature of the assessment of individual needs and the population needs, will not make such arrangements easy.

TABLE 3.1
Purchasers and providers of care (simplified)

Service	Purchasers	Providers
Primary care	Central Government (via the GP contract) FHSAs	GPs (and primary health-care teams) GP fundholders (GPFHs)
Secondary and community care	DHAs and GPFHs	Hospital and community psychiatry, private and voluntary sector.
Social care	Local authorities	Local authority services, housing associations, private and voluntary sector.

This chapter looks at the information requirements of purchasers of psychiatric hospital and community care in the role created for them by the National Health Service (NHS) review. It considers the context of this work, i.e. the NHS review, and the purchaser's role; it then examines the main areas of information required: population needs assessment, service description and specification, and service monitoring. It concludes with an overview of the development of current routine information and a recommendation for a wide-ranging district intelligence facility.

The term 'purchasers' refers, principally, to district health authority planners, managers, and public-health doctors, and the term 'providers' to hospital and community-care clinical staff and managers.

The National Health Service review

The NHS review which culminated in the NHS and Community Care Act 1990 (House of Commons, 1990) revolved around a single dominant theme: the separation of *purchaser* and *provider* roles of health care, that is, the separation of DHA medium-term planning from the day-to-day management and provision of hospital and community-care services.

This was accompanied by the introduction of arrangements for funding each DHA – the principal purchaser – to purchase services for its *resident* population rather than funding providers for their *catchment* populations; and a system of contracting for health care between purchasers and providers. Providers of care have the option to gain increased freedom in managing their own affairs by obtaining NHS Trust status.

While DHAs are the main purchasers of secondary health care, primary care continues to be purchased (but with little freedom of manoeuvre, given the central framing of the GP contract) by the FHSAs. The division of purchaser and provider functions for primary, secondary and social care is outlined in Table 3.1. Better integration of primary and secondary care has been given a stimulus as DHAs and FHSAs are now both accountable to regional health authorities (RHAs). Some group practices (with a list size greater than 7000) have opted to become 'GP fundholders' (GPFHs). Fundholders are able to purchase certain hospital services on behalf of their patients. These services include not only various specific surgical procedures, but also out-patient visits, and so include psychiatric out-patients (but not referrals to community mental-health teams).

Both the new arrangements and the old (pre-1991) arrangements are shown in Fig. 3.1 which also illustrates the links with local authorities.

The purchaser's role

If the purchaser's aim is to respond to the population's health needs "to achieve the optimum improvement in the health of the population they serve" (National Health Service Management Executive, 1989), they need to know what those needs are, and to know what services are already provided. The most significant constraints on purchasing are the current pattern of services and overall finance; the total budget is outside the purchaser's control, allocated by Parliament, the Department of Health and the RHAs in turn. DHAs, in theory, may move money between services (e.g. from surgery to mental health) and between providers, but in practice such changes are likely to be at the margin.

Five stages of purchaser activity have been identified, each affecting the DHA's information requirements as follows:

(a) the *assessment of the health needs* of the local population, including a perspective on the views of that population

(b) the *appraisal of service options* for meeting those needs, including close cooperation with FHSAs and GPs, both in the short term and strategically

(c) the specification of the *chosen pattern of service provision*

(d) *choosing between providers and placing contracts* compatible with the district's cash limits

(e) *monitoring* the provision of contracted services and the health of the population (National Health Service Management Executive, 1989).

These rational and methodical stages will often be blurred in the real world. In practice there are three activities for which information is required:

(a) needs assessment

(b) service description, specification and associated costs

(c) monitoring.

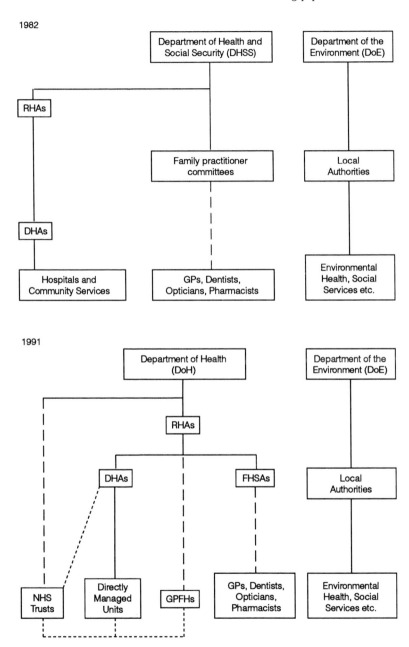

Fig. 3.1. Accountability and linkage in health-care provision in Britain before and after the NHS review (Direct accountability ——, rule-setting accountability ———, and contractual relationships -----)

These activities demand a number of skills within district health authorities: the district general manager is responsible for the overall performance of the DHA. He or she is assisted by a number of executives and non-executive directors (the latter bringing a range of interests from outside the NHS and from local medical schools). The purchasing team comprises public health (needs assessment, interpreting the service), finance, and contract management. All are supported by the district information department. The roles of needs assessment and contract management are closely related and should work in parallel but with a respective bias to the *content* of purchased package of health care and the *process* of achieving it (Fig. 3.2).

Information and population needs assessment

The assessment of health needs of the local population is considered from a variety of angles in this book. From the purchaser's point of view the appropriate definition of need is:

> "The population's ability to benefit from health care."
> (National Health Service Management Executive, 1991*a*)

Each component of this definition is important. First, the *population's* ability to benefit is the aggregate of individuals' ability to benefit but, for any health problem, depends on the incidence and prevalence (of different degrees of severity) of the condition and its effects and complications; secondly, *ability* to benefit does not mean that every outcome is guaranteed to be favourable, but it does mean that there is only a need where the intervention and/or the care setting is effective; thirdly, the *benefit* measured should include not only clinical status and well-being compared with that without the intervention, but also reassurance, both to the individual and professional, that avenues of potential benefit have been explored, for example, confirming

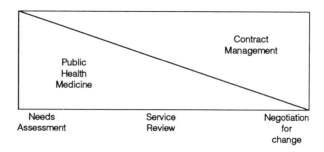

Fig. 3.2. Roles of public health medicine and contract management in purchasing care

the diagnosis, and supportive care and the relief of pressure on other carers; finally, health *care* includes prevention and promotion, diagnosis, treatment, continuing care, rehabilitation, and terminal care.

Given this definition, it is worth distinguishing need from efficacy and outcome.

Need is the population's *ability to benefit* from health care
Efficacy is the intervention's/care setting's *potential to benefit* recipients
Outcome is the actually *achieved benefit* in the local setting.

Need, defined in this way, forms the basis for the epidemiological assessment of need. In practice, two other approaches are common: the comparative approach, and the corporate approach (National Health Service Management Executive, 1991a).

The epidemiological assessment of need

Measuring the population's ability to benefit from health care generates two very specific information requirements.

(a) The local prevalence and incidence of disease, ranged by severity. Prevalence – the number of cases per unit population at a point in time, or over a period – is usually the appropriate measure for chronic disease; and incidence – the number of new cases per unit time – is usually appropriate for measuring acute disease.
(b) The efficacy of the care and care settings available or potentially available to cope with it.

Together these measurements form the basis of the epidemiological approach to needs assessment. Both incidence/prevalence and efficacy present formidable information problems. *Local* data are almost never available.

The only exceptions to this are:

(a) the rare occasions where the local district has been the site of an epidemiological survey or study
(b) those instances where diseases are so definite and so certain to present to hospital services that they are fully recorded in the hospital data systems, e.g. certain fractures or full-blown acquired immune deficiency syndrome (AIDS).

For most diseases, however, some national estimates can be made on incidence and prevalence. Such data can be applied locally if interpreted in the light of knowledge of factors accounting for local variation. Examples of work of this kind are the NHS Management Executive sponsored needs reviews on a variety of topics including: alcohol abuse, severe mental illness, dementia, and learning difficulties (National Health Service Management Executive, 1992).

The collection of these and similar secondary sources of *ad hoc* data suggests the need for each DHA to have a selective library facility as well as a routine information facility (see District Intelligence Facility, p. 59).

Information on the efficacy of health care and health-care settings is at least equally hard to come by. The development of health care has often been characterised by the adoption of procedures and dogmas with poor accompanying evidence of their efficacy. Some excellent examples of summaries of efficacy are available in other fields, for example, in obstetrics and perinatal care (Chalmers *et al*, 1989) and for some preventive strategies (US Preventive Services Taskforce, 1989). The latter adopts a commendable twin scale of efficacy assessment. One scale, A to E, describes the strength of a recommendation that a procedure be adopted; the other, I–III, is on the quality of the evidence. Purchasers who manage to define the care procedures and settings on this sort of scale will have accomplished half the preparatory work for purchasing.

The epidemiological approach to needs assessment, although the ideal for purchasers, is not the only approach. In reality, district purchasing activity is much more influenced by two other approaches: comparative assessments and the corporate approach (National Health Service Management Executive, 1991*a*). Strictly, neither measures the ability to benefit from health care, but each can give clear pointers to priorities for change.

The comparative assessment of need

The comparative approach involves no more than making comparisons between districts, or even within districts of:

(a) morbidity and mortality, for example, in the Public Health Common Data Set (Department of Health, 1991), and in the General Practice Morbidity survey (Royal College of General Practitioners, 1986)

(b) service utilisation and provision, for example, in the Health Service Indicators (HSIs) (National Health Service Management Executive, 1991*b*) and, until 1986 the Mental Health Enquiry (Department of Health and Social Security, 1986)

(c) costs and outcomes (some crude data for each appear in the HSIs and the Common Data Set but mostly this will be available only through local data and measurement).

The comparative approach gives insights into possible priorities for change by exploring differences both within and between districts. Morbidity and mortality data may reveal local black spots of either need or performance.

To the degree that they are responsive to health-service performance, they serve as outcome indicators of the local health services. In the field of mental health the Public Health Common Data Set exposes exceptional suicide rates and liver cirrhosis mortality (Department of Health, 1991). Home Office statistics add further clues in drug-abuse notification rates. The Health Service Indicators include, for example, the proportion of patients compulsorily admitted to hospital. Both of these latter indicators are morbidity information of a sort.

Data on service utilisation and provision, compared between districts, expose the relative differences in supply across the country. High levels do not necessarily mean 'overmet need' nor low levels 'unmet need' but both can trigger scrutiny on whether the levels of provision might be adjusted. The Health Service Indicators (Department of Health, 1991) with 72 indicators in Mental Health Services are the key source of this information, although they have been bedevilled by the complexities and changes in the way mental health activity data have been collected (see Development of current routine information, p. 58).

Comparative-cost data are elusive because of the variety of methods used to calculate costs, but crude measures such as costs per in-patient day or per clinic attendance can indicate any major divergences. To be meaningful, costs must relate to defined activities. Although purchasers will know, for contractual reasons, how much an entire district service for the care of the elderly mentally ill costs, they will also need to know the *unit cost* of the range of services such as for a residential place, an in-patient episode for acute care and assessment, or a year's community care.

Of course, value for money implies a measure of value – hence the need for outcome measurements. In theory, it is only when outcomes are included that comparisons of cost-effectiveness are valid. In practice, comparative-cost data provide clear prompts for purchasers, both to question the value of services purchased, and to decide when not to do so because the cost is trivial. Arguments put by providers to justify greater than average or expected cost, not explained by restructuring costs for example, must put the onus on the provider to demonstrate that the additional cost is justified, that is, by getting down to the collection of adequate outcome data.

The corporate approach to needs assessment

The 'corporate' approach to needs assessment involves the purchaser synthesising the views of interested and informed parties in local health care. These will include:

(a) the purchasing team, advisers, and experts
(b) local people
(c) GPs (including GP fundholders)

(d) providers and clinical staff
(e) other local agencies (FHSAs, LAs etc.)
(f) the regional health authority and the NHS Management Executive.

Inevitably some of these will reveal as much about demand (local people, GPs) and about supply bias (providers, other local agencies) as they do about need. However, demand assessment is part of the purchaser's role, and the National Health Service review was partly predicated on greater responsiveness to both patients and GPs. In practice, many of these sources, particularly providers, i.e. the local psychiatrists and GPs, are in a position to alert purchasers to major crisis areas, reflecting unmet needs, much more quickly than a formal needs assessment would. After over 40 or so years of health-service organisation in which this formal population assessment of need was absent, many crisis areas of unmet need will arise in this way.

Service description and specification

The assembly of this mosaic of information is only the first step in engineering change on the basis of needs. Agreement about priorities requires negotiation and an understanding of the relative costs and benefits of various options. Achieving change requires protracted negotiation and information exchange between purchasers and providers throughout the annual contracting process. Year-on-year such change is likely to be marginal, and will focus on areas where there are the best opportunities for relatively painless shifts in the balance of care. The key information set required is a clear description of the local mental health services contracted and paid for.

A full service description would include details of costs and expected performance, that is, expected outcomes. Since both costs and outcome specifications are relatively new ideas to the health services, neither is yet on a firm enough footing for service specification to use at present, the development of resource management (Clifford, 1991) and various outcome initiatives will improve matters (Jenkins, 1990). Meanwhile, service specification relies on descriptions of facilities and levels of activity. The level of service description required is not universally agreed, but might include staff, equipment, estate, accreditation standards, rules, and protocols. Under estate might be included beds and places, through wards and other settings to entire service systems. Purchasers will want to have an intelligible description of service, but will restrict the level of detail in order to allow providers autonomy to organise the service as they see fit (provided they achieve the desired outcomes), and also because of the cost of collecting and interpreting detailed data.

A variety of levels of description can be outlined from crude to fine as shown below.

(a) Total cost and capacity of a district mental health service. This will have been the 1991 starting level for the block contract used by most purchasers of mental health care. Quality will have been based on provider reassurances of satisfactory services (possibly true but an abdication of purchaser responsibility); or comparisons of cost elsewhere for the same population base (likely to encourage changing quantity up or down, but without any intrinsic rationale).

(b) Cost and capacity of subsections of a district mental health service such as adult mental health; elderly mental health; child mental health; substance misuse; forensic (if not part of adult); and psychotherapy (if not part of adult). This refinement of (a) marks the first step in the direction of recognising the heterogeneity of the service. Value for money, however, remains impossible to judge without more detail on the type of settings in which patients are cared for.

(c) Cost, capacity, activity and staffing of services might be further disaggregated to more specific services, as shown in Table 3.2. Such a specification would include the unit costs for components of the service, defined as the largest homogeneous service units feasible; locations, types of wards, community mental health teams, etc. Since staffing levels are currently measured reasonably well (even if poorly allocated to this level of activity base) they can measure the scale of service and hence check the accuracy of the costing.

This level of information, while more sophisticated than currently compiled in this way either by purchasers or by providers anywhere, is the crudest level at which any meaningful judgement of the service can be made. The contract Minimum Data Set (Information Management Group, 1990) from 1993/94 will, however, provide much of the necessary data (see below). In the interim, a focus on high-cost services, such as long-stay patients, will enable purchasers to begin to monitor their major expenditures.

While greater levels of detail than in Table 3.2 are possible, they are not recommended for the reasons given above (provider prerogative and time considerations). The function column could be expanded, for example, to show the use of agreed protocols, admission thresholds etc., but the basic format is probably sufficient for purchasers to understand the services specified. Meanwhile, it is likely that many purchasers will be operating at a cruder level of specification than this for some time.

Contracts in the mental health services, as for other services, have been predominantly block contracts in 1991–92, with cost per case for extra-contractual referrals. Block contracts have enabled services to be provided as before by aggregating services up to the level at which budgets were previously set. As contracting develops, purchasers will want more detailed accounts of both activity and finance.

Specification of service quality

Quality can be divided into broad fields: clinical and non-clinical, each of which can be assessed according to its structure, processes and procedures, and outcome (Table 3.3).

TABLE 3.2
Detailed service specification

Location or non-locational service e.g.	Function	Capacity	Activity level	Staffing	Cost	Unit cost[1]
In-patient ward (1)	Acute assessment	16 beds	150 consultant episodes	10 wte[2]	£·000	£000 per episode
In-patient ward (2)	Acute assessment	18 beds	120 consultant episodes	10 wte	£·000	£000 per episode
District Community Mental Health Team	Maintenance of e.g. mild dementia at home and primary care support	125 open cases	2250 visits	10 wte	£·000	£ per case
Long-stay ward	Long stay	20 beds	20 patient years	8 wte	£·000	£ per patient
NHS Nursing Home etc.	Long stay	12 places	12 patient years	8 wte	£·000	£ per patient

1. Including pro rata proportion of overheads.
2. wte = whole time equivalent.

TABLE 3.3
Examples of quality measures

	Non-clinical	Clinical
Structure	Environmental quality	Staff accreditation
Process and procedure	Waiting times Information given to patients	Use of clinical protocols Medical audit procedures
Outcome	Patient satisfaction	Improvements in health

The quality of service is generally, often exclusively, taken to mean aspects of quality other than its clinical success and appropriateness. Most purchasers have made much greater progress with these, for example, 'hotel' quality and measures of patient satisfaction than they have with clinical quality. Among the quality items in which progress has been most rapid are:

(a) waiting times (for an appointment, in out-patients etc.)
(b) information given to patients, informal carers, and GPs (both informally and by leaflets)
(c) evidence of their involvement in care plans
(d) facilities for particular groups (translations and advocacy for ethnic minorities, physical facilities for the elderly or physically disabled)
(e) speed and quality of communication with GPs
(f) evidence of communication with voluntary groups, local authorities, etc.
(g) patient satisfaction questionnaires and complaints procedures
(h) inspection of the physical environment.

Progress on clinical quality (other than direct outcome measurement) includes:

(a) evidence of the use of clinical protocols and care plans
(b) satisfactory medical audit–the peer group cyclical setting of standards and review of cases, was given a major boost by the NHS review and has been widely adopted since then. Whether it will generate any management information for purchasers of health care is, as yet, unclear.

Service monitoring

The purchaser's interest in the service is in both sides of the chart:

chart 1.   Resources   - - - - - - - - -> Health care (quality and quantity)

Partly because the purchasers have a responsibility to the whole resident population, and partly because the relevance of health care depends on to whom the care is given, chart 1 can be made slightly more complicated:

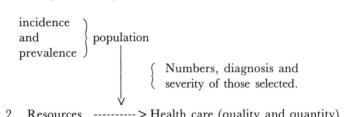

```
incidence  ⎫
and        ⎬ population
prevalence ⎭          │
                      │        ⎧ Numbers, diagnosis and
                      │        ⎨ severity of those selected.
                      │        ⎩
                      V
chart 2.   Resources  ----------> Health care (quality and quantity)
```

It is necessary to measure the characteristics of the population treated vis à vis the population at large to take into account issues of equity and appropriateness, that is, to ensure that care given was to the people with greatest need.

Furthermore, the purchasers' real interest should not be confined to the health *care* received but include the health *gain* achieved (for the resources put in) as in chart 3:

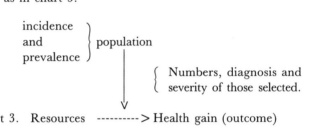

```
incidence  ⎫
and        ⎬ population
prevalence ⎭          │
                      │        ⎧ Numbers, diagnosis and
                      │        ⎨ severity of those selected.
                      │        ⎩
                      V
chart 3.   Resources  ----------> Health gain (outcome)
```

Thus, the key information required pertains to outcome accompanied by severity measurement (on the same scale) of patients on admission. Ideally this should also be known for those not admitted, to measure unmet need.

Of course, such measurements are not routine, least of all in psychiatry, partly because outcome measurement is still in its infancy. The outcomes most easily monitored and most relevant to different areas of health-care activity are usually measured on different scales; for example, non-relapse in schizophrenic care and respite care for people with dementia. Pioneering experiments in the use of measures such as the 'global assessment of function' (Endicott *et al*, 1976), offer scope for generalised measurement of health gain but their widespread adoption will require slow and careful movement towards consensus among practitioners. The requirement that outcome measures be easy to employ, sensitive to health change due to care, and reliable between users will be difficult to meet. Jenkins (1990) has suggested a wide range of psychiatric outcome measures which might be included in contracts. Similarly, *Health of the Nation* (Secretary of State for Health, 1991) put forward a number of outcome and preventive targets for consultation. In the meantime, future purchasers (via contractual arrangements with providers) will measure very few outcomes, for example of rates of schizophrenic relapse, or of patient and carer satisfaction with long-stay care.

The providers of care should, however, be encouraged into linking medical audit to the development of outcome measures which can be used explicitly to commend their services to purchasers.

Meanwhile, purchasers need to measure the structure and process of health care. Measuring structure means maintaining a knowledge of the provider's service as decribed in Table 3.2 and above. As regards monitoring process, this may sometimes be a close and satisfactory substitute for monitoring outcome, that is where research demonstrated a close relationship between process measures and outcomes. Thus although chart 3 summarises the purchasers' idealised interest, there is a wider range of things the purchaser would wish to monitor.

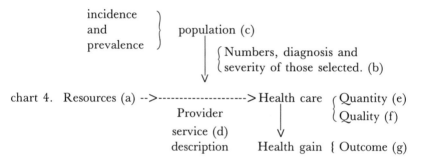

In summary, the measurements are as outlined below.

(a) *Resources, i.e. cost.* This is not necessarily monitored routinely. The annual contract, if specified carefully, can allocate all the risk of overspends to the provider at the beginning of a contractual year. In practice, the risk tends to be shared between purchasers and providers by means of clauses in block contracts which are triggered by activity and cost deviations from planned levels.

(b) *Number and characteristics of patients treated.* Both the number of people treated (which is what is usually, albeit crudely, contracted for), and their medical characteristics, require measuring. Logically, outcome might be measured as the difference between the patient's starting condition (or rather expected untreated end condition) and the actual end condition. In practice, the best that is currently recorded for in-patient care is diagnosis (without severity) and often even that is missing. With the advent of contracts, purchasers will be in a position to insist on diagnostic coding, or at the very least, say, a crude distinction between a primary diagnosis of neurosis and one of psychosis. This will at least allow some eventual mapping of the appropriateness of treatment, even if health gain goes unmeasured.

Another potential approach is the measurement of *casemix*. The experience in the US with Diagnostic-Related Groups (Mitchell *et al*, 1987) suggests that diagnosis is of little help in attempting to measure prospectively the resources required by individual in-patients. Although casemix groups, such as English casemix groups, may enable cases to be grouped in ways that are clinically meaningful and homogeneous in their resource requirements in the acute sector, this is not promising in psychiatry.

Many alternative approaches are being pursued, such as attempting to cross-reference diagnoses with types of individual requiring admission because of the likelihood of them doing injury to themselves or others (Wing, 1992).

(c) *Population not treated.* Purchasers will wish to know about those who might be treated, but in fact have not been. Purchasers could make estimates of unmet need by measuring the difference between prevalence, incidence, and activity. In psychiatry this is probably insufficient because the risk is that the most severely ill, and not the mildest, may fail to receive treatment. Such a position would be extremely rare in general medicine or surgery, because the most severe are the most likely to seek care and to be considered the most rewarding to treat. Neither of these conditions is met by severe schizophrenics and people with challenging behaviour. Purchasers therefore must insist on the monitoring of the most severely psychiatrically ill. In practice, registers and active case-management policies may enable follow-up of the most needy to be maintained.

(d) *Provider–service description.* The provider–service description provides the framework for monitoring the service. The purchaser's understanding of what is monitored depends on separating out the measurements of the service into relatively homogeneous units such as acute in-patient beds, elderly long-stay places, community-team visits, etc. (see Table 3.2).

(e) *Health Care–quantity.* Since the activity levels in the secondary health care are now mainly measured in terms of consultant in-patient episodes, this, in all specialities is at best a very crude measure of quantity and fails to measure quality at all. In mental health care the poverty of this measure is exacerbated by a number of characteristics:

(i) in-patient care is a small and diminishing part of mental health care

(ii) in many respects in-patient care actually represents an alternative model of care to that practised (i.e. community based) for certain patients

(iii) the chronicity and episodic nature of mental illness means that episodes are often part of a longer sequence and vary in length and intensity

(iv) there is a diversity of health-professional contacts – psychiatrists, psychologists, community psychiatric nurses (CPNs), occupational therapists, etc.

A number of other routine process measures also give information of doubtful value on the service to be purchased. The CPN contact rate says nothing about what happened, how long for, or to what end; nor does the day-hospital attendance rate.

Until the new contract minimum data set is in place (see next section) purchasers will have to negotiate with providers for more useful information. Two principles are important. The first is to measure data which is sufficiently well defined to be interpretable. This means measuring not just a patient contact, begging the questions what type of patient (psychiatric, neurotic) and what type of contacts (e.g. new, repeat). The second is to measure different care settings comparably. Measuring interpretable data is obviously vital, but given the contortions that health-care information systems have had to undergo with each review of the NHS, the requirements for change should be modest. Data on patient flow will be most informative if there is a measurement of both the capacity of the part of the system being monitored (cf Fig. 3.2), and the activity level; the activity data must distinguish new from total contacts.

This allows purchasers to get a feel for what they are purchasing (capacity), as well as how much it is used, and also the number of patients (as opposed to episodes) actually cared for.

The different secondary-care settings to be measured are of three broad types:

   (i) acute in-patient care
  (ii) out-patients, daycare, and community contacts
 (iii) residential care.

As there is a tendency for these to be alternatives to each other in many situations (i.e. intensive community care may keep someone out of hospital), they need to be measured comparably. Therefore, the three-way measurement of capacity (e.g. number of open cases a community team can manage), activity level (total admissions in the case of in-patients or contacts elsewhere) and new cases seen should apply to each. Furthermore, in the case of out-patients or community care they should be recorded irrespective of whether contact is with a psychiatrist or with another member of the team.

(f) *Health Care – quality.* A representative list of non-clinical quality items was suggested (p. 53). Some of these are open to routine monitoring at different intervals, for example, GP communication and waiting times. Other quality measures can be constructed for particular parts of the service, and the items suggested can be tailored to the service, for example, on patient satisfaction. Whatever measures are preferred locally, monitoring is essential if they are to mean anything.

(g) *Health Care–clinical, quality and outcome.* Although outcome measurement will be fragmentary for a long time to come, local experiments will both act as a stimulus to recognise that it is positive outcomes which are the ultimate aim of health care, and to increase the portfolio of usable measures. Most progress is likely to be made by experimenting with measures specific to each care group (e.g. relapse with schizophrenia, periodic rating scores with depression, etc.); and also accepting process measures where these are known to be associated with better outcomes. Examples include the measurement of the time interval between addiction and the first treatment in opiate services (Strang, 1991), or the proportion of schizophrenics whose cases have been reviewed according to a care programme.

The development of current routine information

From 1964 to 1986 the Mental Health Enquiry (Department of Health and Social Security, 1986) provided the main data on the activities of the mental health sector, with annual accounts of admissions, discharges, and deaths, and on resident patients, with cross tabulations by variables such as age, sex, diagnosis, length of stay. Data on unit costs (per in-patient day, out-patient and day-patient hospital attendance) were provided in Health Service Costing Returns (Department of Health and Social Security, annual to 1986-87). Each of these sources, along with a range of similar sources referring to the acute hospital sector were discontinued in 1987 with the Körner reorganisation of NHS information.

The Körner information structure (Steering Group on Health Services Information, 1985) which was designed to facilitate management of provider units, led to acute (short-stay) psychiatric activity data being treated as one speciality among many. In addition, Körner recommended that an annual census should be carried out of all patients who have been in mental illness or mental handicap units of hospitals for a year or more, and on all detained patients. New Financial Returns FR11 and FR12 (Department of Health and Social Security, 1987) were developed which provided data on speciality costs without the overheads being allocated.

Although the aims of the Körner reorganisation made good sense at the time, the subsequent NHS reforms of 1991 meant that new and different demands were being placed on the fledgling information system before it became fully established, and new systems are planned to meet the requirements of contracting the Contract Minimum Data Set (Information Management Group, 1990). Partly as a consequence of the changed demands for information, the Körner system has failed to achieve the level of data capture that might otherwise have been obtained.

The Contract Minimum Data Set, which becomes operational within contracts from 1993/94 offers the best prospect for information becoming more structured to meet the requirements of purchasing with data on the main types of activity (although not on needs) and their associated prices. In relation to mental health services, the Contract Minimum Data set follows Körner's recommendations, with acute psychiatric admissions dealt with as one medical speciality among many and with an annual census to cover those in longer-stay institutions. In addition, efforts were made to include data on the diversity of types of service and locations that apply to the mental health services.

The Mental Health Service Indicators (HSIs), formerly performance indicators, have provided accessible data to districts, based on the changing national data sources. Provided on computer diskettes to each district health authority and to provider units, these are a potentially useful source of comparative data. Local and national admission rates, length of stay, with various breakdowns (such as by age, sex, legal status) are provided, with a similar set of data on costs. The supporting raw data are also available so that the methods can be checked and adjusted as appropriate.

The Contract Minimum Data Set should improve the basic data recorded from 1993–94, with the HSIs thus becoming the key source of comparative data for DHAs to use.

The district intelligence facility

In health-service discussions the word 'information' seems to have lost its wider meaning of information in the round. It increasingly refers only to this routine service-operation data. Although the most accessible parts of the monitoring information discussed fit into this category, the service description information and the three categories of needs-assessment data do not. The consequence is that such information has traditionally been all but ignored in district health authority information departments.

In their new role as needs assessors and purchasers of health care, DHAs are starting to realise that this will pose a problem for them, and some are starting to develop broader 'intelligence' facilities to access the wider range of information necessary (National Health Service Management Executive, 1991c).

The intelligence they require includes anything that helps throw light on the local population's health-care needs and the services they receive. The intelligence is not only numerical, but also textual, not only local but also national, and not only routine but also *ad hoc*. These dimensions and the types of information involved are illustrated in Table 3.4.

The intelligence facility is thus a combination of a routine data facility and a library requiring the skills of both an information technology expert and a librarian. The library will need access to a basic range of texts: government circulars, Royal College reports, epidemiological research, etc.

TABLE 3.4
Broad categories of intelligence for purchasing – with examples

| | Local | | National | |
	routine	ad hoc	routine	ad hoc
Numerical	Minimum data sets, population register	Local surveys (DHA,LA, FHSA)	Health Service indicators, common data set, general household survey	Epidemiological study data
Textual	Contracts, DHA minutes	Local reports (DHA,LA, FHSA)	Government circulars	Royal College reports

and also access to other local and national collections and databases. An important component of this will be the mutual access to information of DHAs, FHSAs and local authorities to avoid reinventing local studies and insights which may already have been gathered. Certainly the national sources both of data, for example, on epidemiology and effectiveness, and of text in the form of expert recommendations, offer purchasers of health care a firm starting point for their work.

Conclusion

The new purchasers of health care clearly have major new information needs. These include the collection of information on disease incidence and prevalence and service effectiveness.

The Contract Minimum Data Set will lead to improved information provision, which, combined with the diffusion of information technology, will greatly facilitate the provision and analysis of data. The main challenge will be the collection of cost data and activity or capacity data for the same components of service.

Perhaps the biggest challenge remains the measurement of outcomes in psychiatric services, and the inclusion of the same in the routine data sets. A menu of outcome measures has been outlined by Jenkins (1990). The challenge will be to deliver that menu.

References

CHALMERS, I., ENKIN, M. & KEIRSE, N. (1989) *Effective Care in Pregnancy and Childbirth*. London: Oxford University Press.

CLIFFORD, P. (1991) *The FACE Project, a Research and Development Programme in Mental Health Resource Management*. London: Quality Development Unit.

DEPARTMENT OF HEALTH (1990) *Community Care in the Next Decade and Beyond: Policy Guidance*. London: HMSO.

────── (1991) *Public Health Common Data Set*. 14 Regional Volumes. London: DoH.

DEPARTMENT OF HEALTH & SOCIAL SECURITY (1986) *Statistics of Mental Illness and Mental Handicap Hospitals in England*, various years and subsequent booklet series. London: DHSS.

────── (1987) *Health Service Costing Returns 1986/1987*. London: HMSO.

ENDICOTT, J., SPITZER, R. L., FLEISS, J. L., *et al*, (1976) The Global Assessment Scale, a procedure for measuring overall severity of psychiatric disturbance. *Archives of General Psychiatry*, **33**, 766–771

HOUSE OF COMMONS (1990) *National Health Service and Community Care Act*. London: HMSO.

INFORMATION MANAGEMENT GROUP, NHSME (1990) *Framework for Information Systems: The Next Steps*. London: HMSO.

JENKINS, R. (1990) Towards a system of outcome indicators for Mental Health Care. *British Journal of Psychiatry*, **157**, 500–514.

MITCHELL, J., DICKEY, B., LIPTZIN, B., *et al* (1987) Bringing psychiatric patients into the medicare prospective payments system: alternatives to DRGs. *American Journal of Psychiatry*, **144**, 610–615.

NATIONAL HEALTH SERVICE MANAGEMENT EXECUTIVE (1989) *Role of District Health Authorities – Analysis of Issues*. London: DoH.

────── (1991a) *Assessing Health Care Needs*. London: DoH.

────── (1991b) *Health Service Indicators Directory*. London: DoH.

────── (1991c) *Purchasing Intelligence*. London: DoH.

────── (1992) *Epidemiologically Based Needs Assessment Series*. London: DoH (in press).

ROYAL COLLEGE OF GENERAL PRACTITIONERS (1986) *Morbidity Statistics from General Practice*. Third National Study. London: HMSO.

SECRETARIES OF STATE (1981) *The National Health Service and Community Care Act*. London: HMSO.

SECRETARY OF STATE FOR HEALTH (1991) *The Health of the Nation. A Consultative Document for Health in England*. London: HMSO.

STRANG J. (1991) Injecting drug misuse. *British Medical Journal*, **303**, 1043–1046.

STEERING GROUP ON HEALTH SERVICES INFORMATION (1985) *First Report to the Secretary of State*. London: HMSO.

US PREVENTIVE SERVICES TASK FORCE (1989) *Guide to the Clinical Preventive Services*. Baltimore: Williams & Wilkins.

WING, J. (1992) *Epidemiologically Based Needs Assessment. Report 6: Mental Illness*. London: NHSHE DHA Project Research Programme.

4 Statistical models to predict district psychiatric morbidity

BRIAN JARMAN and STEVEN HIRSCH

This chapter is concerned with estimating the expected psychiatric admission rates for a health district population from the district's demographic, health, and social characteristics. In April 1991 the NHS moved to a new basis of financial resource distribution via Regional Health Authorities in the UK based on the size of the regional population, its age structure, and a measure of the level of health in each region (the square root of the standardised mortality ratio to age 75 was used as the measure of health). A fixed sum is allocated according to the numbers of residents in each of a number of age groups, and the overall sum is multiplied by the measure of health. Subregional allocations to District Health Authorities are expected to follow a similar method with a weighted capitation formula "funded broadly on the same basis as Regions" but allowance can be made for social and other factors (Department of Health and Social Security, 1989). The allocations for psychiatric services are lumped in with all other hospital- and community-health services in the costs per head for each age group.

We have carried out a total population study of psychiatric admission rates to all health districts in England in order to determine their relationship to more than 150 social, demographic, health status, and provision service variables, including various established social deprivation indices, indicators of poverty and isolation, and indicators of health-care supply and availability. We have developed a model which can be used by planners to predict a level of psychiatric service provision for the residents of district health authorities.

Background

In their report on Bed Norms and Resources, the Working Party of the Royal College of Psychiatrists (1988) found a high correlation between social and demographic factors based on national census data, and psychiatric admission rates for the populations within electoral wards of the previous health district of South Hammersmith and within the districts of the North West Thames Regional Health Authority.

In reviewing previous work they found a well established literature which suggests that the prevalence of psychiatric disorders correlates with various social and demographic variables (Ödegård, 1932; Faris & Dunham, 1939; Buglass *et al*, 1980; Goldberg & Huxley, 1980; Richman *et al*, 1984; Miller *et al*, 1986). The majority of work finds a strong relationship between the prevalence of specific disorders such as schizophrenia (Shepherd, 1957; Goodman *et al*, 1983; Cooper *et al*, 1987), and alcoholism (Goodman *et al*, 1983), suicide (Durkheim, 1952; Sainsbury, 1955), and parasuicide (Burke, 1976; Platt & Kreitman, 1985) and various social and demographic factors. However, the working party also identified five studies which showed a relationship between admission rates and rural or urban status of the population served, poverty, isolation, ethnicity, unemployment, and owner-occupied housing. Thornicroft, in his paper on psychiatric admission rates in the South East Thames region (Thornicroft, 1991), gives an excellent review of the literature on this subject.

Initially the aim of the Royal College Working Party was to explain the large variation of psychiatric bed provision among health districts by studying 20 psychiatric units in district general hospitals with high, medium and low bed turnovers. A significant factor which affected bed use was length of stay, but variations in length of stay could not be explained by differences in the amount, or type, of service available. Their finding of a correlation $r = 0.67$ between underprivileged area (UPA) scores (Jarman, 1983, 1984) and psychiatric admission rates across the electoral wards of South Hammersmith was their first strong indication of the influence of social factors.

The variables which constitute the UPA score were chosen by a survey of one in ten general practitioners (GPs) in the UK (with a 77% response rate) to obtain their opinions and relative weightings of factors which they considered were likely to increase their workload or pressure on their services when present in their areas. The factors finally used for the UPA score were the proportions of:

elderly alone
children under 5
people living in one parent families
unskilled workers
unemployed (as a % of the economically active)
people living in overcrowded households
people who had moved house within the preceding year
people in ethnic groups (New Commonwealth and Pakistan).

To calculate the UPA score for electoral wards, these eight census variables were (a) transformed with an angular transformation to make their distribution more symmetrical, then (b) standardised by subtracting the mean and dividing by the standard deviation of the transformed values, and then (c) weighted by the average weighting of each variable from the national GP survey. The values so obtained were used to give the UPA score of a ward or other area such as a district health authority (DHA). For Scotland, postcode sectors (with roughly the same populations as electoral wards, about 6000) were used.

A correlation, similar to that found for the wards of South Hammersmith, of $r = 0.76$ between UPA scores and admission rates for the Health Districts of the North West Thames RHA, further supported the impression that social factors could be powerful predictors of psychiatric hospital use which would be of importance if confirmed for larger and more extensive population groups. If a strong relationship between social and demographic factors and admission rates holds for other population groups, theoretical issues arise regarding the direction of causality. Equally important are the implications for health-care planning.

The relationship between actual service use and the need for services is difficult to determine because of the problems in defining need and the paucity of accurate and reliable data regarding the prevalence of psychiatric illness in each DHA. One indication of a relationship between the prevalence of psychiatric illness and service use was the association of the district standardised mortality rates (SMRs) for suicide plus other unspecified injury, averaged from 1982 to 1986 with the crude psychiatric admission rate of district residents, which showed a correlation coefficient of 0.51 ($P < 0.0001$).

The Royal College's report suggests that admission rates may be taken as a proxy for the psychiatric service requirements of a district.

Method

Our purpose was to study acute general psychiatry. It is possible to calculate the rate of admission to psychiatric hospitals from data collected annually up to 1986 for the Mental Health Enquiry (MHE) (Department of Health and Social Security, 1986). The district of residence and district of treatment of patients admitted to hospital for treatment by a psychiatrist are recorded as part of the MHE data. From this it is possible to calculate the total admissions for the *residents* of the district health authorities of England. A wide range of data is available from other sources regarding the demographic, social, and health status of the residents of these districts and the extent and availability of services from hospitals, GPs, and community psychiatric and non-psychiatric services and nursing homes (although little information is available regarding private psychiatric hospital provision). These data can be used to study the associations of these variables with psychiatric admission rates, which in turn may be used as a proxy indicator for levels of service provision required.

Of all psychiatric admissions recorded by the MHE, those for mental handicap (18%) and psychogeriatrics (11%) were excluded from further study as were any other admissions with a diagnosis of senile dementia (ICD–9 code 290; World Health Organization, 1978). For the years before 1986, the district of residence was not well recorded on the MHE returns and the data were inadequate for studying the admission rates of the residents of each district. However, for 1986 the data were relatively complete: only 779 (0.46%) of the 168 652 admissions remaining after removal of mental handicap and psychogeriatric admissions were coded only to a region of residence and not to a district of residence. There were 7784 (4.62%) admissions which were not coded to either a region or district of residence. The admissions where the district of residence was not recorded were allocated to each district in proportion to the total number of district admissions.

As a check on accuracy and completeness, the MHE data extracted from the original tapes were compared with data from two other sources for 1986. The SH_3 (a head count of people on the ward used as a check on other recorded data) returns which record the numbers of patients treated in each district for all speciality groups were obtained, and from these the returns for psychiatry (excluding mental handicap and psychogeriatrics) were calculated. In addition, the NHS Performance Indicator MI3 for the age/sex standardised psychiatric admission rate of district residents for April 1985–86 was obtained. In six of the 191 districts (Paddington & North Kensington, Camberwell, Wandsworth, North Birmingham, Preston, and West Lambeth) there were substantial differences in standardised admission ratios between the MHE data for 1986 and the Performance Indicator data for 1985–86 and/or the SH_3 data. Therefore, the data from these six districts were excluded from the analyses, leaving 185 districts. It is worth noting that the West Lambeth district standardised rates were nearly three times the national average and notably higher than for any other district.

It is important to realise that the MHE data for 1986 may turn out to be a unique data set regarding psychiatric services in England. These data were not recorded in this form after 1986 (when the MHE was discontinued) and the data for the years before 1986 are of such poor quality (because of non-recording of district of residence, probably for reasons of confidentiality) that they can not be used for reliable studies. One of the most useful aspects of the MHE data is the ability to study psychiatric in-patient hospital usage for both residents and for the districts in which patients are treated – this giving a very accurate idea of district cross-boundary flows (as this is a 100% sample of psychiatric admissions and discharges). Another aspect which is very valuable, because of its influence on psychiatric admission rates, is that marital status is recorded in addition to age and sex.

For our study, the national admission rates by age and sex, and by age, sex and marital status were calculated from the Mental Health Enquiry data

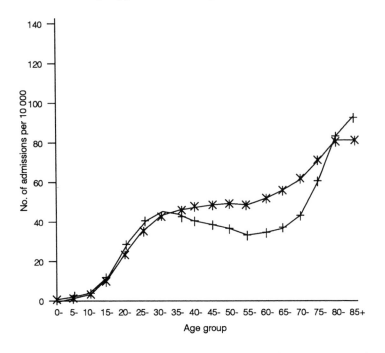

Fig. 4.1. Psychiatric admission rates per 10 000 population for males (——+——) and females (——✳——) in 1986

for the whole of England (see Figs 4.1 and 4.2). They were then applied to the age, sex and marital status structures of each district to calculate the numbers of admissions in each district which would have been expected if the national rates had been applied. An overall crude national admission rate (without allowance for age, sex or marital status) was also used to give an expected number of admissions based on the total population rate alone. The *actual* utilisation rates can be compared with these *expected* utilisation rates to produce an estimate of under (or over) utilisation of services by district resident populations. The actual number of admissions for the residents of each district divided by the expected number of admissions, calculated as described (× 100), gave the standardised psychiatric admission ratio (SPAR) based on population alone ($SPAR_{popn}$), age and sex standardisation ($SPAR_{as}$), and age, sex and marital status standardisation ($SPAR_{asms}$) respectively.

The Pearson correlation coefficients of 169 independent variables with the standardised psychiatric admission ratios, $SPAR_{popn}$, $SPAR_{as}$, and $SPAR_{asms}$ for 1986 for the 185 districts were calculated. These variables included a wide range of social, health status, and health-service provision factors including those reflecting hospital and GP provision,

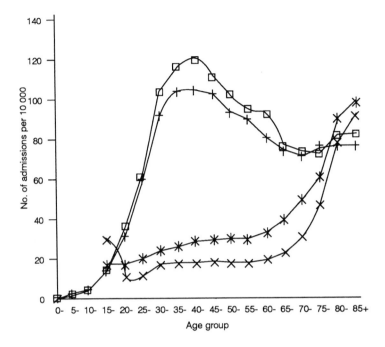

Fig. 4.2. Psychiatric admission rates per 10 000 population for married males (—✕—), married females (—✱—), unmarried males (—☐—) and unmarried females (—+—) in 1986 (Department of Health and Social Security, 1986)

community-based psychiatric and non-psychiatric health service and nursing-home provision, and the supply of community based and hospital medical and nursing staff, as well as psychiatric beds (but not private psychiatric-service provision). They are given in Appendix 1.

Finally, after standardising the admission rates for age, sex and marital status, as described above, in order to control for the effects of these variables, a stepwise regression analysis was used to determine which combination of these independent or explanatory variables most economically explained the variation of the standardised psychiatric admission ratios.

Results

The national psychiatric admission rates of males and females varied by age but were fairly similar, the rates for females being one-third greater than for males in the 45–70 age group (Fig. 4.1) However the unmarried of both sexes have much higher psychiatric admission rates than the married up to about age 75 (the maximum difference being for unmarried males

TABLE 4.1
Correlations between actual and expected number of admissions

Expected number of admissions	Correlation coefficient with actual number of admissions	% variance explained
Expected admissions based on population size alone	0.78	61
Expected admissions based on age and sex	0.79	62
Expected admissions based on age, sex and marital status	0.83	69

compared with married males where the unmarried rates are about six times the married rates for the 40–44 age group) – Fig. 4.2. As a result, expected psychiatric admissions calculated using the age, sex and marital status structure of a district were found to differ by up to 30% from the values based only on the age and sex structure alone. Differences in marital status structures therefore account for an important source of variation in the admission rates between health districts.

Correlations between actual and expected number of admissions

We first calculated the association between the actual (observed) numbers of admissions for the residents of the 185 districts of England and the expected numbers based on population alone, on age and sex, and on age, sex and marital status. These are indicated by the Pearson product–moment correlation coefficients between them (Table 4.1).

By comparison, a correlation coefficient of 0.89 was found between the actual number of admissions and the number predicted with the best-fit regression analyses (described below). If a model using the more easily available underprivileged area (UPA) score and crude admission rates is used, the correlation between the actual and predicted admissions is 0.84. Regression analyses were also carried out using the crude psychiatric admission rates per 1000 resident population as the dependent variable and the UPA score as the independent variable. Appendix 3 shows the relationship between these variables for the DHAs of England. The district UPA score explains 23% of the variation of district crude psychiatric admission rates (excluding mental handicap & psychogeriatrics).

Using Körner data for 1988–1991, in one Regional Health Authority (about 800 wards), the ward UPA score (ward UPA) explained 14% ($P < 0.0001$). The relationships found were:

Ward psychiatric admission rate (/1000 resident popn) = 3.99 + 0.095 (± 0.0085) × (ward UPA score)
Ward psychiatric admission rate (/1000 resident popn) = − 0.496 + 0.047 (± 0.0027) × (ward SMR75)

Correlation between standardised admission ratios and other variables

The values for each district of 169 variables (see Appendix 1), which it was thought might be associated with psychiatric admission rates, were correlated with $SPAR_{popn}$ (the standardised psychiatric admission ratio based on population alone and national overall admission rates). The strongest correlation coefficients (given in brackets) between different types of factors were (see also Appendix 2):

(a) indicators of isolation: percentage of single-person households, old people living alone, and unmarried (0.57 to 0.55)
(b) illegitimacy (0.53)
(c) composite measures of social deprivation: the Department of the Environment (DOE) index (Department of the Environment, 1983) UPA score, and the Townsend index (0.53 to 0.48) (Townsend *et al*, 1986)
(d) indicators of poverty: households lacking a car, personal service workers – socioeconomic group 7, and unskilled workers – socio-economic group 11 (0.54 to 0.45): unemployment (0.37)
(e) first and total notifications of drug misusers in 1988 (0.53 and 0.51)
(f) the availability of non-psychiatric hospital services: non-psychiatric bed availability, total consultants (and consultants plus junior doctors) per head of the population (0.52 to 0.42)
(g) levels of mortality and morbidity: SMR to age 65, SMR all ages, proportion of the population temporarily sick (0.50 and 0.47)
(h) high population density: population density, overcrowding of households (0.40 and 0.36).

One of the highest correlations of $SPAR_{popn}$ was with the percentage unmarried (0.55). This illustrates the importance of controlling for marital status by calculating for age, sex, and marital status in standardising psychiatric admission ratios – $SPAR_{asms}$.

In order to examine the association between psychiatric admission rates after taking account of age, sex, and marital status, the values of $SPAR_{asms}$ were correlated with the wide range of variables. The highest correlations were with SMR to age 65 (0.50), percentage of the elderly who live alone (0.48), illegitimacy (0.47), and SMR for bronchitis and emphysema, ischaemic heart disease, and circulatory system diseases (0.47 to 0.39), (see Appendix 2).

All the correlation coefficients cited above were highly significant ($P < 0.0001$).

TABLE 4.2
Regressions between dependent and explanatory variables

Dependent variables	Explanatory variables significant at $P < 0.0001$ level in stepwise regression analyses	
SPAR$_{popn}$	% unmarried, 1986 +	
	% born in UK, 1981 +	
	% socioeconomic group 7, personal-service workers, 1981	$r^2 = 0.44$
SPAR$_{asms}$	rate of notifications of drug misusers, 1988 +	
	% illegitimacy, 1986 +	
	SMR86	$r^2 = 0.33$
	(or + SMR86 for ischaemic heart disease $r^2 = 0.35$)	

Regression analyses

As shown above, the proportion of the variation of the actual number of admissions of district residents which was explained by the numbers expected based on population size alone, population age/sex structure and population age/sex/marital-status structure (and national admission rates) were 61%, 62%, and 69% respectively. Further regression analyses of the ratio of the actual to the expected admissions were carried out to determine how much additional variation could be explained by social, health status, and service factors.

The regression analyses using, in turn, as dependent variables, SPAR$_{popn}$ and SPAR$_{asms}$ gave models in which the following independent, or explanatory, variables were found to contribute most strongly to the explanation of the variance at the $P < 0.0001$ level of significance (the results for SPAR$_{as}$ were similar to those for SPAR$_{popn}$) (Table 4.2).

The model using age, sex, and marital status standardised ratios as dependent variables together with drug-misuser notification rate and SMR or SMR for ischaemic heart disease, SMR(IHD), as independent variables was used to calculate the values of SPAR$_{asms}$ which would be predicted from the regression equation for the 185 districts. Using SMR(IHD) with the rate of drug misuse first notifications (without the illegitimacy variable) explained almost as much ($r^2 = 0.34$) of the variance of SPAR$_{asms}$ as the full model ($r^2 = 0.35$) and was used in the final model shown in Appendix 3.

The final model was used to predict the numbers of psychiatric admissions for each district. The relationship between these and the actual number of admissions for each of the 185 districts is shown in Fig. 4.3. The predicted admissions correlated, $r = 0.89$, with the actual admissions. There was no significant difference in the model if the districts of inner London were removed from the analyses (in order to investigate whether the high admission rates in inner London have an unduly large influence).

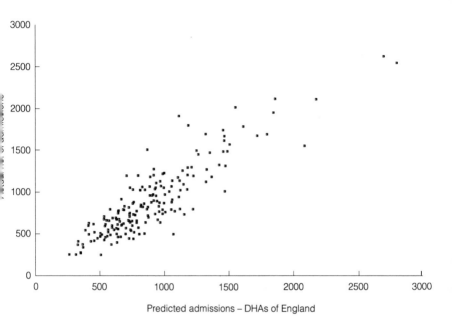

Fig. 4.3. Actual v. predicted psychiatric admissions (using SPAR_{asms} and recommended model, 1986)

TABLE 4.3
Actual/expected or actual/predicted admissions × 100 in various regions

Region	Actual divided by expected admissions from age/sex/marital status structures and national rates × 100 ($SPAR_{asms}$)	Actual divided by predicted admissions using the full model × 100
Northern	113	100
Yorkshire	120	107
Trent	89	91
E. Anglia	89	101
N.W. Thames	92	98
N.E. Thames	94	93
S.E. Thames	104	116
S.W. Thames	106	121
Wessex	100	111
Oxford	75	90
S. Western	87	96
W. Midland	93	94
Mersey	125	99
N. Western	116	95

Table 4.3 shows the ratios (× 100) of the actual admissions for the regions of England to the predicted psychiatric admissions, using this model. Also shown are the ratios of the actual admissions for the regions of England to the expected number of admissions based on district residential population age, sex, and marital-status structures, and national admission rates ($SPAR_{asms}$).

With many of the models, the proportion of mental-illness nurses working in the community was also significant at the $P<0.05$ or $P<0.01$ levels: the higher the proportion of mental-illness nurses working in the community, the lower the admission rates, after allowance for the other factors included in the model. Similarly, the proportion of mental-illness nurses in training was associated with higher admission rates.

Regression analyses were also carried out using the crude psychiatric admission rates per 1000 resident population as the dependent variable and the UPA score as the independent variable (see Appendix 3).

Discussion

National psychiatric admission data for one year (1986) were analysed in order to determine the relationship between admission rates and social, demographic, health, and service-provision indices.

The analysis reveals interesting relationships with all these influences and provides a useful tool for identifying resource needs. However, when interpreting the results of regression analyses of the relationship between psychiatric admission rates and social factors, the problems of multi-collinearity and linearity of the model must be borne in mind. Furthermore, studies based on the relationship between variables which are the averages for populations in geographical areas (as opposed to those based on individuals) suffer from the possibility that the relationships found between the area-based averages may not exist to the same degree between individuals within the populations in the areas on which the averages are based (the ecological fallacy) (Thornicroft, 1991).

The importance of the influence of marital status on psychiatric admission rates has been shown. The Resource Allocation Working Party (RAWP) recommended that marital status be used for calculating the allocation of psychiatric resources and these recommendations were followed. This paper gives support for the wisdom of this judgement and, in addition, suggests that the number of psychiatric admissions for a district can be predicted using a regression model which standardises for the effects of age, sex, and marital status and makes an allowance for the drug-misuser notification rate and standardised mortality ratios.

The current national formula for allocation of resources to hospital and community health services

From April 1991, as a result of the Review of the National Health Service (NHS) (Department of Health and Social Security, 1989) and the Resource Allocation Working Party (RAWP) (Department of Health and Social Security, 1988) formula, the revenue resources allocated to Regional Health Authorities for all hospital and community health service (H & CHS) provision for their resident populations have been calculated as the sum of a number of costs per age group (age groups 0–4 to 85 +) multiplied by the numbers of the resident populations in each age group in the region, all multiplied by the square root of SMR to age 75 (SMR75) (averaged from 1985 to 1989) for the region.

The expenditures per head related to age group on the third line of Table 4.4 are from DHSS data for 1986–87. They do not include the costs of births but do include a 'modification for dependency' which is applied to the costs of acute in-patient and out-patient services (which has since been changed). This modification has the effect of increasing the relative resource allocations for young and elderly residents.

These allocations include the resources for psychiatric hospital in-patient services which represent about 10% of the total costs (Department of Health and Social Security, 1987, 1990). Psychiatric out-patients constitute about 0.5% and day cases about 0.9% of the total H&CHS costs. No allowance is made in this allocation, at the regional level, for the important factors influencing the use of mental illness in-patient services such as marital status. However, regions, in their sub-regional allocations to district purchasing authorities, are able to take these factors into account. Doing so in one region with low levels of social deprivation would make up to about 3% difference to district H&CHS revenue allocations within the region (with an average change over all districts in the region of about 1% difference). We know of no region which specifically allocates resources to districts for mental illness services separately from the rest of H&CHS, nor of any region which takes account of the factors discussed above which our analyses and previous studies indicate are likely to influence the use of psychiatric in-patient services.

In the regression analyses, the only psychiatric service variables which added significantly to the explanation of variance in district admission rates were the proportions of psychiatric nurses in a district working in the community (more CPNs was significantly associated with lower admission rates) and the proportion of psychiatric nurses in training (higher values associated with higher admission rates). Although this finding was not very important for the predictive models (because it only added a small amount to the proportion of the variance explained), it is relevant in view of the reduction in the provision of psychiatric hospital beds which has continued

TABLE 4.4

Calculation of revenue resources for all hospital and community health service provision in a Regional Health Authority

Steps	Age groups							
	0–4	5–14	15–44	45–64	65–74	75–84	85 +	
Summary								
Step 1 Age group	0–4	5–14	15–44	45–64	65–74	75–84	85 +	
Step 2 Population	p1	p2	p3	p4	p5	p6	p7	
Step 3 × Expenditure/head	c1	c2	c3	c4	c5	c6	c7	
Step 4 × (SMR75)$^{0.5}$ = S	S	S	S	S	S	S	S	

Total allocation £ = Sum $(p_i.c_i.S)$ over the seven age groups.

Example								
Age group	0–4	5–14	15–44	45–64	65–74	75–84	85 +	Total
Resident population 1000s	24.35	43.99	161.53	79.25	33.88	21.81	6.75	371.56
Expenditure/head £	196.60	97.17	89.27	148.66	414.76	926.88	1452.35	
(SMR75)$^{0.5}$	0.949	0.949	0.949	0.949	0.949	0.949	0.949	
Product £1000s	4543	4056	13 683	11 179	13 334	19 182	9302	75 279

District sum = £75 279 000

in a steady way since about the time (1954) of the introduction of phenothiazine drugs for treating psychotic illnesses (Department of Health and Social Security, 1990). Our analyses suggest that, although social and demographic factors such as the proportions of the population living alone or unmarried, illegitimacy, and the levels of drug misuse, together with measures of general ill health, are likely to be the major factors associated with psychiatric hospital usage, there is some indication that health authorities may be able to compensate for lower levels of psychiatric bed provision by providing more CPNs.

When the actual numbers of psychiatric admissions (excluding mental handicap and psychogeriatrics) in each region are compared with the numbers expected based on national admission rates and the age, sex, and marital status structures of the districts in each region, without taking account of any other factors, Mersey and Yorkshire regions have higher admissions than expected and Oxford region lower than expected. When, in addition, allowance is made for the levels of drug misuser notification rate and standardised mortality ratios in the regions by regression analysis, then the predicted admissions for Mersey region approximate more closely to the actual numbers of admissions (i.e. the ratio of actual/predicted admissions approaches 1). On the other hand, the South West Thames region falls out of line (see Table 4.3). When these analyses are repeated at the district health authority level the differences between districts are more marked than the differences between regions. Assuming that regional health authorities are unlikely to allocate resources to districts specifically for mental illness service provision, it seems probable that there could be major differences between the resources which our analyses would indicate to be appropriate for some districts and those which are actually provided.

It would be possible, and probably more satisfactory, to separate the current district allocations for psychiatric services from the total of H&CHS and to determine an allocation for psychiatric services based on the model described above. This would involve dividing the allocation to the region for psychiatric services in proportion to the predicted numbers of psychiatric admissions for each district to arrive at district allocations for psychiatric services.

Variations within districts

The model using UPA scores and crude admission rates, although it explained less of the variation of psychiatric admission rates than the more complex model described above, is nevertheless more powerful than using only population size and age/sex structure. This simpler model could be useful for predicting crude psychiatric admission rates at Census electoral ward level because the age, sex, and marital status structure of the ward populations, and the drug modification rates needed for the more detailed model are usually not known at ward level whereas tables of UPA scores are available. This could be helpful when calculating service requirements within local or health authority boundaries.

Summary

We have shown the relationship between a wide variety of social, demographic, health care and services variables and the number of psychiatric admissions for 185 of the 191 health districts in England in 1986. A simple regression model explains 79% of the variation of the number of admissions per district. The five-fold difference in crude admission rates observed among health districts (or twelve-fold if West Lambeth district is included) is largely explained by differences in the health and social characteristics of the district populations. Differences in health-care delivery policy may account for some of the remaining unexplained variation.

The approach which we have adopted highlights certain factors such as drug misuse, illegitimacy, measures of general illness, and a variety of social conditions, such as social isolation, which are associated with higher rates of admission in certain populations. The formulae derived from the regression analyses which can be used to calculate the predicted numbers of admissions for a district are given in Appendix 3. The more complex model could be used where the age, sex, and marital status, expected numbers of admissions, and drug misuser and SMR data are available. The slightly less powerful model using crude admission rates and UPA scores can be used in the UK, based on UPA score data which are available for electoral wards from the first author and published for districts elsewhere (Jarman, 1985). We would recommend that the simple or full model be substituted for the model proposed in the Royal College of Psychiatrists (1988) report.

Acknowledgements

We would like to thank Pat White, Madhavi Bejekal, Rick Driscoll and Susan Dolan for the help which they have provided for the analyses described in this paper which is based on a similar paper published in the *British Medical Journal* (Jarman *et al*, 1992).

Appendix 1   Summary of independent variables used for correlation and regression analyses
(a full list of the variables used is available on request)

For each DHA for various years:

Health status

infant mortality rates
perinatal mortality rates

neonatal mortality rates
postneonatal mortality rates
proportions of births under 2500 g
standardised mortality ratios, full age range and to 65, 75 and 85
SMRs for each ICD group and for common causes of death
childhood death rates

Social

Composite social indices:

UPA – underprivileged area score
Vera Carstairs deprivation index
Townsend deprivation index
N.E. & N.W. Thames socioeconomic group bed use weighting (excl. geriatrics)
N.E. & N.W. Thames socioeconomic group bed use weighting (incl. geriatrics)
DOE social index

Individual variables:

% population single, widowed or divorced 1981
% total population aged 65 + 1981
% total population elderly alone 1981
% total population aged under 5 1981
% total population in lone parent family 1981
% total population unskilled -scv, seg11 1981
% economically active population unemployed 1981
% total population lack basic amenities 1981
% total population overcrowded > 1/room 1981
% total population moved house in year 1981
% total population New Commonwealth/Pakistan 1981
% total population born outside UK 1981
% total population born Pakistan 1981
% total population born New Commonwealth 1981
% total population Europe 1981
% total population Caribbean 1981
% total population Ireland 1981
% 17 yr olds not in education 1981
population density 1983 pers/hectare
% economically active & residential population permanently & temporarily sick 1981
% households with no car 1981
% households not owner-occupier 1981
% households single-occupier 1981
% social class I to V, 1981
% socioeconomic group 1 to 17, 1981
illegitimacy index 1986
drug misusers 1st notification/100000 1988
drug misusers renotification/100000 1988

Supply variables

Hospital services – non-psychiatry & psychiatry:

wide range of supply data relating to consultants, junior doctors, bed availability, mental-illness nurses in hospital

Community services:

mental-illness nurses in day hospitals and community
general practice average list size, group practices, general practitioners' ages, community health services expenditures
nursing homes: private bed supply, beds for elderly.

Appendix 2   Six highest Pearson correlation coefficients with the 169 independent variables

Correlation coefficients with $SPAR_{popn}$ and $SPAR_{asms}$.

$n = 185$, all correlation coefficients significant at $P < 0.0001$

$SPAR_{popn}$ – *Standardised admission ratio based on district population size and national overall rate*

% households single-occupier 1981	0.573
% over 65s living alone 1981	0.559
% population single, widowed, or divorced 1981	0.546
% households with no car 1981	0.545
average illegitimacy index 1982–1987	0.536
% residential private households with no car 1981	0.533

$SPAR_{asms}$ – *Standardised admission ratio based on district age, sex, marital status composition*

SMR for ages under 65, 1986	0.503
SMR for ages under 75, 1986	0.487
% over 65s living alone 1981	0.481
SMR 1981–85 bronchitis, emphysema + asthma	0.474
average SMR 1981–87	0.471
illegitimacy index 1986	0.467

Appendix 3   Regression equations used for district models
(standard error of coefficient shown in brackets)

Full model

$$SPAR_{asms} = 12 + 0.66 \times DRUG1STN + 0.82 \times SMR(IHD) \quad r^2 = 0.34 \text{ (model used)}$$
$$\phantom{SPAR_{asms} = 12 + } (\pm 0.10) (\pm 0.11)$$

where:

$SPAR_{asms}$	= standardised psychiatry admission ratio
	= actual admissions/age, sex, marital status expected admissions of residents, 1986 × 100
DRUG1STN	= drug misusers, 1st notifications/100 000 resident population, 1988
SMR(IHD)	= SMR averaged 1981–85 for ischaemic heart disease

The predicted admissions for each district are calculated as the predicted value of $SPAR_{asms}$ times the expected admissions based on the district's age, sex, marital status structure and national psychiatric admission rates by age, sex and marital status.

The model used explains 34% of the variation of $SPAR_{asms}$ values between districts. The predicted values of $SPAR_{asms}$ are calculated and multiplied by expected values to give predicted numbers of admissions.

The predicted admissions explain 79% of the variation between districts of actual admissions.

Simple model

$$Crude\ rate = 3.65 + 0.034 \times UPA\ score$$
$$(\pm 0.0046)$$

where:

crude rate = psychiatric admissions/1000 resident population
UPA score = district underprivileged area score

Notes:
1. Psychiatric admissions do not include mental handicap or psychogeriatrics
2. Figures apply to districts for 1986.

References

BUGLASS, D., DUFFY, K. & KREITMAN, N. (1980) *A Register of Social and Medical Indices by Local Government Area in Edinburgh and Lothians*. Edinburgh: Scottish Office Central Research Papers.

BURKE, A. (1976) Attempted suicide among the Irish born population at Birmingham. *British Journal of Psychiatry*, **128**, 534–537.

COOPER, J. E., GOODHEAD, D., CRAIG, T., *et al* (1987) The incidence of schizophrenia in Nottingham. *British Journal of Psychiatry*, **151**, 619–626.

DEPARTMENT OF THE ENVIRONMENT (1983) *Urban Deprivation*. Information note No. 2. London: Inner Cities Directorate.

DEPARMENT OF HEALTH AND SOCIAL SECURITY (1976) *Sharing Resources for Health in England, Report of the Resource Allocation Working Party*. London: HMSO.

—— (1986) *In-Patient Statistics from the Mental Health Enquiry for England*. London: HMSO.

—— WELSH OFFICE (1987) *Health services costing returns. Year ending March 1987*. London: Department of Health and Social Security.

—— (1988) *Review of the Resource Allocation Working Party Formula*. Final report by the NHS management board. London: Deparment of Health and Social Security.

—— SECRETARIES OF STATE FOR HEALTH, WALES, NORTHERN IRELAND AND SCOTLAND (1989) *Working for Patients*. Command 555. (The White Paper on the review of the NHS.) London: HMSO.

—— (1990) *Health and Personal Social Services Statistics for England: 1990 edition* (and earlier editions). London: HMSO.

DURKHEIM, E. (1952) *Suicide*. (Published 1897, translated 1952.) London: Routledge & Kegan Paul.

FARIS, R. E. L. & DUNHAM, H. W. (1939) *Mental Disorders in Urban Areas*. Chicago: Hafner.

GOLDBERG, D. & HUXLEY, P. (1980) *Mental Illness in the Community. The Pathway to Psychiatric Care*. London: Tavistock Publications.

GOODMAN, A. B., SIEGAL, C., CRAIG, T., *et al* (1983) The relationship between socio-economic class and prevalence of schizophrenia, alcoholism and affective disorders treated by inpatient care in a suburban area. *American Journal of Psychiatry*, **140**, 166–170.

JARMAN, B. (1983) Identification of underprivileged areas. *British Medical Journal*, **286**, 1705–1709.

—— (1984) Underprivilegd areas: validation and distribution of scores. *British Medical Journal*, **289**, 1587–1592.

—— (1985) Underprivileged areas. *Medical Annual*, pp. 224–243. Bristol, John Wright & Sons.

——, HIRSCH, S., WHITE, P., *et al* (1992) Predicting psychiatric admission rates. *British Medical Journal*, **304**, 1146–1151.

MILLER, G. H., DEAR, M. & STREINER, D. L. (1986) A model for predicting the utilisation of psychiatric facilities. *Canadian Journal of Psychiatry*, **31**, 424–430.

ÖDEGÅRD, O. (1932) Emigration and insanity: a study of mental disease among Norwegian born population in Minnesota. *Acta Psychiatrica et Neurologica Scandinavica* (suppl. 4).

PLATT, S. & KREITMAN, N. (1985) Parasuicide and unemployment among men in Edinburgh 1968–82. *Psychological Medicine*, **15**, 113–123.

RICHMAN, A., BOUTILIER, C. & HARRIS, P. (1984) The relevance of socio-demographic and resource factors in the use of acute psychiatric in-patient care in the Atlantic Provinces of Canada. *Psychological Medicine*, **14**, 175–182.

ROYAL COLLEGE OF PSYCHIATRISTS (1988) *Psychiatric Beds and Resources; Factors Influencing Bed Use and Service Planning*. Report of a Working Party of the section for Social and Community Psychiatry. London: Gaskell.

SAINSBURY, P. (1955) *Suicide in London*. London: Institute of Psychiatry.

SHEPHERD, M. (1957) *A Study of Major Psychosis in an English County*. Maudsley monograph No. 3. London: Chapman Hall.

THORNICROFT, G. (1991) Social deprivation and rates of treated mental disorder. *British Journal of Psychiatry*, **158**, 475–484.

TOWNSEND, P., PHILLIMORE, P. & BEATTIE, A. (1986) *Inequalities in Health in the Northern Region*. Northern Regional Health Authority and the University of Bristol.

5 Case registers and mental health information systems

TOM FRYERS and IAN GREATOREX

Psychiatric case registers (PCRs) have played a prominent part in the recent history of British research in psychiatric epidemiology but there are few left and little chance of others being re-established. The experience gained, however, should not be lost, and is peculiarly relevant to the new National Health Service (NHS) created by recent government reforms. In this chapter, a brief review of the characteristics, history and limitations of PCRs leads to a discussion of practical issues facing all service-use information systems. We examine the current context in the UK, particularly regarding assessment of health needs, collaborative commissioning, and community participation, and then discuss how information service use can be used in a wide variety of ways, whatever the system. Finally, we consider to what degree routine, collaborative, networked, and computerised population-based systems in the new NHS might be able to reproduce the benefits of PCRs without a separate system.

Features and history of case registers

Although 'register' is used widely and variably, 'case register' has been used specifically for 30 years to mean a prospective cumulative, population-based aggregate of linked records of individual-orientated data, collected in a systematic and standardised form (Fryers, 1984). Unlike traditional event-orientated health-service information systems, a case register is person-orientated. Unlike disease registers, which aim to record everybody with a particular diagnosis in a population, psychiatric case registers (PCRs) record only users of particular services from a population. Unlike 'at-risk' registers, which define at-risk status by screening, they record people only after making contact with a specialist mental health service. Nevertheless, there are elements of all these within a PCR; event data can be analysed to compare with routine sources; if it encompasses a sufficiently comprehensive range of services, it will catch virtually all cases of some diagnostic groups, such as chronic schizophrenia; and some patients can be awarded 'at-risk' status because of certain types of service contact, such as discharge from long-stay in-patient care.

Population-based registers started in the 1950s and 60s in the USA and UK, but many succumbed to loss of funds after a few years. British registers suffered withdrawal of government funding in the 1980s, and only four long-established registers survive: Aberdeen, Nottingham, Oxford, and Salford. Both the organisational and technological contexts have fundamentally changed and alternatives have arisen (Wing, 1989). In Europe and elsewhere there is increasing interest and activity, with many systems of varied form (ten Horn *et al*, 1986).

Figure 5.1 illustrates the social, political, professional and technological factors motivating their original development (Fryers, 1987). There was widespread interest in alternatives to large mental hospitals and in-patient care, and the potential of community mental health programmes (e.g. Caplan, 1961). This was fuelled by ideas of human rights as well as therapeutic optimism associated with the first generation of psychotropic

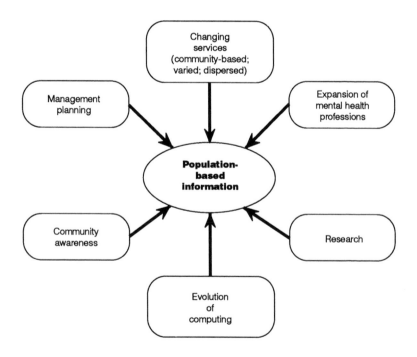

Fig. 5.1. Factors influencing the formation of case registers

drugs. There was a large expansion of care professionals working in mental health and interested in research, and new types and patterns of care were rapidly emerging in an atmosphere of experimentation involving both public-health and clinical personnel (Susser, 1968).

Greater emphasis was being placed on management and planning, and, as in other medical fields, high-quality information was desired to plan, monitor and evaluate these new services, as well as to facilitate epidemiological research. The advent of computers raised expectations of sophisticated and easy data processing from the early 1960s, stimulating and facilitating these developments; from the mid-1980s the technical expectations have been more or less fulfilled!

All district PCRs accumulated data on residents' use of a defined range of mental health services, but the agencies, facilities and personnel encompassed varied. All included contacts with consultant psychiatrists and specialist psychiatric in-patient and out-patient contacts, but day care, community facilities, and other health professionals were not always recorded. Only Salford routinely collected data from social services (Fryers & Wooff, 1989).

The data set also varied: generally, the larger the population base, the smaller the data set; national person-orientated records tend to be in-patients only; small sectors, as in South Verona, can cope with detail for a comprehensive service. Efforts in the 1980s to harmonise eight British registers met with considerable success (Gibbons *et al*, 1984; Wing, 1989). Data collection varied in the degree to which it was integrated into routine information systems: Aberdeen is closely integrated into medical records; Oxford is part of the wider Oxford Record Linkage Study. Storage and processing usually used mainframe or minicomputers, but analytical conventions grew up differently and also had to be harmonised.

Extra-district users of district services have usually been included, but district residents' use of out-of-district services was seldom complete. District information was used by public health physicians, managers and researchers, but care staff often wanted sector or patch information, especially for multidisciplinary and multiagency teams. PCRs can provide information for such service situations, but only if a 'clinical record' is included, data turnaround is fast, and the team has immediate access.

These conditions were difficult to meet with large systems and early computers, but microcomputers encouraged an alternative development of sector registers with direct data input and access by the clinical team, and serving operational rather than strategic needs. The principle has been outlined by Rohde (1986), but financial constraints have limited developments in the UK. If a whole district were covered by sector systems feeding into a central base, strategic functions could also be served, data quality control being handled not by dedicated 'register' staff, but by reward feedback of information needed by the team (Wing, 1989).

Problems and limitations of case registers

Some limitations of registers have already been touched on. Data on service use cannot tell us directly about demand, even less need. But they can tell us something, and register information is a better starting point for these than most alternatives. Registers monitor services and facilitate evaluation, but only for those agencies, facilities and personnel they cover; a substantial study in Salford comparing and evaluating the work of psychiatric community nurses and mental health social workers could not be repeated elsewhere because relevant data were not recorded (Wooff *et al*, 1988).

No PCR includes coverage of primary-care data, which in the case of mental illness represents a significant gap in milder cases, early stages, chronic disease, and rehabilitation. Computer systems are rapidly increasing in general medical practice, and linkage is possible in the future. This might be particularly relevant to psychiatric sector teams working with specific primary health care (PHC) teams. Out-of-district service contact by district residents is not easily solved by PCRs, but new routine systems will be able to link across districts to record cross-boundary flows.

All information systems need a perpetual focus on data-quality control; NHS routine systems have a poor record, and registers have provided much better quality information by ensuring that data are accurate, comprehensive and up-to-date. But some personal and social data cannot be guaranteed: for example, changes in marital status may only be up-dated incidentally at a much later service contact.

Diagnosis remains a problem in psychiatry; available means of standardising diagnosis are not much used in daily clinical practice, and PCRs have had to accept the diagnostic variation and ambiguity they get. This is a serious issue for research, but is not so important in district strategic planning. Denominator data to understand the characteristics, history and dynamics of the local population are needed for both, but are not always available: for example, inter-censal data on migration and unemployment for small areas.

These difficulties affect the ability of a PCR to produce reliable, relevant and timely information, and they have often been accused of doing so, and of being little used. There is justification for this, but bare statistics from data banks are rarely used; they need interpretation if managers, planners, clinicians and politicians are to use them. Resourcing has often left out the epidemiological skills or time to provide this, leading to a waste of expensive technology. Unfortunately there is a powerful tradition of decision-making in health care without good information, and there is a major task ahead if this is going to change.

This is crucially important; all high-quality information systems are expensive, and the cost must be justified in terms not of the output *per se*, but the use made of it. Good information is expensive because it requires high-level skilled personnel, paid appropriately. Reliability and accuracy are only achieved by rigorous procedures, dedicated staff and sophisticated computing (Fryers, 1989).

Privacy, confidentiality and data protection are all important issues (Wing, 1986). In some countries, recent laws have virtually precluded epidemiology and health-service research. In the UK, experience has been more encouraging. Wing considered that "the Data Protection Act of 1984 has safeguarded the confidentiality of the subject without imposing impossible conditions on research"; the same applies to public-health and management uses. The new 1991 NHS will require much more sophisticated linked information systems which may come to resemble PCRs. As long as access is restricted to people with legitimate service interests, data protection seems unlikely to be too problematic in the UK.

Practical issues in information systems

Most practical issues are common to all information systems, and are concerned with maximising the quality of data and minimising the cost. Routine information systems require the same epidemiological skills, rigour, and interpretive caution as research, and these cannot be bought cheaply, but NHS systems have often had little access to epidemiological, statistical and information technology (IT) expertise unless linked to research units.

Relationships between information staff, public-health doctors, management and clinicians must be worked at continually; information is a powerful resource and must be guided by someone with appropriate expertise, status, and time. In the current ferment of change in the NHS, there may be an unusual opportunity for public-health departments to provide this. The key role of information broker also calls for higher level skills. The technology of data storage, retrieval and analysis now poses few problems, but data quality is most prejudiced where data are generated. PCRs mostly coped with this by using dedicated staff to collect, check and chase up data, but this is expensive. If NHS routine systems are to compete, they must show the same commitment to input quality control. Where clinical teams input data, the incentive is their own need for high quality output; access and feedback must be designed in. Appropriate incentives for institutional clerical staff must be found or information systems will fail.

Output also needs attention; it should not normally be data, but information, and that which fulfils an overt need. To serve users' needs it must be negotiated repeatedly (Hamers *et al*, 1986), although sometimes information must be 'marketed' as users do not always know what can be provided, or what they could use.

Although few UK Registers continue, their rationale remains, and indeed, gains weight with recent Health and Social Service changes. The standard 'Körner' data set has not satisfied the demand for information in a developing, multi-disciplinary service situation. The greater autonomy of districts, and their overt role in determining and evaluating contracts on the basis of assessed population needs, requires information of quality and extent rarely achieved before.

Registers could offer this, linked into hospital and district patient-administration systems, family health service authorities' (FHSAs') systems and, to a limited extent, social-service systems. In the UK, new PCRs are very unlikely to be funded; however, the new Health Service offers an opportunity for getting the benefits of PCRs from routine information systems, and this is discussed later. Applications of PCR type service-use information apply equally to similar information from routine sources if they can provide it.

The UK context: the NHS and Community Care Act (1990), needs-led commissioning and mental health

During the 1980s, the UK government issued three White Papers on the health and social services. *Promoting Better Health, Working for Patients*, and *Caring for People* (Department of Health, 1987, 1989a, b) led to the *NHS and Community Care Act* (House of Commons, 1990), and fundamental changes in philosophy, structure and function of all services, intended to increase professional accountability, tighten financial control, and make explicit decisions about priorities.

Two major changes have been largely welcomed by public-health doctors as consistent with traditional public-health approaches; a requirement that services will reflect assessed needs for health-related services in a community, instead of the uncontrolled aggregation of individual decisions by professionals providing care; and a separation at district level of purchasing or commissioning authorities representing the population, from contracted provider units such as hospitals. However, commissioning presents conceptual and practical problems, not least in mental health. What are mental health needs in a district population? How can they be assessed, quantified, and translated into service contracts? What are the implications for information systems?

DHAs must seek a balanced provision of services, securing the greatest health benefit from their resources. The range of care options as well as the total capacity of the service must reflect community needs, as must the balance between prevention, treatment, rehabilitation and care. All should be seen to promote mental health. Present imbalances and inequalities should be addressed by redistribution of resources. The Department of Health's definition of 'need' as ability to benefit from health care emphasises that services must be effective, but is insufficient. It is not only health care which fulfils health needs, but environmental change, social support, housing, education, employment, income support, and so on. Moreover, where lack of resources results in unmet need, DHAs have the responsibility to assess it so that resource issues can be addressed.

Assessing needs

Unfortunately, perceptions of health needs are neither objective nor value free. They are conditioned by health knowledge, experience of health care, risk-taking propensity, the balance of short-term and long-term views of benefits and dis-benefits, importance of autonomy, and other personal and cultural factors. Professional assessment of need will often differ from personal assessment. This has encouraged adoption of a 'care management' approach to those with long-term problems; it combines multidisciplinary assessment, client participation, an agreed structured individual 'care plan', coordination by a key worker, and systematic review.

On this model, individual needs are combined within a 'patch' by a 'Care Manager', who must balance needs and commission services within a budget. Rationing, always present, will be more overt, with more explicit criteria. Evidence of unmet need from care managers will aggregate at district level to justify arguments for more resources. However, it seems likely that care managers will be fully occupied providing services for the clients they know, and needs of people not in contact will not be known. Assessment of population needs cannot be limited to a highly selected group, but must relate to the whole population at risk.

This requires thorough epidemiological investigation; there is much available in the literature but much more to do in both basic research and reviews collating what is known about the occurrence and determinants of disease in relevant populations. This can provide guidelines for districts to modify with local factors for purchasing services. Needs-led commissioning also requires information on effectiveness, and relative costs and benefits of interventions, but currently our knowledge is very limited. The epidemiological approach is more difficult for mental health needs; case definitions, therapeutic options, and outcomes are all diverse, client perceptions are often prejudiced by the nature of the condition, and diagnostic groups may not be the best focus.

Other perspectives will qualify the public-health perception of population needs. Managers will emphasise limited resources, the media will raise particular needs to prominence, and politicians will respond without recourse to comparative epidemiology! Traditions within health and social care may be very resistant to change. For district populations, assessing mental health needs will be complex and difficult, subject to varied views and judgements, and based on limited information, especially about unmet needs.

The potential for collaborative purchasing/commissions

DHAs are now responsible for commissioning provider units to meet the health needs of their population. Especially for mental health, this will necessarily include non-health service providers, but other purchasing authorities – FHSAs and social services – will also be commissioning from the same range of providers. There is, therefore, potential for collaborative commissioning, offering greater effectiveness in promoting mental health.

For example, resettlement of long-stay in-patients into the community involves housing, community psychiatric nursing, social work, sheltered employment, occupational therapy, primary-health care, day care, and a variety of other support and caring services. Goodwill and cooperation, upon which development depended in the past, will still be needed, but it is now possible for purchasing authorities, through contracts or service agreements, to combine their resources through care managers who can access a variety of providers for their client group.

This will require harmonising 'patch' arrangements and sharing of information to allow purchasers collectively to understand current provision and agree a shared health agenda for service improvement, directions of development, and redistribution of resources to be pursued through contracts with providers.

Involving communities in decisions affecting services

Perhaps the biggest challenge to DHAs and FHSAs in commissioning services on behalf of their community, is to know and to take account of the views of local people, who are not formally represented on the authorities. The process and techniques of consultation are not clear, for a district of 250 000 people, and in some ways community participation is antithetical to representative democracy. But in representing local needs we cannot ignore local opinion. Authorities need the support of local people in decisions on priorities, and need to optimise acceptability of services.

From a public-health perspective, significant health gains can only be realised for disadvantaged communities, with poor health across a wide range of health indicators, if they are involved in decisions and developments. A 'medical', or even a 'health-behaviour' approach may be rejected if a community perceives its main problems to be low income, housing, unemployment, crime, and a prejudiced environment. Closer involvement of Community Health Councils and Councils for Voluntary Service may help, GP teams may be able to reflect many patient preferences, self-help groups can be encouraged, and community development projects supported.

In some areas, a 'mental health forum' has established open debate about mental health issues.

In all these contexts, information, its content, relevance, and presentation, is crucial, if we are to achieve community participation and inter-sectoral collaboration in addressing inequalities in health. Few districts have psychiatric case registers, and if what they offer is really important, routine information systems must achieve similar standards and encompass equivalent functions.

Applications of service-use information such as that provided by psychiatric case registers

Mental health information systems are justified only if they facilitate promotion of mental health in communities; Fig. 5.2 illustrates strategic and operational uses. Strategic uses represent a public-health perspective, concerned with the occurrence and determinants of health and ill-health in populations at risk, the needs of communities for services, and the distribution of resources. This means assessing population needs for service planning and commissioning; evaluating and developing services to promote mental health; facilitating community participation; and long-term research. Operational uses represent a clinical perspective concerned with the needs and experiences of individual patients, and include coordinating multidisciplinary and multiagency work, facilitating continuity of care, triggering follow-up and review, and providing information to members of the community about service options.

Assessment of population needs, for planning or commissioning

Population needs related to mental illness can rarely be measured directly; we usually have only proxies. Some groups have well researched epidemiological data, but many lack firm foundation and at best we may derive generalised indicators. Demand as a proxy is also difficult to measure, and service-use data may be the only proxy for demand. Nevertheless, comparative descriptive analysis and careful interpretation of patterns of service use, with sound denominator data, and the known epidemiology, may prove useful for strategic planning.

Service use may indicate minimum demand for services, if: services are comprehensive in extent and range, data show trends over a substantial period, referring agencies such as GPs and social workers can quantify their view of unmet demand, and evaluation data can show to what extent services match individual clinical and felt needs of patients and families. These conditions are rarely fulfilled, but we can work towards them starting with

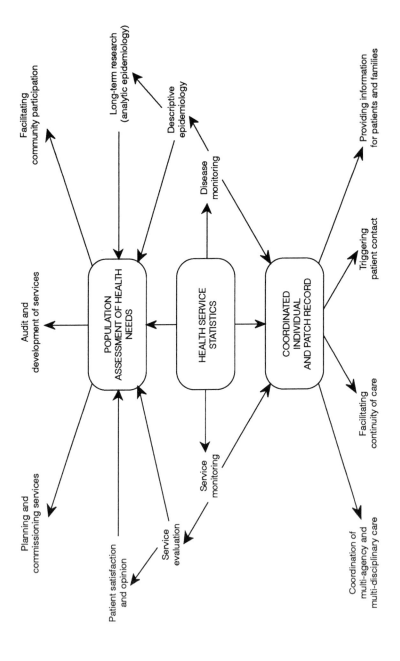

Fig. 5.2. Uses of mental health information systems

good data on service use (Wing & Fryers, 1976; Gibbons *et al*, 1984; Wing, 1989).

The value of data is greatly enhanced by comparative analysis; differential use by population subgroups, and changes over time may reveal gaps in provision, access or take-up, or greater use which might indicate greater need. Care must be taken with denominator data, especially for small areas or specific age, sex, ethnic, or socioeconomic subgroups; population ratios, the only basis for comparison, are sensitive to denominator inaccuracies as well as numerator inaccuracies. Comparisons between populations and over time are especially demanding on denominators whose variations may be insecure, and long-term studies of long-stay patients need very careful handling because of the effects of differential migration (Der, 1989).

'Needs' are many sided. Equitable and reasonable access to a full range of mental health care specifically requires comparative service-use data, combined with social, demographic and epidemiological information. For example, day-care facilities for older people can be related to small-area age structures, public-transport routes, expected rates of dementia by age and sex, and levels of family and neighbourhood support. Inequalities may then be addressed.

Information on service use may also guide development of, for example, mental health centres or multidisciplinary sector teams. Appropriate populations and the range of services best sited together can be identified, to be supplemented by local surveys involving communities in the planning process.

Need for one type of service may also be predicated upon the use of others. For example, the long-stay in-patient population may indicate need for supported housing; individual need for a particular type must then be assessed clinically. Aggregated for whole populations, individual assessments may then inform future commissioning and contracting for services in both hospital and community.

These applications of information on service users might be greatly enhanced for specific diagnostic groups if standard protocols were used; if clinicians want high quality information relating diagnosis to particular regimens or service arrangements, they must guarantee accurate and consistent input data. This would also facilitate local research to identify determinants of high or low service use and unmet perceived need. Service data can be supplemented by local survey data, and should be related to known epidemiological information, and compared with national, regional and other district data.

Evaluation and development of services to promote mental health

Health information must assist the promotion of mental health in the community. A principal means will be by facilitating evaluation of services, facilities, and personnel to inform continuing planning and development.

Evaluation is an imperative, but not all can be evaluated; some issues are technically too complex, and constraints on time demand decisions about priorities. Comprehensive information systems can ensure the widest range of practical options, and person-based, whole population, longitudinal data, whether in PCRs or routine systems, offer most.

Administrative audit is one starting point for evaluation, and registers have contributed to this. For example, detailed monitoring of long-stay in-patient populations over 20 years has fed into community-service development in Salford, stimulated changes in consultant practice, and raised important issues of equity in resource allocation to provide for the excess of long-stay patients due to vast population diminution (Gibbons *et al*, 1984; Giel, 1986; Wing, 1989). Monitoring the extramural long-stay population is much harder, but registers offer some experience (Wing, 1982).

Clinical audit is another starting point for evaluation, and registers can provide follow-up data and linkage across episodes of care and agencies. Comparative data for consultants or units may stimulate discussion of admission and discharge policies, treatment protocols, and so on. Aggregated data can do the same for sectors, client groups, or staff cadres. Related to cost data, cost-effectiveness and cost-benefit studies may indicate development required to promote mental health.

In new services, data collection protocols should be built in to facilitate evaluation; this is easy for small residential units but difficult for something as complex as a community mental health centre. Clear service objectives must be set, against which to measure performance, and to direct changes in the light of progressive evaluation. In the current field situation in health and social services it is particularly important to evaluate professional performance, and this needs precise, longitudinal data; a good example from register data is the study of training, attitudes and work of community psychiatric nurses and mental health social workers in Salford, which provides essential information for planning community services (Wooff *et al*, 1988; Wooff, 1987).

Conventional single-service information systems provided no insights into interactions between different professions, facilities and agencies. PCRs offered the necessary additional dimension to study, for example, total day care received by people with recent mental illness; or follow-up of discharged patients in residential homes. From 1991, the UK requirements for routine information in new DHAs, FHSAs and LAs may enforce the linkages to this without a PCR, but PCRs represent one of few traditions of collaborative information systems and it is hoped that the experience will be used.

Community participation

Health and social care for people with mental illness have changed beyond recognition in 30 years in most communities, not least in the humaneness and openness of care. Legislation has increasingly recognised the need to respect human rights, but more needs to be done to involve patients, relatives, and potential patients who constitute the community, in inescapable choices about the extent, type, style, location, and content of care. There are opportunities for this in the new UK authorities, purchasers, and providers, in collaboration with patient support organisations and other voluntary bodies.

In spite of the emphasis on community participation in the WHO Health for All strategy and the 38 European targets, effective involvement of communities in developing local health care has been very limited in the UK. However, there is growing awareness of the potential for this, and growing experience of community development methods. Sharing information is an important element; where possible, information should be held in common 'ownership'. Medical data pose problems of confidentiality and privacy, particularly in mental illness, but aggregated population data do not, and it is in these that PCRs offer a peculiar contribution to the process of participation. Information in public-health annual reports is a useful start, but needs supplementing with more localised, accessible, and widely disseminated information.

A 'mental health forum' where local public discussion can explore perceived needs for and problems of mental health care may be located with primary care or a sector mental health team, especially in a community mental health centre. Shared information between professionals, patients, families, and the public will include local service-use information, but other types of information will also be needed if clinical, legal and ethical issues are to be demythologised, and mental illness and psychiatric treatment are to continue to grow in acceptance, stigma to be diminished, and issues of mental *health* to be placed on the agenda.

Long-term research

Strategic research, offering no immediate local pay-off, has been a major contribution of PCRs. The major current issue in the UK is funding, and this will be no different if PCRs are encompassed by routine systems. DHAs and RHAs can fund little long-term research; government is reluctant to fund any; universities are increasingly dependent on specific outside funds for research. The field is very discouraging in the UK. Registers can be valuable resources but must have financial stability, and researchers must have some career security. The immense importance of mental illness in society, paucity of our understanding of aetiology, and the very limited potential for preventive programmes present a challenge to research which should not be ignored.

Coordination of sector teams

PCRs have seldom provided coordinated information for multidisciplinary teams, but personal computers can be team based, and include standard diagnoses and assessments, projected programmes of treatment and care, and full records of contacts. These data can be aggregated centrally for district applications, and networked to give peripheral access to relevant district and comparative data. Rohde's (1986) system is simple to use and builds in the reward feed-back of immediately up-to-date clinical and historical summaries, documentation required for patient care, and administrative returns. The problems are time, resources and motivation; it needs discipline to ensure standardisation of interviews and assessments, and rigour of recording (Wing, 1989).

Facilitating continuity of care

In ensuring coordination between hospitals, primary care and social services, quality of information is vital, but it must be up-to-date, always a problem for PCRs because of processing time. Networked PC systems with direct data entry can solve this, and could generate, for example, standard discharge letters. Similar advantages might accrue from linkage with FHSA and social-service systems. The objective here is to guarantee that professionals sharing responsibility for the care of individual patients and families have rapid access to the information they need derived from others involved.

Triggering individual patient review

Routine information systems now commonly produce follow-up, domiciliary treatment, or clinical review lists, and invitation letters according to a predetermined pattern, superseding this particular contribution of PCRs, although not yet generally across agency boundaries.

Providing service information for members of the community

Earlier we discussed using information to facilitate community participation but it is also important in individual care. There is growing demand for patients and families to have a say in the choice of health and social-care options. For this to be an informed choice they must have access to good factual information about the range of services, facilities and personnel available, and options appropriate to particular needs; a local community handbook on mental health services needs PCR-type information.

Future developments

Present registers in the UK are still under threat. They represent an invaluable archive of longitudinal data for research which it would be vandalism to destroy, but there is little hope of their gaining sufficient financial support on this basis. If they are to continue, it will be because those districts have found them useful for required district work. The PCR experience was an important one, and the lessons learned are valuable for all health-information systems, but the context is now quite different from 25 or even 10 years ago. At that time, the content and quality of most routine health-service information were so poor that only a separate special system, usually with research funding and high levels of trained staffing, could produce the comprehensive, accurate and reliable information required. It is now possible to conceive of a PCR encompassed within a routine health-service system, and fully integrated within it – a 'virtual PCR'?

One of the necessary concomitants of the new NHS is the extensive redevelopment of basic information systems. The contracting relationship between purchasers and providers has two effects: firstly there is an absolute requirement for a substantial range of data on patient contact and service use to allow contracts to be set, monitored, and continually renegotiated. Secondly, there is the power of the purchaser to write requirements into contracts for specified data and data quality, specified systems with specified characteristics, and guaranteed transfer to population-based, public-health information systems.

Although the current standard data set which has developed from the Körner initiative is still event-based not person-based, and has no linkage built in to record 'patient careers', if all the contracting provider units, hospital and community, conform to the full data-set requirements including NHS number as well as more personal identifiers, it will not be too difficult for district information systems to do their own linkage, and analyse longitudinal person-based records.

Since districts have been left to work out these matters for themselves, only some are well on with this, but others must follow if the contract system is developed in the next few years. There has been a substantial investment in computer hardware, networking systems, and analysis software, and there are currently no serious technical difficulties. The 1990 Act and the directives which support it are forcing DHAs, the new FHSAs, and LA social services to work closely together, driven by contracts or 'service agreements'; this is proceeding variably and with difficulty, but is compelling those working in these bodies to explore ways of sharing information.

It is possible to share the basic population database of the FHSA, now much more reliable than it used to be, and to integrate it with service-use data of health and social services into a single individual longitudinal patient record; it is possible to integrate census and other demographic data from the LA planning department, and to add epidemiological data, comparative data from other districts and regions, social deprivation indices, patient satisfaction survey results, and other research results to bring to bear on the analysis of data. Cohort analysis programmes are available for follow-up analyses, geographical information systems to focus on small areas, GP populations, hospital catchments and so on.

This may sound millennial, but all these are under current discussion in districts, many are already in hand and others are expected in very few years. Within this, a 'virtual CPR' can certainly be created, but many questions remain, reflecting the same problems which plagued CPRs. High-quality data at the collection base of the system will still require appropriately trained staff, constant attention from information brokers or their equivalents, and support and feedback to maintain motivation. On the other hand, direct input of data from service-located terminals promotes accuracy and regularity, and allows built-in checks on data quality and a certain amount of instant feedback.

The staffing issue is wider than data clerks and medical secretaries. Hospital and community units do not generally employ highly trained information staff who can undertake systems development. They could be facilitated and supported by public health/purchaser information units, who must guarantee their own information needs, but many departments have not yet developed their public-health information function. However, they must do so in the future to serve 'assessment of needs' in their populations, so this may change. Whatever the system, we will not have high-quality information without high-quality staff, which means paying appropriate salaries for trained people.

The quality of diagnostic, clinical, and social-assessment data raises a different issue. Is it conceivable now that all clinical psychiatrists in a district could agree to use the same standard diagnostic instrument, the same categories, and the same treatment protocols? Apart from medical diagnosis, there is hope of standardisation of clinical–social assessment because of the requirement that health and social services agree care plans for clients. These will be the basis of the client record at the client-contact points of the services, and can include a standard data set for abstraction to a central database. This allows development of patch or sector information systems which might look like the Waltham Forest CPR model (Fagin, 1986), but similar in every patch, and susceptible to aggregation at district level similar to the model suggested by Wing (1989). This will be particularly relevant where a community-based service is focused upon a multidisciplinary, multiagency mental-health centre.

The confidentiality issue also remains, although it has not featured prominently in the discussion of current changes in the NHS. Sharing information between specialities, units and authorities raises important questions about who has access to data on individual people. This must be clearly sorted out before shared systems are set up; the technology allows the limiting of data transfer to specified users, and the blocking of specified data from specified channels of communication; indeed, this is going to be an intrinsic part of social service and health systems. But, again, the bigger problems are the human ones; can we find consensus and agreement on these matters to allow the systems to develop? This is particularly relevant to the mental health field because of the sensitiveness of many of the data.

There remains the major issue of how much an information system based on service use can be used to assess health needs. This always limited CPRs, but a 'virtual CPR' within a public-health information system will at least have the advantage of a built-in denominator base, which will allow a further epidemiological dimension to be explored. How much of a reality this will turn out to be we must wait and see, but those who perceive it as an important objective should be able to make it happen!

Although the establishment of more traditional registers seems unlikely, the history and experience of psychiatric case registers should not be lost or wasted. They have provided for a particularly difficult specialist service, a high quality, population-based, comprehensive, multiagency and multidisciplinary, person-based, longitudinal database for whole population information over a long period of time, and these are now characteristics required of a good public-health information system for all specialist fields. If we think of the psychiatric case register as a concept rather than a system, perhaps its time has just come!

References

CAPLAN, G. (1961) *An Approach to Community Mental Health.* London: Tavistock.
DER, G. (1989) Population changes and long stay in-patient rates. In *Health Services Planning and Research; Contributions from Psychiatric Case Registers* (ed J. K. Wing), pp. 53–57. London: Gaskell, Royal College of Psychiatrists.
DEPARTMENT OF HEALTH (1987) *Promoting Better Health.* London: HMSO.
—— (1989a) *Working for Patients.* London: HMSO.
—— (1989b) *Caring for People.* London: HMSO.
FAGIN, L. (1986) Development of the Waltham Forest local mental health care register. *Bulletin of the Royal College of Psychiatrists*, **10**, 303–306.
FRYERS, T. (1984) *The Epidemiology of Severe Intellectual Impairment: The Dynamics of Prevalence.* London: Academic Press.
—— (1987) The future of psychiatric case registers. In *Psychiatric Epidemiology; Progress and Prospects* (ed. B. Cooper), pp. 1–14. London: Croom Helm.
—— (ed) (1989) *Practical Issues in the Establishment, Maintenance and Exploitation of Psychiatric Case Registers in Public Health: A Worldwide Inventory, 1960–1985*, pp. 262–306, Amsterdam: Elsevier.
—— & WOOFF, K. (1989) A decade of mental health care in an urban community. In *Health Services Planning and Research: Contributions from Psychiatric Case Registers* (ed. J. K. Wing), pp. 31–52. London: Gaskell, Royal College of Psychiatrists.
GIBBONS, J. L., JENNINGS, C. & WING, J. K. (eds) (1984) *Register Areas; Statistics from 8 Psychiatric Case Registers in Great Britain, 1976–1981.* Southampton: University of Southampton Department of Psychiatry.

GIEL, R. (ed) (1986) The use of a case register in administrative and operational research. In *Psychiatric Case Registers in Public Health: A Worldwide Inventory, 1960–1985* (eds G. H. M. M. ten Horn, R. Giel, W. H. Gulbinat, *et al*), pp. 360–384. Amsterdam: Elsevier.

HAMERS, H., ROMME, M. & DEVRIES, M. W. (1986) Resistance, privacy and technology: comments on the negotiations to establish the case register in Maastricht. In *Psychiatric Case Registers in Public Health: A Worldwide Inventory, 1960–1985* (eds G. H. M. M. ten Horn, R. Giel, W. H. Gulbinat, *et al*), pp. 274–281. Amsterdam: Elsevier.

HOUSE OF COMMONS (1990) *The NHS and Community Care Act 1990*. London: HMSO.

ROHDE, P. (1986) *CRISP: Computer Recorded Information System for Psychiatry*. Consultation paper. London: Riverside Health Authority.

SUSSER, M. W. (1968) *Community Psychiatry: Epidemiologic and Social Themes*. New York: Random House.

TEN HORN, G. H. M. M., GIEL, R., GULBINAT, W. H., *et al* (eds) (1986) *Psychiatric Case Registers in Public Health: A Worldwide Inventory, 1960–1985*. Amsterdam: Elsevier.

WING, J. K. (ed) (1982) Long-term community care. *Psychological Medicine* (suppl. 2).

—— (ed) (1986) Data protection and problems of data confidentiality. In *Psychiatric Case Registers in Public Health: A Worldwide Inventory, 1960–1985* (eds G. H. M. M. ten Horn, R. Giel, W. H. Gulbinat, *et al*), pp. 360–384. Amsterdam: Elsevier.

—— (ed) (1989) *Health Services Planning and Research; Contributions from Psychiatric Case Registers*. London: Gaskell, Royal College of Psychiatrists.

—— & FRYERS, T. (1976) *Psychiatric Services in Camberwell and Salford; Statistics from the Camberwell and Salford Case Registers, 1964–1974*. London: Institute of Psychiatry.

WOOFF, K. (1987) *A Comparison of the Work of Community Psychiatric Nurses and Mental Health Social Workers in Salford*. PhD thesis. Manchester: University of Manchester.

——, GOLDBERG, D. P. & FRYERS, T. (1988) The practice of community psychiatric nursing and mental health social work in Salford; some implications for community care. *British Journal of Psychiatry*, **152**, 783–792.

6 Assessing the need for psychiatric treatment at the district level: the role of surveys

PAUL BEBBINGTON

In an ideal world, psychiatric services should be designed to deal with the needs for treatment in the community. Such needs exist at a whole range of levels, and the extent to which the responsible authorities feel able to meet them is determined by the tension between financial constraints and political imperatives. Although information about levels of need is an essential part of the equation, in practice it is at best sketchy, at worst non-existent.

The development of psychiatric services is never arbitrary. It always depends at some level on an evaluation of perceived need. There are a number of informal sources of this information. It may emerge because general practitioners (GPs) become aware of particular demands for their services – for instance that in an inner-city area they are seeing more cases of schizophrenia in recent residents – and communicate this to their psychiatric colleagues. Psychiatrists themselves may notice increasing demands from particular sorts of patients, for instance young people with eating disorders. Local pressure groups may also voice concerns about the inadequacies of current services for certain conditions.

The fact that services do develop in response to need in this informal way means that there is at any rate some virtue in planners' use of *utilisation data* to evaluate need. However, the consequence of relying on this information is essentially conservative, particularly if analyses are unsophisticated – the implication is that what has been shall continue. Nevertheless, utilisation data can provide insights into the ways that services might develop. One example is our own bed-use audit (Chapter 12, this volume).

Actual needs can only be assessed by surveying the local population, but only about 20 such surveys the world over have been based on adequate methods. Planners have therefore tended to extrapolate information from studies carried out in areas often very different from their own. Even if more community surveys were completed, most areas would lack the resources to carry out one of their own and would therefore have to fall back on data from elsewhere. This extrapolation would be less dubious if the sociodemographic characteristics of each area were known, so that corrections could be made for social differences. It is thus crucial to be able to characterise planning areas, both in terms of raw social attributes, and in terms of composite measures of known worth, such as the Jarman Index (Jarman, 1983). It is the purpose of this chapter to describe the requirements for the evaluation of the need for psychiatric services through the use of community surveys.

Determining the prevalence of psychiatric disorder through community surveys

Among their various functions, community psychiatric surveys enable us to extend and complete our view of the clinical picture, and to determine the frequency of given disorders. These two purposes are inextricably interwined, as where we choose to place the boundaries of a disorder inevitably affects both the values we obtain for prevalence, and the relationship between cases found in the general population and in the clinic. The way we define cases therefore determines what may allowably be inferred from the results of surveys. Comparing the characteristics of people with psychiatric disorder in the community with those of referred patients gives an idea of the influences that shape the *use* of services. However, the question I raise specifically in this chapter concerns the extent to which community surveys have illuminated the *need* for psychiatric treatment and services, and how they might be made to provide better information than they do.

Ideas about psychiatric illness were inevitably formulated around the conditions actually seen by physicians, and these were naturally of some severity. The subsequent movement of psychiatry into the community was therefore bound to change such ideas, and has resulted in a corresponding broadening of disease categories. So, for example, cases of depression in out-patient clinics may have *some* of the features of plain old-fashioned melancholia, but they are unlikely to have a full range of the more severe symptoms.

In the clinic, the referral process colours the recognition that someone is suffering from a medical disorder. Doctors feel duty bound to come up with a diagnosis. It is reassuringly easy to decide that, if people seek help for what they see as a psychiatric problem, they must be suffering from a psychiatric disorder. Those engaged in community psychiatric surveys have no access to this reassurance, and, in consequence, formal techniques for defining cases are absolutely essential. These techniques can in turn be applied to referred patients, and thus permit valid comparison between groups of cases or between studies.

There are problems over the choice of case definition for use in the community, which can be illustrated by considering the affective disorders. The individual symptoms that are the basis of affective syndromes vary in their frequency in the population at large, but most are quite common (e.g. Wing *et al*, 1981). Many people experience a few symptoms, a few experience many. The fewer the symptoms, the less the clinical picture corresponds to cases of affective disorder seen in the clinic. Most authorities are prepared to expand the concept of affective disorder to include some of the milder cases seen in the general population. However, there is clearly a limit beyond which further expansion ceases to be useful. If the definition of affective disorders is too inclusive, the study of community cases no longer illuminates the more severe conditions that are, of necessity, the bread and butter of the treating doctor. For this reason, most workers do use the characteristics of clinical cases as a point of reference. This is then used to decide the threshold below which the number and severity of affective symptoms are regarded as insufficient to justify the identification of a case.

In recent years, great advances have been made in the detection of psychiatric disorder in the community. The current psychiatric surveys have been described as a third generation (Dohrenwend & Dohrenwend, 1982). The two most widely accepted instruments embody very different principles, but each has been used in several studies around the world. The first to be developed was the Present State Examination (PSE) and its attendant computer programs, which together make up the PSE-ID-CATEGO system (Wing *et al*, 1974; Wing & Sturt, 1978). Its developers felt that reliable and comparable measures could be attained if symptoms were specified in detail and the rules for classifying disorders were made explicit and precise.

The CATEGO program provides a classification based on the International Classification of Diseases (ICD–9; World Health Organization, 1978) even in cases with very few symptoms. This means that when it is used in general population surveys case definition is so broad as to be meaningless. This problem was overcome by developing a sub-program, the Index of Definition (ID; Wing & Sturt, 1978). This allocates each case to one of eight levels that reflect the reliance that can be placed on the CATEGO classification. Levels 1 to 4 are non-cases, level 5 is a threshold set deliberately low, and levels 6–8 are held to indicate definite cases. In population surveys, levels 5 and above have generally been taken as the definition of a case. The system has now been used in several such surveys (Brown & Harris, 1978; Orley & Wing, 1979; Bebbington *et al*, 1981; Henderson *et al*, 1981; Costello, 1982; Surtees *et al*, 1983; Mavreas *et al*, 1986; Mavreas & Bebbington, 1987; Vazquez-Barquero *et al*, 1987; Hodiamont *et al*, 1987; Romans-Clarkson *et al*, 1988; Lehtinen *et al*, 1990a; Carta *et al*, 1991). It clearly depends on administration by people of some clinical sophistication, although it has been used as a screening device by lay interviewers (Sturt *et al*, 1981).

The Diagnostic Interview Schedule (DIS; Robins *et al*, 1981, 1985*a*) deliberately incorporates a very rigid structure: it is a list of questions whose form is exactly prescribed, and interviewers are trained not to deviate from the printed format, so that the scope for clinical judgement is reduced to a minimum. This controls variations on the part of the interviewer, but at the cost of failing to exert any control over variations due to the idiosyncrasies of respondents.

The data obtained by the DIS are used to establish lifetime diagnoses using three sets of criteria: those of DSM–III (American Psychiatric Association, 1980), those of Feighner *et al* (1972); and the Research Diagnostic Criteria (Spitzer *et al*, 1978). It was used in the population surveys of the Epidemiologic Catchment Area program (Eaton & Kessler, 1985), results from which have since been extensively published (Myers *et al*, 1984; Robins *et al*, 1984; Blazer *et al*, 1985; Burnham *et al*, 1987; Karno *et al*, 1987; Regier *et al*, 1988; Weissman *et al*, 1988). It has now also been used in population surveys in Puerto Rico (Canino *et al*, 1987), Edmonton, Canada (Bland *et al*, 1988), Christchurch, New Zealand (Wells *et al*, 1989), Taiwan (Hwu *et al*, 1989), and Munich (Wittchen *et al*, 1992). The DIS covers more diagnostic categories than the ninth edition of the PSE, the version so far employed in surveys.

There is now considerable agreement over the prevalence of psychiatric disorders in the community, and this stands in contrast to the position 20 years ago (Silverman, 1968; Dohrenwend & Dohrenwend, 1969). The consensus from studies around the world using the PSE can be illustrated by reviewing the one-month prevalence of CATEGO-derived depressive disorders: the Ugandan figures are really very high (Orley & Wing, 1979), but those apart, the range of values for men is from 2.6% to 4.8%, and for women from 5.9% to 10.1%. This range is of the order that could plausibly be explained by the effects of different local circumstances: it is entirely reasonable that Camberwell, an inner-city area in South London, should have around twice the rates seen in the affluent Australian city of Canberra. The Ugandan values might represent over-rating of PSE items, the insecurity in that country at the time of Amin's excesses, a high prevalence of alcohol-related symptoms, or the unavailability of treatment.

As with the PSE community surveys, those using the DIS display good agreement, especially when it is considered that the populations are not standardised for demographic differences like age. So, for instance, the overall one-month prevalence of major depressive disorder varies from 1.5% to 2.6%. Six-month prevalences are available for more sites, and vary from 1.7% to 3.5% (males 1.3–2.5%, females 3.0–4.6%) (Bebbington, 1990). The high rates in Christchurch and the low rates in Taiwan do raise questions about whether they represent real differences or some local oddity of administration of the DIS: the rate for somatisation disorder in Taiwan does not seem to be raised, as might be expected if, for instance, the subjects were expressing depressed mood in somatic terms (Hwu *et al*, 1989).

The last ten years have therefore seen the publication of community surveys with just about the right level of inconsistency to disarm incredulity. What can be made of the results? The discrepancies between, and the consistencies within, the DIS and PSE studies suggest that CATEGO depression categories of Index of Definition level 5 and above may represent a lower recognition threshold than the category of major depressive disorder elicited through the DIS. Relatively small shifts in threshold lead to appreciable changes in prevalence, as cases in the community will tend to cluster around the threshold.

However, we cannot assume that, because we have instruments that provide a reasonably consistent population prevalence, they will necessarily identify individual cases in a consistent way. There is likely to be disagreement both when two people use the same instrument and when one person uses different instruments (Dean *et al*, 1983; Bebbington *et al*, 1984). Anthony *et al* (1985) cast doubt on the ability of the DIS to identify cases established through a more orthodox style of clinical evaluation. Despite this, results from community surveys can be useful in estimating the likely burden of these disorders in the population and thus for providing indirect evidence of needs for treatment. Indeed, this was a major purpose of the ECA studies (Eaton *et al*, 1981). I have argued elsewhere that the threshold represented by the criteria for major depressive disorder is probably a reasonable one to assess needs for treatment for this condition, and that prevalence so defined is probably 2% – 3% in British communities of average prosperity and resources (Bebbington, 1992). However, I would argue that establishing prevalence can only be regarded as a first step in the assessment of the needs for treatment in the general population. We can probably do better by more direct methods, although these have never been applied in general population studies.

The prevalence of disorder and the need for treatment

To recapitulate, case definitions derive their value ultimately from their relationship to the range of cases seen in clinical practice, although they embody criteria broad enough to include the less severe end of that range. Because of the relationship between the criteria and clinical disorders, the prevalences obtained by applying them in the community have implications for the need for treatment in the population.

However, we cannot assume that subjects in the community need psychiatric treatment merely because they meet symptomatic case criteria. Firstly, most authorities would acknowledge that the need for treatment is related to the persistence of the disorder, and the level of persistence that might be taken to indicate a need for treatment may not be the same as the duration required to meet diagnostic criteria – it is usually greater.

Secondly, there are other features commonly associated with psychiatric illness that do not necessarily form part of the definition of disease. By this I mean social performance. The PSE evaluates the presence of psychiatric symptoms in isolation from the subject's social performance. Some symptoms, for instance subjective anergia or loss of concentration, will often be associated with impaired social functioning, but are nevertheless evaluated on the basis of the respondent's subjective experience. The PSE is designed in this way because its authors felt that definitions of cases of disorder for testing aetiological theories should be couched in terms only of symptoms. Other instruments include criteria relating to social performance, and both the Schedule for Affective Disorders and Schizophrenia (SADS; Endicott & Spitzer, 1978) and the DIS do this. Impaired social functioning should be assessed separately from the central definition of disorder in symptomatic terms because the relationship between the two can then be examined empirically.

Findings from studies of the association between social performance and psychiatric symptoms are inconsistent, probably because of the great variety of measures used. However, the association may be weaker in community samples. In other words, *cases in the community are less consistently associated with social impairment* (Cassel, 1974; Blumenthal & Dielmann, 1975; Hurry et al, 1983). If so, we can again query the assumption that cases in the community identified symptomatically are necessarily in need of treatment.

There have been several studies of the relationship between impaired social performance and the *utilisation* of services. Several authors have argued that poor social functioning is central to people's views of themselves as mentally ill: it may be at the point of social breakdown that they take their symptoms seriously (Herzlich, 1973; Foulds, 1967). If so, one would expect that failure of social functioning is closely involved in the decision to seek treatment, and that it would contribute to this decision over and above the level of symptoms. Our own studies offer little support for this hypothesis (Hurry et al, 1987), but it is possible that the role of social performance is more important at lesser levels of symptom severity (Mechanic & Volkhart, 1961; Mechanic, 1963). It has also been claimed that the impairment of social functioning is a factor over and above straightforward symptom levels in leading the family practitioner to refer patients for psychiatric treatment (Mowbray et al, 1961; Kaesar & Cooper, 1971; Casey et al, 1985).

There is thus evidence that both patients and their doctors see the effects of psychiatric illness on social functioning as grounds for treatment. How prevalent is impaired social performance in the community? The range of measures employed make it impossible to give absolute answers to this question. However, in our own study using the latest version of the MRC's Social Role Performance Schedule (Wing, 1989), only 3.8% of the population scored at levels of impairment exceeded by 50% of an out-patient sample (Hurry & Sturt, 1981).

The relative dissociation between symptomatic and social impairment in cases in the community I think confirms my contention that prevalence as measured in the recent community surveys can only be an approximate guide to the possible need for services. Some authors have acknowledged this, and have attempted to provide improved evaluations of need. Shapiro *et al* (1985) tried to do this by assessing three potential indications of need: a DIS disorder in the last six months, a current GHQ score of four or more, and the respondents' report of being unable to manage their usual activities for at least one whole day in the preceding three months. Not unexpectedly, the indices were all associated with the use of professional services. Although this combined index acknowledges the role of social functioning, the measure is crude, and one is not struck by its face validity.

Lehtinen *et al* (1990*b*) report on an evaluation of the need for treatment in the mini-Finland Health Survey. Need for specialist treatment was judged to be present if the case was *definite* according to the PSE-ID-CATEGO system (i.e. ID level 6 and above), *or* if the interviewer thought that treatment was needed. Interviewers also made judgements about the need for treatment by the GP in cases of a lesser degree of severity. The subject's own judgement about whether they needed treatment was also recorded.

The results of this study are interesting. The need for treatment assessed by the interviewers was less than the prevalence of disorders, and that assessed by the subjects themselves was lower still. The interviewers reckoned that around 9% of subjects were in need of specialist treatment, whereas only 1½% thought so themselves; a further 6%, however, felt that they were 'probably' in need of treatment. Taking all forms of treatment, around 4% of subjects were receiving adequate treatment, and 14% showed an unmet need for treatment, albeit not necessarily specialist. This study is a useful attempt at a more direct measure of need. Its drawback is that it still confuses need with mere prevalence in that an ID level of six or over is taken as an absolute indication of a need for treatment. Moreover, the structuring of the assessment of need is not described and may have been inadequate. Finally, no attempt is made to say exactly *what treatment is needed* or *by whom it might be provided*.

The community surveys described above are immeasurably better than their predecessors, so we can at least place some credence on the reported prevalence of common mental disorders in the general population. However, we remain unsure of the implications of this information for planning mental health services. There is thus a good case for a *fourth generation* of surveys with a direct focus on the evaluation of the need for specific treatments and the services within which they are most appropriately provided.

Direct evaluation of the need for treatment in the community

We can make progress by basing the methods of assessment on explicit and detailed criteria. One possible avenue towards this is by adopting the MRC Needs for Care Assessment. This was originally designed for use with patients suffering from longstanding mental disorders.

The underlying model and rationale of this family of instruments is presented by Brewin *et al* (1987) and by Mangen & Brewin (1991) (see also Chapter 13 by Brewin in this volume). A primary need for care is defined as being present when (a) a subject's level of functioning falls below, or threatens to fall below, some minimum specified level (i.e. there is distress from symptoms, or disablement), and (b) this is due to some potentially remediable or preventable cause. For each area of clinical and social functioning covered, the assessment specifies a minimum level of functioning and a set of appropriate interventions or items of care. Problems are assessed through an evaluation of symptoms and of abnormalities of social behaviour. Details of the timing and effectiveness of treatment are recorded. Needs for care in each area are then determined by comparing the actual items of care provided with an ideal model of what those items of care should be. Because assessments of the needs for care are made within an explicit model of ideal practice, the inevitable value judgements inherent in the procedure have the virtue of being public and consequently accessible to argument.

The community version of the MRC Needs for Care Assessment has been specifically adapted for use with the relatively mild psychiatric conditions seen in general populations. Considerable modification was required, but the underlying principles remain those of the original instrument. It is designed to approximate in an itemised and systematic manner the functioning of well-organised primary care and psychiatric services. The information required is provided by the subjects themselves, but may be backed up by collateral sources such as GPs' notes. The assessment covers the same range of conditions as the short version of the 10th edition of the PSE (Wing *et al*, 1990). A manual has been prepared by Brewin *et al* (1991).

Unlike conventional measures of symptoms and behaviour, this assessment generates data both on level of functioning and on the appropriate actions that should be taken by clinicians. Needs are defined in terms of these actions, that is, have specific items of care been offered? The primary-need status in each area of functioning falls into the categories:*no need* – there is no problem and therefore no appropriate action; *met need* – appropriate action to deal with the psychiatric problems is already in progress; *unmet need* – some action is appropriate now, but has not been undertaken; *no meetable need* – there is a problem but no action is both appropriate and feasible. The assessment also provides information on *overprovision*.

The assessment is designed for use by research teams. Many of the decisions to be made depend on clinical judgement, and hence it is not suitable for use by persons inexperienced in this area. It has been designed primarily for psychiatrists and clinical psychologists. The required information can, however, be obtained by a research worker, and judgements of need are made later by members of the research team. Because of the requirement to evaluate the need for pharmacological treatments, the research team must have ready access to psychiatric opinion.

Needs are in large part *value judgements*, and therefore cannot be objectively defined. We do not claim that the assessment will tell the user what a person's needs are in any absolute sense. Rather, the assessment sets a standard against which to compare the care being given at the time of measurement, and registers any shortfall. The assessment will not cover all eventualities, nor answer every question about the needs of individual respondents. It is limited in the areas it covers, in the interventions it includes, and in the decision rules it incorporates; it does not aim to provide the kind of detailed fact-gathering necessary for planning an intervention, nor has it yet been conclusively demonstrated that the assessment will generate identical results when used by different people. What we do claim is that it represents a first step towards a more systematic and logical approach to assessing need in the community. By using it, judgements can be made about the extent to which individual psychiatric problems are being dealt with or could be dealt with by professional care. The meeting of need depends on many factors, including the availability of appropriate services and the skills and attitudes of family doctors. It will also be affected by individual beliefs about and attitudes towards treatment.

Need is treated by us as a normative concept which is to be defined by experts. We distinguish between needs for specific items of care (such as advice, treatment, shelter, etc.) and needs for services to supply these items of care. It is intended that a separate 'Needs for Services Assessment' will be developed to allow judgements of the most cost-effective agent for a particular form of treatment or care, together with the most appropriate service setting. This information can then be used to evaluate the extent to which the needs for services are being met (see Mangen & Brewin, 1991). However, these procedures are at a very early stage of development.

Because experts will vary in their thresholds for judgements of needs for care, we distinguish between *primary needs*, which are expected to attract the greatest professional consensus, and *secondary needs*. As mentioned above, primary needs are characterised by two main elements in combination: the subject's functioning falling below or threatening to fall below a minimum level; and this being due to a potentially remediable or preventable constraint. These minimum levels are based on the absence of clinical symptoms of moderate intensity and duration, and the ability to carry out the ordinary tasks of daily living. The emphasis on the remediability of the constraints experienced by the subject implies that, in our definition, need is only present so long as some reasonable and generally accepted therapeutic or preventive procedure remains to be tried; if after adequate trial all such procedures have been found to be ineffective, or if they have been refused, then we say that no meetable need currently exists.

For the purposes of community psychiatric surveys, only one type of secondary need has been distinguished. This involves the *overprovision of care*. In general, this is only rated where a subject has already attained the target level of functioning and is not in any apparent danger of relapse or deterioration were care withdrawn, but nevertheless continues to receive it. In the community this is most likely to relate to the provision of medication. It is recognised, however, that clinical judgement about the correct balance between the risks of relapse and of dependency will vary.

Needs for care in the community are evaluated on the basis of clinical and social characteristics, and are divided into the seven specific areas of functioning listed below.

Positive psychotic symptoms
Depressive symptoms
Anxiety and obsessional symptoms
Problems with alcohol
Problems with drugs
Eating disorders
Distress about psychosocial problems (e.g. housing or marital difficulties).

In order for results to be comparable between studies, common thresholds must be determined and standardised instruments employed to measure them. In the Camberwell Community Needs Survey (CCNS) currently being planned, the threshold for most disorders will be taken as the continuous presence of clinically significant symptoms over a period of six weeks, although psychotic symptoms would be seen as worthy of medical attention if they are present at all.

We recommend that the clinical significance of symptoms be identified from several types of evidence. First, a clinical interview using a standardised psychiatric assessment is required. The CCNS will employ the short version of the 10th edition of the Present State Examination and associated instruments, together known as SCAN, to assess psychotic and neurotic symptoms (Wing *et al*, 1990). PSE–10 requires raters to assess severity using such criteria as the frequency and intensity of symptoms. SCAN also allows consideration of the clinical history. This enables the recorder to ascertain whether there is a threat of other symptoms recurring that are not currently present. The information is occasionally required to establish the appropriateness or otherwise of preventive measures, such as long-term treatment with lithium, an antidepressant or a major tranquilliser.

SCAN also has sections devoted to substance abuse and to eating disorders. These disorders are defined in terms of the criteria underlying the DSM–III–R (American Psychiatric Association, 1987) and ICD–10 (World Health Organization, 1992) classifications. The presence of an eating disorder or of hazardous use of or dependence on alcohol or other drugs will itself be taken as sufficient to warrant treatment. In addition, information is collected about the consumption of substances that may potentially be abused. Where alcohol has been consumed at more than recommended levels for one year, needs for treatment will be considered, even when the subject does not meet criteria for dependence or hazardous use.

Secondly, the tendency for symptoms to result in social disability should be assessed through the use of measures of social functioning. In the original MRC Needs for Care Assessment, the evaluation of social functioning was based on the Social Behaviour Schedule (SBS; Wykes & Sturt, 1986; Wing, 1989). The social performance of subjects in the community, even those with psychiatric disorders, is likely to be relatively unimpaired, and a more sensitive instrument is thus required. In the CCNS, information about social functioning will be provided by the MRC Social Role Performance Schedule (SRPS; Hurry & Sturt, 1981; Hurry *et al*, 1983). While the SBS is designed to record the gross abnormalities of social behaviour that may be seen in patients with longstanding psychiatric disorder, the SRPS is used to quantify failures to match the expectations associated with given roles – the sort of impairment that may, for instance, reflect relatively mild disturbances in mood.

To determine the presence of a moderate problem one must evaluate both the medium-term threat to well-being and the social impact of symptoms on subjects. Symptoms that are mild by ordinary clinical standards may occasionally be quite disruptive to the respondent's life, and thereby qualify as a moderate or severe problem. Clinical judgement is essential, as in evaluations of this type in population surveys we argue that social disablement is only relevant in so far as it derives from the presence of psychiatric symptoms.

Long-term mental illness is associated with many disabilities. These may be the direct result of the illness process, or may have other causes, but even so they must be managed as part of the competent management of longstanding mental illness. Failure to do this has immediate impact on the course of the illness. This situation lends itself to relatively straight-forward decisions about what is to be done for the patients with these illnesses, although it emphasises the difficulty of making an ideological split between medical and social care.

Psychiatric disorders in the community are not like this. They may well have social concomitants so those affected are unable to continue with their employment, their household responsibilities, or even their self-care. However, there is generally little doubt that these social features are the direct consequence of the psychiatric conditions, even though they may linger after the symptoms have apparently improved (Weissman & Paykel, 1974). Accordingly, the primary thrust of treatment, whether pharmacological or psychological, is towards the psychiatric symptoms, and dealing with the social consequences may merely involve a holding operation of the sort often left to the family.

At the same time, within the community there are those who get into difficulties they find hard to deal with. Sometimes this will be through no action of their own, sometimes it is a result of not being very socially competent. They may have significant psychiatric symptoms as a result and, if so, the thrust of treatment is towards the resolution of both symptoms and social problems, through practical assistance and encouragement of the individual's own coping resources.

In the large majority of cases, it will probably be easy to distinguish between the psychiatric domain and the province of the social worker. In designing the community version of the Needs for Care Assessment, it was necessary to come to clear decisions about the limits to the appropriateness of psychiatric care. Accordingly, we chose psychiatric symptoms as the focus of the assessment, taking account of social difficulties only in so far as they generate or amplify symptoms. In the CCNS we will have access to information about social difficulties through the use of the Life Events and Difficulties Schedule (Brown & Harris, 1978). In the context of the community version of the Needs for Care Assessment, this will be used to evaluate the requirement for help with problems that are clearly associated with the generation of symptoms. Psychosocial problems not associated with psychiatric symptoms fall outside the scope of the assessment.

In each area, the rating of *primary-need status* follows logically from the ratings that have already been given to the level of functioning and to the individual items of care.

Met need is rated when there is a current or recent problem or the threat of a problem occurring, and a potentially effective item of care is being offered. Met need may therefore imply either that a current problem is being effectively treated, or that preventive measures are successfully being employed to guard against relapse, or that some form of care is being provided to ameliorate a long-term disorder or deficit. Met need also describes the situation in which there are only partially effective items of care available, but these are worth continuing and the criteria for unmet need are not satisfied.

Unmet needs for assessment are rated when there are impairments in level of functioning and further observation or specialist testing is required.

In all cases of *unmet need for treatment*, the current level of functioning is below the acceptable threshold. Raters must satisfy themselves that current treatments have been ineffective in dealing with the problem and the subject is not continuing to show marked improvement. They must also be confident that alternative interventions have not been recently refused or proved ineffective, and are appropriate to try *now*. If the family doctor has made a referral for an appropriate intervention but it has not yet begun (for example, the subject is on a waiting list), the item of care is rated as potentially effective and the need is met.

Unmet needs are always rated in preference to met needs, if the criteria for both are satisfied. In addition, it is important not to rate the same unmet need twice in different sections of the schedule. For example, if people have significant depressive symptoms and are rated as having an unmet need for counselling, they should not be given a separate rating of unmet need for counselling to deal with symptoms of distress. They might, however, be legitimately rated as having an additional unmet need for welfare advice to overcome distress arising from a separate cause such as housing difficulties.

No meetable need is rated when there is a current or recent problem, but no intervention seems likely to be even partially effective. Any item of care still being offered is thus likely to be an overprovision.

Not applicable ratings are used when needs have already been rated under another subsection.

A rating of *overprovision* indicates that an item of care is being provided unnecessarily. It is used in two different situations. In some cases the level of functioning will be below threshold, and overprovision then implies that an item of care being provided is ineffective or inappropriate.

However, where the current level of functioning is adequate, it should not be assumed that corresponding items of care are not being provided, and so users of the schedule must always be careful to consider possible overprovision.

For overprovision to be rated, the item of care should usually have been offered for a period of at least three months with no demonstrable benefit. This period may be extended to as much as three or four years where the subject suffers from a regularly recurring condition such as manic–depressive psychosis for which the item of care is a specific and effective preventive measure like lithium therapy. Overprovision may also be rated if an item of care is provided at *an excessive level* despite being worth continuing. In this case it will usually have been provided for three months or more at the level judged to be unnecessarily high. Overprovision is not rated, however, if adequate but unsuccessful attempts have been made to reduce provision.

Overprovision of medication may be rated when drug levels have not been reviewed for some time. This implies that, once symptoms had been brought under control, psychotropic medication should be steadily reduced wherever possible. Because benzodiazepines are known to be ineffective after three months, and because there is a risk of dependence, most instances of benzodiazepine use lasting for longer than three months should be rated as overprovision.

Some subjects may have problems not covered in the assessment. Interventions required for these may be rated as *additional needs*. In other cases, investigators may wish to rate an unmet need even though the person's level of functioning is still currently satisfactory, for example because they can anticipate a need for preventive action. Finally, they should rate additional needs when within the same area of functioning, there are separate problems requiring separate intervention.

In the original Needs for Care Assessment, account had to be taken of cultural constraints when it was used outside Britain or outside the mainstream of British culture. For example, in Verona (and presumably in other parts of Italy) it appears to be inappropriate to expect men to have demonstrated competence in cooking and other household chores. These are not part of the accepted male role, and hence were not accepted as needs either by professionals using the instrument or by service users (Lesage *et al*, 1991). Some people, of course, feel that cooking is not part of their role, even in the absence of general cultural constraints. However, in the community version of the instrument, these cultural constraints are taken into account in the Social Role Performance Schedule itself.

Another environmental constraint to be considered is that of policy and resources. Obviously, services differ enormously in their philosophy of care and in the resources available for family intervention, remedial education, etc. It is worth emphasising that our procedure sets normative standards of care, and does not take these differences between individual services into account. For the sake of comparability between studies, unmet needs should therefore be rated without considering whether particular items of care are routinely provided, or whether the manpower and expertise exists to provide them.

Conclusion

The community version of the Needs for Care Assessment depends upon detailed information of good quality. The process of evaluating the needs for care in the general population is therefore likely to require considerable resources. Nevertheless, I would argue that the resulting advances in our detailed knowledge of the burden of mental illness in the community and of the requirements for specific treatments justifies this cost. Without it, only the vaguest judgements of the adequacy of services can be made.

Assessing needs for care directly through community surveys will result in a quality and range of information previously unavailable to planners. What should they do with it? It is unlikely to be reassuring, since it will probably identify more underprovision than overprovision, with the implication that services fall short of meeting overall needs. Much of the need is likely to require action by family practitioners, and thus the findings of needs surveys will underline the requirement, already well supported by other evidence, that GPs should be adequately trained to recognise and deal with psychiatric problems. More resources and support may need to be given to general practice psychiatric services.

The number of people picked up in surveys with more serious mental illness requiring treatment will be small. Although specialist services deal only with a minority of those with psychiatric difficulties, the latter may nevertheless represent a significant shortfall in services if they are inappropriately failing to receive specialist treatment. The pattern of unmet need may itself give vital information about the ways in which services might be run more effectively.

Apart from the requirements of planners, community surveys of the needs for psychiatric treatment should have benefits for the professions of psychiatry, as they provide an empirical basis for justifying service developments whose appropriateness is initially suggested by clinical experience.

Community surveys in short are likely to identify unmet need, and this will require decisions on the future direction of psychiatric service development. These decisions will be coloured by three considerations: *the financial constraints* that must apply to any service; *the principle of equity* – that those with equivalent disorders have an equal right to treatment; and *the principle of proportionality* – that the greatest suffering merits the greatest effort by the treating professions. Equity itself demands the best possible information, based on needs rather than utilisation: a complacency based on ignorance of our services' failings is inappropriate. Service planners will also have to take account of the *reasons* why people are not getting the services they require. This in turn may lead to a greater emphasis on public education and designing services to be more acceptable and more accessible.

As indicated above, it is unlikely that funding can be found for more than a few surveys, and extrapolation will still be necessary. Nevertheless, the validity of extrapolation increases with the number and geographical proximity of the surveys (some British planners have used data from the ECA surveys as the basis of their decisions). In my view there is thus a good argument for mounting surveys of this type in areas that together cover a range of social settings. They are expensive, but their results would be invaluable.

References

AMERICAN PSYCHIATRIC ASSOCIATION (1980) *Diagnositc and Statistical Manual of Mental Disorders* (3rd edn) (DSM–III). Washington, DC: APA.
—— (1987) *Diagnositc and Statistical Manual of Mental Disorders* (3rd edn, revised) (DSM–III-R). Washington, DC: APA.
ANTHONY, J. C., FOLSTEIN, M., ROMANOSKI, A. J., *et al* (1985) Comparison of the lay Diagnostic Interview Schedule and a standardized psychiatric diagnosis. *Archives of General Psychiatry*, **42**, 667–676.
BEBBINGTON, P. E. (1990) Population surveys of psychiatric disorder and the need for treatment. *Social Psychiatry and Psychiatric Epidemiology*, **25**, 33–40.
—— (1992) The epidemiology of depressive illness. In *The Psychopharmacology of Depression* (ed. S. Montgomery). BAP Monograph Series. Oxford: Oxford University Press.
——, HURRY, J., TENNANT, C., *et al* (1981) The epidemiology of mental disorders in Camberwell. *Psychological Medicine*, **11**, 561–580.
——, STURT, E., TENNANT, C., *et al* (1984) Misfortune and resilience: a community study of women. *Psychological Medicine*, **14**, 347–364.
BLAND, R. C., NEWMAN, S. C. & ORN, H. (1988) Epidemiology of psychiatric disorders in Edmonton. *Acta Psychiatrica Scandinavica*, **77** (suppl. 338).
BLAZER, D., GEORGE, L. K., LANDERMAN, R., *et al* (1985) Psychiatric disorders: a rural/urban comparison. *Archives of General Psychiatry*, **42**, 651–656.
BLUMENTHAL, M. D. & DIELMAN, T. E. (1975) Depressive symptomatology and role function in a general population. *Archives of General Psychiatry*, **32**, 985–991.
BREWIN, C. R., WING, J. K., MANGEN, S. P., *et al* (1987) Principles and practice of measuring need in the long-term mentally ill: the MRC Needs for Care Assessment. *Psychological Medicine*, **17**, 971–982.
——, BEBBINGTON, P. E. & WING, J. K. (1991) *The Needs for Care Assessment – Community Version: A Manual*. London: Social and Community Psychiatry Unit, Institute of Psychiatry (unpublished manuscript).
BROWN, G. W. & HARRIS, T. (1978) Social origins of depression: a reply. *Psychological Medicine*, **8**, 577–588.
BURNHAM, M. A., HOUGH, R. L., ESCOBAR, J. I., *et al* (1987) Six month prevalence of specific psychiatric disorders among Mexican Americans and non-Hispanic whites in Los Angeles. *Archives of General Psychiatry*, **44**, 687–694.
CANINO, G. J., BIRD, H. R., SHROUT, P. E., *et al* (1987) The prevalence of specific psychiatric disorders in Puerto Rico. *Archives of General Psychiatry*, **44**, 727–735.
CARTA, M. G., CARPINIELLO, B., MOROSINI, P. L., *et al* (1991) Prevalence of mental disorders in Sardinia: a community study in an inland mining district. *Psychological Medicine*, **21**, 1061–1071.
CASEY, P. R., TYRER, P. & PLATT, S. (1985) The relationship between social functioning and psychiatric symptomatology in primary care. *Social Psychiatry*, **20**, 5–9.
CASSEL, J. C. (1974) Psychiatric epidemiology. In *American Handbook of Psychiatry (2nd Edition)* (eds S. Arieti & E. Caplan). New York: Basic Books.
COSTELLO, C. G. (1982) Social factors associated with depression: a retrospective community study. *Psychological Medicine*, **12**, 329–339.
DEAN, C., SURTEES, P. G. & SASHIDHARAN, S. P. (1983) Comparison of research diagnostic systems in an Edinburgh community sample. *British Journal of Psychiatry*, **142**, 247–256.
DOHRENWEND, B. P. & DOHRENWEND, B. S. (1969) *Social Status and Psychological Disorder: A Causal Inquiry*. New York: Wiley.
—— & —— (1982) Perspectives on the past and future of psychiatric epidemiology. *American Journal of Public Health*, **72**, 1271–1279.
EATON, W. W., REGIER, D. A., LOCKE, B. Z., *et al* (1981) The NIMH epidemiologic catchment area program. In *What is a Case? The Problem of Definition in Psychiatric Community Surveys* (eds J. K. Wing, P. E. Bebbington & L. Robins), pp. 99–106. London: Grant MacIntyre.

—— & KESSLER, L. G. (1985) *Epidemiologic Field Methods in Psychiatry: The NIMH Epidemiologic Catchment Area Program.* Orlando, Fl.: Academic Press.

ENDICOTT, J. & SPITZER, R. (1978) A diagnostic interview: the schedule for affective disorders and schizophrenia. *Archives of General Psychiatry*, **35**, 837–844.

FOULDS, G. A. (1967) *The Hierarchical Nature of Personal Illness.* London: Academic Press.

HENDERSON, A. S., BYRNE, D. G. & DUNCAN-JONES, P. (1981) *Neurosis and the Social Environment.* Sydney: Academic Press.

HERZLICH, C. (1973) *Health and Illness.* London: Academic Press.

HODIAMONT, P., PEER, N. & SYBEN, N. (1987) Epidemiological aspects of psychiatric disorder in a Dutch Health Area. *Psychological Medicine*, **17**, 495–506.

HURRY, J. & STURT, E. (1981) Social performance in a population sample: relation to psychiatric symptoms. In *What is a Case? The Problem of Definition in Psychiatric Community Surveys* (eds J. K. Wing, P. E. Bebbington & L. Robins), pp. 202–216. London: Grant MacIntyre.

——, ——, BEBBINGTON, P., *et al* (1983) Socio-demographic association with social disablement in a community sample. *Social Psychiatry*, **18**, 113–121.

——, BEBBINGTON, P. E. & TENNANT, C. (1987) Psychiatric symptoms and social disablement as determinants of illness behaviour. *Australian and New Zealand Journal of Psychiatry*, **21**, 68–74.

HWU, H.-G., YEH, E.-K. & CHANG, L.-Y. (1989) Prevalence of psychiatric disorders in Taiwan defined by the Chinese Diagnostic Interview Schedule. *Acta Psychiatrica Scandinavica*, **79**, 136–147.

JARMAN, B. (1983) Identification of underprivileged areas. *British Medical Journal*, **256**, 1587–1592.

KAESER, A. C. & COOPER, B. (1971) The psychiatric patient, the general practitioner, and the out-patient clinic an operational study and a review. *Psychological Medicine*, **1**, 312–325.

KARNO, M., HOUGH, R. L., BURNHAM, M. A., *et al* (1987) Lifetime prevalence of specific psychiatric disorders among Mexican Americans and non-Hispanic whites in Los Angeles. *Archives of General Psychiatry*, **44**, 695–701.

LEHTINEN, V., LINDHOLM, T., VEIJOLA, J., *et al* (1989) The prevalence of PSE-CATEGO disorders in a Finnish adult population cohort. *Social Psychiatry and Psychiatric Epidemiology*, **25**, 187–192.

——, JOUKAMAA, M., JYRKINEN, E., *et al* (1990) Need for mental health services of the adult population in Finland: results from the Mini Finland Health Survey. *Acta Psychiatrica Scandinavica*, **81**, 426–431.

LESAGE, A. D., MIGNOLLI, G., FACCINCANI, C., *et al* (1989) Standardised assessment of the needs for care in a cohort of patients with schizophrenic psychoses. *Psychological Medicine*, suppl. **19**, 27–34.

MANGEN, S. & BREWIN, C. R. (1991) The measurement of need. In *Social Psychiatry: Theory, Methodology and Practice* (ed. P. E. Bebbington), pp. 163–182. New Brunswick, NJ: Transaction Press.

MAVREAS, V. G., BEIS, A., MOUYIAS, A., *et al* (1986) Prevalence of psychiatric disorder in Athens: a community study. *Social Psychiatry*, **21**, 172–181.

—— & BEBBINGTON, P. E. (1987) Psychiatric morbidity in London's Greek Cypriot community. I. Association with socio-demographic variables. *Social Psychiatry*, **22**, 150–159.

MECHANIC, D. (1962) Some implications of illness behavior. *New England Journal of Medicine*, **269**, 244.

—— & VOLKHART, E. A. (1961) Stress, illness behavior and the sick role. *American Sociological Review*, **26**, 51–58.

MOWBRAY, R. M., BLAIR, W., JOBL, L., *et al* (1961) The general practitioner's attitude to psychiatry. *Scottish Medical Journal*, **6**, 314–321.

MYERS, J. K., WEISSMAN, M. M., TISCHLER, G. L., *et al* (1984) Six month prevalence of psychiatric disorders in three communities: 1980–1982. *Archives of General Psychiatry*, **41**, 959–967.

ORLEY, J. & WING, J. K. (1979) Psychiatric disorders in two African villages. *Archives of General Psychiatry*, **36**, 513–520.

REGIER, D. A., BOYD, J. H., BURKE, J. D., *et al* (1988) One month prevalence of mental disorders in the United States. *Archives of General Psychiatry*, **45**, 977–986.

ROBINS, L. N., HELZER, J. E., CROUGHAN, J. L. *et al* (1981) The NIMH Diagnostic Interview Schedule: its history, characteristics and validity. In *What is a Case? The Problem of Definition in Psychiatric Community Surveys* (eds J. K. Wing, P. Bebbington & L. N. Robins), pp. 79–98. London: Grant McIntyre.

——, ——, ORVASCHEL, H., *et al* (1985a) The Diagnostic Interview Schedule. In *Epidemiologic Field Methods in Psychiatry: The NIMH Epidemiologic Catchment Area Program* (eds W. W. Eaton & L. G. Kessler), pp. 143–170. Orlando, Fl.: Academic Press.

——, ——, WEISSMAN, M. M., *et al* (1984) Lifetime prevalence of specific disorders in three sites. *Archives of General Psychiatry*, **41**, 949–958.

ROMANS-CLARKSON, S. E., WALTON, V. A., HERBISON, G. P., *et al* (1988) Marriage, motherhood and psychiatric morbidity in New Zealand. *Psychological Medicine*, **18**, 983–990.

SHAPIRO, S., SKINNER, E. A., KRAMER, M., *et al* (1985) Measuring need for mental health services in a general population. *Medical Care*, **23**, 1033–1043.

SILVERMAN, C. (1968) *Epidemiology of Depression*, Baltimore: Johns Hopkins University Press.

SPITZER, R. L., ENDICOTT, J. & ROBINS, E. (1978) Research Diagnostic Criteria: rationale and reliability. *Archives of General Psychiatry*, **35**, 773–782.

STURT, E., BEBBINGTON, P. E., HURRY, J., *et al* (1981) The Present State Examination used by interviewers from a survey agency: report from the Camberwell Community Survey. *Psychological Medicine*, **11**, 185–192.

SURTEES, P. G., DEAN, C., INGHAM, J. G., *et al* (1983) Psychiatric disorder in women from an Edinburgh community: associations with demographic factors. *British Journal of Psychiatry*, **142**, 238–246.

VAZQUEZ-BARQUERO, J.-L., DIEZ-MANRIQUE, J. F., PENA, C., *et al* (1987) A community mental health survey in Cantabria: a general description of morbidity. *Psychological Medicine*, **17**, 227–242.

WEISSMAN, M. M. & PAYKEL, E. S. (1974) *The Depressed Woman: A Study of Social Relations*. Chicago: University of Chicago Press.

——, LEAF, P. J., TISCHLER, G. L., *et al* (1988) Affective disorders in five United States communities. *Psychological Medicine*, **18**, 141–154.

WELLS, J. E., BUSHNELL, J. A., HORNBLOW, A. R., *et al* (1989) Christchurch Psychiatric Epidemiology Study: methodology and lifetime prevalence for specific psychiatric disorders. *Australian and New Zealand Journal of Psychiatry*, **23**, 315–326.

WING, J. K. (1989) The measurement of 'social disablement': The MRC social behaviour and social performance schedules. *Social Psychiatry and Psychiatric Epidemiology*, **24**, 173–178.

——, COOPER, J. E. & SARTORIUS, N. (1974) *The Measurement and Classification of Psychiatric Symptoms*. Cambridge: Cambridge University Press.

—— & STURT, E. (1978) *The PSE-ID-CATEGO System: a supplementary manual*. London (mimeo): Institute of Psychiatry.

——, BEBBINGTON, P., HURRY, J., *et al* (1981) The prevalence in the general population of disorders familiar to psychiatrists in hospital practice. In *What is a Case? The Problem of Definition in Psychiatric Community Surveys* (eds J. K. Wing, P. Bebbington & L. N. Robins), pp. 45–61. London: Grant MacIntyre Ltd.

——, BABOR, T., BRUGHA, T., *et al* (1990) SCAN: Schedules for Clinical Assessment in Neuropsychiatry. *Archives of General Psychiatry*, **47**, 589–593.

WITTCHEN, H.-U., ESSAU, C. A., VON ZERSSEN, D., *et al* (1992) Lifetime and six-month prevalence of mental disorders in the Munich Follow-up Study. *European Archives of Psychiatry* (in press).

WORLD HEALTH ORGANIZATION (1978) *Mental Disorders: Glossary and Guide to their Classification in accordance with the Ninth Revision of the International Classification of Diseases* (ICD-9). Geneva: WHO.

―― (1992) *International Classification of Diseases (10th edn) (ICD–10). Chapter V.* Geneva: WHO.

WYKES, T. & STURT, E. (1986) The measurement of social behaviour in psychiatric patients: an assessment of the reliability and validity of the SBS schedule. *British Journal of Psychiatry*, **148**, 1–11.

7 Setting priorities during the development of local psychiatric services

ELAINE MURPHY

Health policy will always reflect the values of those who create it. The process of setting priorities in health-care planning brings sharply into focus the conflicts between organisational and professional groups whose aspirations are founded on differing philosophical values. Over the past 30 years services for mental health care have been especially vulnerable to planning 'blight' as a result of a failure to reconcile differences between the professions, statutory agencies, voluntary organisations, the general public, and those who use the services. The planning process is hindered further by the fact that there is no easy way of discerning, still less proving, that there is a clear causal link between levels of health care expenditure and states of health. Mental health professionals have been poor advocates for the development of their services because they have been unable to articulate a coherent vision of the specific outcomes they were aiming at for individuals beyond the traditional goals of improvements in symptoms, behaviour, and social independence. Priorities arise out of specific service objectives which have their roots in a clear vision of the service's aims. This chapter describes the process by which a district can decide on its own local priorities.

Doctors, and others educated in a rational, scientific tradition, sometimes have difficulty with the concept of health-policy planning as a process of decision-making which accommodates multiple conflicting interests. Planning has two parts to it: first a rational, scientific judgement is made about what service is required based on hard information gleaned from local demographic data, epidemiological studies, case registers, and current usage of services, but the second, more difficult, part of planning is concerned with making a political judgement about what is realistically achievable locally given the existing dominant influences, the funds available and the time to achieve the objectives. Setting priorities is a fundamental part of the planning process in which explicit choices are made; it involves a political and social process for reconciling goals and objectives.

Health services have generally adopted an 'incrementalist' approach to planning. The first assumption underlying this approach is that what now exists must remain and that as extra growth money becomes available, there will be marginal improvements by the addition of an extra consultant here, a couple of community nurses there, a new day centre perhaps, and so on. These marginal improvements are usually determined by local influential people within the service system such as a group of consultant psychiatrists. Each year a set of disjointed decisions muddles up through the planning hierarchy to senior managers who choose from the assorted menu of excessive bids presented to them. In lean times, when public expenditure drops or the service falls out of favour locally, an equally *ad hoc* converse process of expenditure cuts are proposed which will have the least impact on the most influential people in the service. Under these circumstances, reduced funding nibbles around the edge of the service, creating internal staff resentment but rarely influencing the overall pattern of care.

A contrasting style of planning is the 'rationalist' approach. Those who are impatient with incrementalist shuffling of existing services may aim instead at comprehensive, rational problem solving, and try to tackle the important issues at one fell swoop in a short series of strategic planning meetings, assuming capacities of analysis and powers of implementation that do not exist within public health and social care organisations. In the health service 'incrementalism' has consistently won out over 'rationalism' because of low expectations of real change, the influence of senior professionals in the health service, who have very good reasons for resisting major change, and the continual disappointments afforded to 'rationalists' by the ever-changing economic and organisational climate in which planning is carried out.

However, there are feasible ways of achieving significant changes within public-sector services if priorities can be agreed on and a cultural change effected across the service to support the chosen priorities. One of the most effective ways to achieve the necessary cultural and attitudinal changes is to use the planning process itself as a vehicle for change (Nichol, 1986). Plans are merely statements of preferred options at a given point in time and must change in response to the changing environment. It is possible to keep options fairly flexible to accommodate change and to adopt a pragmatic approach to changing specific plans as new circumstances arise, as long as the overall service priorities remain steady and are universally acknowledged and 'owned' by those who will implement them.

The final practical task of planning is to appraise no more than three or four carefully costed options for local action against a set of criteria which are believed to best describe the priority objectives. The manner in which the technical task is achieved, through widespread participation, consultation, and education of the local community is at least as important as interpreting local information correctly.

In this chapter, the task of priority-setting has been divided into the following key areas:

(a) understanding the current focus of the service
(b) establishing principles and goals, developing a vision
(c) interpretation of local information
(d) participation and consultation, joint planning, neighbourhood planning
(e) the impact of the *NHS and Community Care Act, 1990* (House of Commons, 1990)
(f) maintaining flexibility and responsiveness.

Understanding the current focus of the service

An important barrier to change is the tendency of service providers to believe their own rhetoric about the characteristics of their own service. Almost all districts now claim to provide a 'community-orientated psychiatric service' but the pattern of allocation of financial resources tells a different story. The first step in accepting that change must occur is accepting the reality of the present focus of the service.

All services have an existing philosophy of care, usually unstated but implicit in the way the services are delivered. Over the past 30 years, since the policy of community care was officially adopted, two linked themes have been emphasised in government policy documents. The dominant theme was a plan for short-term treatment of mental illness in district general hospital units, out-patient clinics, day hospitals, and community mental health centres. The second theme, played *sotto voce* and much less forcefully presented, was the plan for local government to provide a network of hostel and home accommodation, social-work support, day care, and sheltered work for chronically disabled people, to provide a real alternative to the back wards of the mental hospital. The first theme grew into a major symphonic work, the second theme was scarcely audible until the 1980s.

District health authorities have shifted very large amounts of money originally invested in care for chronically disabled people living in large old mental hospitals into the development of acute psychiatric services for the local community which focused mainly on those patients with short-term, treatable conditions. The change of focus of the health-service component of mental health services can be measured along two dimensions. The first dimension is the distribution of services between acute short-term patients and those in need of long-term care. The second dimension is the proportion of services devoted to providing specific health-care services for diagnosis, treatment, and rehabilitation, and the proportion of the service devoted to 'social care', that is meeting patients' basic human needs for adequate financial resources, a home, work, and friendships, and ensuring that all the daily activities of normal life are satisfactorily achieved. This latter distinction is extremely important since a large part of community service development in the last 30 years has been concerned solely with promoting health care through the appointment of community psychiatric nurses, psychologists, occupational therapists and other therapists, and there has been much less investment in comprehensive social care, for example by providing welfare rights officers, accommodation and home finders, work-development schemes, staff to develop befriending and leisure schemes, and personal and domestic care staff.

The analysis of the division of services between acute, short-term patients and long-term chronic patients is not quite so straightforward as the above paragraph might suggest. There are many patients with long-term problems who suffer intermittent episodes of acute psychiatric illness which may recur as frequently as every few weeks, or may occur with a gap of several months or years. The phrase 'the revolving door' refers to those patients who at one time would have remained continuously in hospital for many years but are now readmitted frequently to acute psychiatric units but are rapidly discharged again once the acute phase of the illness is settled. It is therefore necessary to take account of the acute health-care needs of long-term patients in addition to their social-care needs.

In 1990, approximately £2 billion was spent by the National Health Service directly on mental health services, some 10% of total health-service expenditure. In addition to this, social-services departments spent £50 million on residential and day-care services. A further £100 million from the Department of Social Security was spent on supplementary benefit for board and lodgings payments in the private and voluntary sector and, finally, a considerable but difficult to estimate amount of money is expended by the courts, prisons and the police. A further £500–600 million was spent supporting elderly people with dementia in private residential-care homes and nursing homes. Approximately £3000 million in total from the public purse is spent on disabling mental disorder. Out of every £1, 7 pence is spent by local authorities, 27 pence is spent on supplementary benefit from the Department of Social Security and 66 pence is spent by the National Health Service, of which 83% (55 pence) is spent on in-patient beds. Two-thirds of all spending is within the health service. This is a high proportion but significantly less than before the mid 1970s when a new government initiative made high levels of welfare benefit from Social Security funds available for board and lodgings payments. This enabled the transfer of patients from state institutions into private residential care.

In the 1960s and 70s it was assumed that as long-stay hospital beds closed money would transfer from the health service to local authorities in order to provide alternative facilities. But all bureaucracies have a tendency to hang on to their own funds and the NHS successfully retained mental health funds to cover the rapidly growing costs of in-patient beds and new acute services.

Health managers and professionals have potent reasons for wishing to retain funds within services directly under their own control. The larger the unit budget, the greater the pay and status of its managers, but also the more flexibility can be created within the budget. An expanding budget in general acute psychiatry attracts personnel to extend professional departments; large professional departments attract trainees and postgraduate students; professional esteem is enhanced and the influence of the professional group grows within the local health service. It is not surprising then to find that during a period when thousands of long-stay beds closed, mental health's share of the NHS cake has remained steady and the proportion of funds for mental health spent on in-patient beds and professional services has remained much the same with very little movement of resources into local authority and other community services. However, over this period the cost of an in-patient bed for a mentally ill person doubled.

There are two main reasons for the rise in proportion of costs attributable to the 'acute' arm of mental health services. In part it was due to increased staffing levels on acute psychiatric wards and improvements in community psychiatric nursing and other professional services, and in part to a direct shift of resources out of long-stay care beds into new acute units in district general hospitals, the growth of community health centres and community assessment teams. An example taken from my own home health authority in south London shows how during the first five years of the strategic planning period 1984 to 1989, long-stay care places were closed in order to fund the growth of assessment beds and increased numbers of professional community assessment teams (Table 1). The realisation of this shift in resources has led to a reappraisal of the strategic plan in this district but

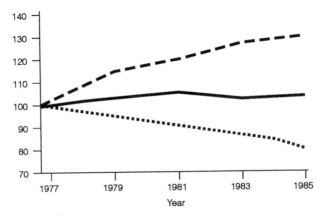

Fig. 1. Mental illness in-patient costs in England and Wales (cost per in-patient — — — —, in-patient numbers ------, and total cost ———). Index: 1977 = 100. Adapted for Audit Commission (1986)

TABLE 7.1

Mental health services for elderly people, strategic plan, 1984 to 1994, Lewisham and North Southwark Health Authority

	Services in 1984	Strategic target 1994	Progress by 1989
Number of acute assessment beds in hospital	27	60	50
Number of long-stay care places in hospitals and homes	170 (in Bexley, Cane Hill, and New Cross Hospitals)	144 (in small nursing homes)	66 (24-bed unit open, 42 domus places being built in 3 homes)
Community teams for assessment and treatment	1	3	3

similar major shifts in districts across the country have not always been recognised or tackled.

A major problem has been that as long-stay patients have died or left hospital there have been only marginal savings on the overall costs of running a hospital and as a consequence the unit costs of each long-stay patient have risen. The overall cost of in-patient beds has risen both because of the rising cost of long-stay beds and the cost of new in-patient services.

The result of the gradual shift in the use of health-service resources is that most health districts in Britain now spend approximately half of their total mental health service budget on those parts of the service which can broadly be designated as 'health care' rather than 'social care', that is on funding doctors, psychologists, occupational therapists, other therapists, nurses on acute psychiatric wards and catchment-area community psychiatric nurses, whereas in pre-closure days, before the 1960s, approximately 20% of funds were spent on direct health care, the rest on social care. As a consequence of this shift of resources, the vital social-care aspects of the service such as providing assistance with welfare benefits, supported accommodation, day care, work opportunities, leisure, education, and improvements to the quality of daily life have not been able to grow at the required pace because of the diminishing proportion spent on social care.

'Health care' and 'social care' are not easily defined. I use the term health care to describe specific diagnostic, investigatory and treatment interventions designed either to reduce or eliminate symptoms and signs of mental disorder or to rehabilitate an individual to maximum social and occupational function. Thus the specific interventions of health-care professionals such as prescribing drugs, giving psychotherapy, providing social retraining groups and behaviour modification treatment are all 'health care'. Social care, on the other hand, is the provision of assistance to individuals to sustain activities of daily life which are common to all humanity – assistance with provision of an adequate income, shelter, food, and clothing, protection from physical and mental harm, a means of daily occupation and the opportunity for emotional, spiritual, and social fulfilment. In long-term hospitals, social care is provided largely by people called 'nurses' but in the transition of care into the community, 'hands-on' personal and domestic social care is not provided by nurses but by home helps, home-care aides, social workers, welfare-benefits rights officers, housing workers and so on.

This distinction between health care and social care is not clearly defined in practice. An individual's progress in responding to treatment is often measured by an improvement in the performance of social-care tasks and everyday activities. Specific rehabilitation programmes frequently use a therapeutic approach which practises and rehearses ordinary activities so as to help people manage everyday life. In other words, therapy itself may be of a social-care nature. Nevertheless, the distinction between health and social care is a helpful one in understanding the focus and objectives of a service.

It is clear that in recent years there has been a very strong priority given to professional health-service treatment aimed at short-term treatment and care. Districts vary a great deal in the degree to which they have begun to move away from this health-care focus. Consequently, the first task for a district considering its future priorities is to understand the baseline pattern of care out of which the strategic plan must develop, and to gauge the overall shift in the balance of acute/long-term care and health/social-care division of resources which will be needed to achieve their vision of the future service. Stein & Test (1980) argued that 85% of resources for mental health services should be allocated to community-based services rather than hospital in-patient services and perhaps this is broadly correct. The proportionate allocation will depend on the *relative values* afforded to health and social care. What is needed is an explicit consideration of the balance of care, how the balance has come about and what degree of shift, if any, is desirable. A further crucial decision is the proportion of the allocation of community-based resources to health and social care respectively.

Establishing principles and goals, developing a vision

Developments will tend to be unplanned and haphazard if there is no target to aim for, so this section is placed before the section on participation and consultation, but the two processes must be closely linked. There is no point in a local mental health service developing its own vision in isolation from other key 'stakeholders' in the service. Following the *NHS and Community Care Act, 1990*, the responsibility for developing a vision of the future service lies jointly with the two purchasing agencies, the district health authority and the corresponding local authority, and the authorities therefore carry a joint responsibility for ensuring that real participation of community groups occurs.

A vision must be rooted in values and moral principles. Clinicians tend to view 'mission statements' with distaste, probably rightly if they have not been involved in developing them. Too often 'mission statements' are full of grandiose notions of good intent to 'care' but have no recognisable hard content. But it is important to be explicit about principles if only because they are so rarely shared at the outset by all the interested parties inside and outside the service. To give examples, a service which has as its main aim:

> 'the alleviation of mental distress by accurate diagnosis, assessment and treatment; the provision of shelter, asylum, safety from harm; a service which is readily accessible twenty four hours a day'

may end up looking very different from one which

> 'aspires to provide individuals with as fulfilling and rewarding a life as possible and provides for the ordinary needs of life – a home, daily occupation, emotional support through friendships and social contacts, and recognises individuals' rights as citizens'.

And yet both mission statements contain legitimate principles in which services can be rooted. Many districts will wish to target as their first priority those patients who experience the greatest personal burden of mental illness for long periods of their lives and, secondly, those who impose the greatest emotional burden and distress on relatives, neighbours and the community at large. Inevitably, those individuals who pose the greatest economic burden on their families and statutory agencies will also be a priority for consideration because setting priorities is an explicit rationing and control procedure aimed at containment of costs and getting better value for money. Locally, therefore, a district may decide to prioritise, for example, any one or more of the following groups:

(a) people with life-threatening acute disorders
(b) people with acute disorders who pose a threat to other people's health or safety
(c) people detained under the Mental Health Act legislation and their aftercare
(d) adults with severe chronic mental disorder
(e) elderly people with dementia living at home and in institutions
(f) adolescents and young people with severe behavioural problems
(g) mentally abnormal offenders in need of secure accommodation
(h) people with markedly distressing long-term neurotic symptoms.

The choice of setting local priorities between these needy groups is undoubtedly difficult but essential. The issue of treatability and the contribution that specific health interventions can make are irrelevant for planning the total comprehensive health and social care service, but they become important in assessing the emphasis which service planners should give to funding specific treatment activities for each of their priority groups. The health service traditionally has funded those parts of the service which its existing staff of doctors, nurses and therapists felt most able to treat or cure. Future plans need to take a broader view of the needs of mentally disordered people across the total local population. Specific medical and nursing interventions may form a relatively small part of the requirement for many priority groups.

Priorities need to be described in detail for the district as a whole and also for different localities within the district. The following descriptive dimensions are useful:

target groups – age range; sex; income group; ethnic or cultural group; geographical area within district

client groups – diagnostic group; type of illness or disability; short term/long term; severity level

type of function needed – preventive and educational work; treatment; social support; financial-benefit assistance; accommodation; work opportunities; education; leisure; family support.

Interpretation of local information

There is a wealth of data available on the epidemiology of mental disorders in the community and in institutions, and a good deal of information about existing patterns of service use. Unfortunately the former is unhelpful in predicting demand or highlighting current need for specialist services and the latter only reflects historical and current patterns of service provision. Goldberg & Huxley (1980) demonstrated that referral 'filters' modify the decision of individuals with psychiatric morbidity to attend general practitioners (GPs) and further selection factors determine which GP patients will be directed to psychiatric services. Many potential patients will not seek help from their GPs, for example, members of certain ethnic groups, for fear of acknowledging mental disorder within the family. Factors such as the patient's age, sex, social class, and type of disorder heavily influence patterns of referral by GPs. Furthermore, community surveys are often flawed methodologically from the point of view of assessing the prevalence of relatively rare conditions. Community surveys in which as many as several thousand of the population have been surveyed or interviewed will reveal only a handful of individuals in need of the specialist mental health services.

Even for common conditions such as senile dementia, where perhaps 3% or 4% of the population over 65 years may be expected to suffer from the condition, local surveys are rarely large enough to produce statistically significant results with anything but very broad confidence limits, which when applied to the whole resident population of a district may be too broad to be useful. Furthermore, demand for specific psychiatric treatments from professionals is notoriously hard to predict from surveys. Individuals with short-lived episodes of disorder may be severely disabled and require expensive treatments for a short time, only, but a point-prevalence survey is unlikely to detect such cases.

Current patterns of service use will be influenced by the accessibility of the service to local users, the willingness of the service to accept referrals of certain categories of patients, the availability of in-patient beds and treatment facilities, the existence of specialist services such as services for drug misusers or old-age psychiatry and the popularity of the service with local GPs and social workers. The one area where data on current usage of services are useful is about need for treatment and care for individuals with the most severely disabling acute disorders, since these individuals have a high likelihood of being admitted to hospital and therefore usage may reflect need. But even for this group, local prisons may be providing containment for seriously disturbed people if local hospital services are insufficient to meet the need, so information on current usage would have to be supplemented by information from the local criminal-justice system and prison medical service. Current data on bed usage also highlight where in-patient resources are being used, perhaps inappropriately, for example to provide long-term accommodation for those in need of further rehabilitation and support.

For detailed planning, a district mental health information system is required which performs three separate tasks: firstly, it provides managers with the information they need to assess and monitor service performance against objectives, secondly, it provides clinicians with relevant information for delivering the clinical service to individuals and, thirdly, it provides social services authorities with relevant information on social-care needs of the population. However, information systems are expensive to develop and maintain and while districts should invest in the right technology and systems in order to help them deliver an efficient service, the practical process of planning and priority setting can rarely wait for the systems to be established and, furthermore, the perfect information system will still mainly reflect the existing pattern of service use and will not provide guidance on future planning of priorities. Planning nearly always has to be done using imperfect information. Other chapters in this book focus on methods of assessment of mental health needs and the interpretation of information; all that needs to be repeated here is the vital importance for every district of developing a strategy for long-term information gathering.

In practice, a very rough and ready estimate of local-district needs can be made using the following written sources of information:

(a) Department of Health policy guidance
(b) Regional Health Authority (RHA) planning guidance and norms
(c) Royal College of Psychiatrists policy statements and guidance
(d) Royal College of Nursing, College of Occupational Therapists and British Psychological Society documents
(e) published epidemiological survey data of mental disorder in community populations with similar demographic profiles
(f) local social and demographic data and social-deprivation factors
(g) small-area statistics within local electoral wards
(h) case-register information on current usage, where available
(i) existing service profile data – Körner statistics, national and local comparative performance indicators
(j) policy documents from national voluntary organisations such as MIND and Good Practices in Mental Health
(k) local Health Advisory Service reports
(l) annual reports of Mental Health Act Commission visits to local institutions and national Biennial Reports of the Commission
(m) information from the Special Hospitals Service Authority and Regional Secure Units about local need for mentally abnormal offenders.

The above list is not exhaustive. All these sources of information, particularly policy guidance from professional and voluntary organisations, are laden with the values of the organisations which produced them and must be appraised accordingly.

In addition to the sources listed above, local 'political' information about needs should also be sought. Local organisations and individuals who are in close touch with the impact of the service on local users and their families will often express very clear views on their own priorities based on information they receive directly, often in the form of complaints. The Community Health Council (CHC), local councillors, local Members of Parliament, the police, local ethnic-community leaders, church leaders, and local voluntary organisations all have important information on the way the services are perceived and the gaps they believe should be filled. The CHC in particular, because it often comprises individuals who reflect the prevailing local dominant political influences, is a valuable source of information about perceived unmet needs from the point of view of local people, but again information must be appraised in the light of knowledge about local political aims and intentions.

Gathering and interpreting local information should not be a sterile exercise carried out in isolation from the rest of service planning. Ideally, it should be an integral part of the process which includes communication with and education of local people and underpins the participative planning process which leads to priority setting.

Participation and consultation, joint planning, neighbourhood planning

Health-service planning has conventionally been a centralising process which concentrated control over priority-setting in the hands of a few senior personnel. It is natural that those who hold the purse strings should wish to retain sovereignty over the way money is spent. A central planning approach in development of mental health services is almost bound to lead to widespread conflicts at the official consultation stage when other agencies and the local population are confronted with documents which reflect only the attitudes and values of existing senior health-service staff. Loosening the reins of control over priority-setting by a participative planning process both improves the quality of decision making and fosters the local commitment needed to implement plans. A 'democratic' participation approach can also be seen as promoting ideals of social justice, redressing in part the balance of power between the community of people on the receiving end of the service and those who control its delivery. Whether or not senior managers espouse an underlying philosophy which underpins commitment to participative planning, a pragmatic realisation of the practical benefits should encourage districts and local authorities to adopt a participative approach.

Who should participate and how? Joint planning teams are usually made up of officers from the health authority and local authority with perhaps a local GP, a token representative from the CHC, perhaps someone from a voluntary organisation, rarely also a single representative of the users and/or a person representing relatives and carers. Two common problems emerge. First, the group is too big to do any real work and, second, there is no mechanism by which the individuals representing the 'community' can effectively tap the views of their 'constituents'. Furthermore, official joint-planning structures often founder on the difficulties outlined below.

(a) Health and local authorities will not talk to each other until they have worked out their own approach and solutions. ('Let's get our own house in order first.') Districts and social-services departments must have the courage to acknowledge their own ignorance, state of disorganisation and uncertainty.

(b) The two statutory authorities concentrate on aligning their two separate written plans on paper simply to get the plan accepted by the central Joint Consultative Committee and the RHA.

(c) Planning focuses only on bids for new money, for example, mental illness specific grant or joint finance, and no consideration is given to changing the shape and form of existing services.

(d) Existing professional and organisational boundaries and management structures are left untouched.

(e) Those who exert the strongest influence on how the service is delivered, such as consultant psychiatrists and local GPs, delegate the joint planning task to one or two colleagues and then ignore the process completely.

(f) Local 'power brokers' who have a reputation for being reactionary or awkward, for example, a local consultant, the nearby university professor of psychiatry, the director of a local voluntary organisation, the senior nurse manager, are excluded from the process with the consequence that they later effectively sabotage the implementation of plans.

Avoiding the pitfalls is not easy but the process can be made easier, as outlined below.

(a) Recognise that the practical administrative work of planning can only be done by one or two people with the help perhaps of an inner circle of five or six key players.

(b) Ensure that there are mechanisms for involving on a continuing basis the following groups, in addition to the health-service and social-services staff.

(i) *Family Health Service Authority.* FHSAs are an essential part of the planning structure with health authorities and local authorities because they are now responsible for the strategic development of primary-care services.

(ii) *Service users*, through a current users' forum. Give professional support, take users' views seriously, consider paying users for the time they spend on planning work. Where users are added to formal professional committees they should be in large enough numbers not to be daunted or dominated by professionals.

(iii) *Relatives/carers*. Relatives have a different perspective from users. They should be represented in a planning group in large enough numbers to feel confident of expressing their views when professionals are also present. Support groups for carers exist in many districts and are a good place to start the process of recruitment.

(iv) *Housing*. Local housing authority, housing associations and any locally focused building society.

(v) *General Practitioners*. GPs should be invited through their local medical committee, if that mechanism has been found to be constructive in the past or, if not, a separate forum of influential local GPs can be assembled.

(vi) *Voluntary organisations*. MIND, the National Schizophrenia Fellowship and the Alzheimer's Disease Society now operate nationwide and are supported by vigorous national central policy departments. But in addition to these agencies, in most districts there are influential local voluntary organisations providing services for specific groups, for example, for homeless people, alcohol misusers, and drug misusers, and also self-help groups, for example a local benzodiazepine-withdrawal group.

(vii) *Education authority*. Local education authorities and those responsible for developing higher education and further adult education locally could play a larger part in many mental health services but are rarely involved at the planning stage.

Locally there may be other key groups within a district who should be involved in the process, for example Members of Parliament, major local employers, and private-sector companies who provide a significant proportion of local residential care places and so on.

A perspective of change can be encouraged by starting unusual meetings which cut across existing structures and boundaries. Seminars, local conferences, small working group 'away days' are all useful vehicles for tapping views and providing opportunities for consultation, feedback, and developing new ideas, but they cannot substitute for groups being formally asked to participate in a process which gives them rights to be heard and to have a say in decision making. The process must be made legitimate by the commitment of authority members from local government and the health authority to respect the decisions of these groups and to incorporate the groups into the formal planning structure.

District health authority areas usually comprise a miscellany of neighbourhoods with differing social and demographic characteristics. The pattern of mental health services appropriate to these neighbourhoods may differ considerably. Consequently, many districts have developed *locality or neighbourhood planning groups* which encompass a population of between 10 000 and 50 000 people. The district and local authorities have the responsibility jointly to create a foundation of strategic priorities and to agree the allocation of resources to different service groups. They should also agree the allocation of resources to differing localities and neighbourhoods and agree priorities within neighbourhoods. Locality planning is in some ways easier to organise than district-wide planning since there will usually be only a handful of key professionals and because GPs, local councillors, tenants associations, voluntary organisations, local church leaders and other spiritual, ethnic and cultural organisations are usually more interested in participating in planning activities which will be visible in their own 'back yard'. Locality planning groups must be clear at the outset about how much flexibility and discretion is within their remit to set their own priorities and how much will be determined by the district planning strategy.

The impact of the NHS and Community Care Act, 1990

From 1 April 1990, district health authorities' role is to establish local priorities, decide on the shape of local services and then to purchase a spectrum of services from whatever 'providers' can best match their requirements for the lowest cost and the highest quality. In theory the local District Health Authority, local authority and Family Health Services Authority should agree jointly a set of strategic planning priorities for mental health services for their resident population and then decide from which statutory agencies, hospitals, community services, and independent-sector organisations they will purchase services. In reality, much of the local expertise and the enthusiasm, drive, and commitment required to change mental health services lies with existing service providers. To make matters more complex, the senior officers responsible for long-term planning within the local authority have traditionally engaged in direct discussions with people on the provider side of the health service divide. Joint care-planning teams at present usually contain representatives of both health service 'purchasers' and 'providers'. This kind of structure may well prevent too much local turbulence and sudden change in the first years of the NHS reforms but may not provide the most suitable structure for achieving significant strategic change of direction of services. District health authorities need to develop their own expertise in the field of mental health or their plans will inevitably be over-influenced by the views of existing local service providers.

The Community Care part of the 1990 Act is now due to be implemented in 1993. While, as mentioned above, the health service currently controls two-thirds of all spending on mental health services, and the local authority only 7%, following the implementation of the community-care proposals, local authorities will become responsible for spending one-third of the budget through their new role of controlling the allocation to individuals of social-security welfare benefits for board and lodging. The role of the local authority under the new arrangements will be to assess the needs of their resident population for community-care support, set local priorities and service objectives, and arrange the required care by designing, organising and purchasing care. To allow them to do this effectively, social-security benefit and existing community-care grant monies are to be channelled via social services. These funds will be available to support people at home as well as in institutions.

Joint planning of mental health services will be fostered by the allocation of a small extra grant, the Specific Grant, which local authorities can spend only with the agreement of their district health authority. Health authorities are also required to provide every mentally ill patient discharged from long-term hospital care with a plan for his or her future care, agreed with the local authority. Unfortunately, there is no designated person responsible for implementing these proposals for individual care-planning and unless

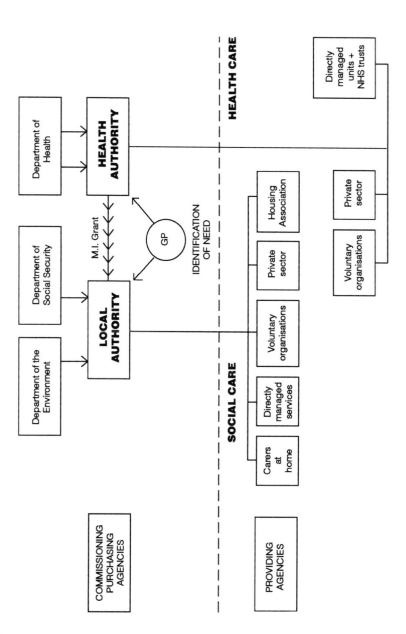

Fig. 7.2. Organisation structure, NHS and Community Care Act, 1990

health and social services agree jointly who will be responsible, progress is likely to be slow.

The new community-care plans do not, however, directly link together the health service and local authorities in order to improve coordination of services. Figure 7.2 shows how few direct links exist between the two authorities. The plans exhort those responsible to bridge the gulf but do not, themselves, bridge it. Griffiths (1988) in his report to the government on the funding and organisation of community care suggested that rather than try to create new bridging structures by organisational change, it would be better for both statutory authorities to have clearly defined responsibilities and roles which did not overlap. He suggested that the health service should confine itself to 'health care' and local authorities should be responsible for 'social care'. Thus, most long-term care for people who require a lot of daily support would be the responsibility of the local authority rather than, as formerly, the health service. The idea, under the new plan, is that, over a number of years, the local authority will contract with a wide range of voluntary and private agencies to provide a spectrum of different services which the local authority pays for. It will purchase the total range of care needed by local people with mental disorder and, meanwhile, the health service will restrict itself to providing a psychiatric service to these individuals in whichever is the most appropriate setting.

These proposals are, however, made much more complex by the existence of old long-stay wards in hospitals whose main function, quite clearly, is social care, yet for many years these are going to be run by the health service. Griffiths realised that this situation could not be changed overnight, so the health service will still be allowed under the new regulations to carry on providing long-term care if it wishes.

A further problem is that there are no satisfactory definitions of *health* care and *social* care, as has been noted earlier in this chapter. An individual's progress in responding to treatment is often measured by an improvement in the performance of social-care tasks and everyday activities. Under such circumstances, it is not at all clear which statutory agency should take the leading role in developing such therapeutic houses and homes, something perhaps which explains the government thinking underlying the proposed specific grant for mental health services in the community which can only be spent by the *joint* agreement of local health and social services. The specific grant, introduced in April 1991, should encourage authorities to plan together so that a broad spectrum of services is developed and there are no gaps for individual patients to fall between.

In some parts of Britain health services and local authorities are beginning to work together to develop an overall plan for services in their area. Fortunately, the National Health Service reforms and the community care changes share some unifying principles which should encourage the two statutory authorities to work together more closely.

(a) The role of the responsible local statutory authority is to develop an overall strategy for the shape of services for the local population in a defined geographical area. The authority must develop a plan for the design and development of a service, set priorities, and determine the most appropriate set of services for its residents, within the constraints of its resources. The authority will be purchasers and enablers, but not necessarily providers, of care.

(b) The management of services will be via contracts. Authorities will develop specifications for services and then reach contractual agreements with provider agencies such as voluntary or private organisations. Public authorities have, however, minimal expertise in this area, although they have 'cut their teeth' by developing 'specifications for contracts' for non-clinical and non-care services such as cleaning and catering. Developing an effective contractual style of management is a challenge which has, in the main, still to be faced across the public sector. One major difference between the authorities, however, is that health authority 'contracts' with NHS providers will not be legally binding contracts in the same way as local authorities will have contracts with the independent and voluntary sector.

(c) A 'mixed economy of care', with care being provided on similar terms by public and independent sectors, is not particularly new to local authorities, although the contracting of care from multiple organisations has not been a key policy in the past, more an *ad hoc* response to specific local problems. Getting the right balance of 'in house' provision and 'contracted out' services will vary from one locality to another and will reflect local authorities' employment policies as well as the availability of effective local voluntary organisations. It will also reflect the propensity or otherwise of the private sector to invest in the provision of care services. Clearly, both statutory authorities will need to develop new attitudes and approaches to the 'other world' of the independent sector.

(d) Local authorities will need good information on the costs, quality and volume of services needed and provided. While the health service has been developing its computerised databases and information systems for general hospitals with astonishing rapidity, community-care services lag far behind. Both authorities will need to invest substantially in information systems over the next decade if they are to maximise the amount of care they can squeeze out of their constrained budgets.

(e) Last, but possibly most important, both public-sector services are moving towards more 'explicit' accountability for the use of their resources. While the health service has become increasingly concerned with ensuring that there is a hierarchy of individuals with responsibility for achieving certain objectives, and an increasing commitment by individual doctors, nurses and therapists to agreed aims, local-authority staff too have come under increasing pressure from elected council Members and behind them, the voting electorate, to demonstrate that their service departments have effective management structures and are truly accountable.

These common features should therefore enable health and local authorities to develop a common philosophy about the style of delivery of mental health services. They also highlight the relative inexperience of both authorities in certain key areas, although benefits of cooperation between authorities, such as in the development and sharing of computer information systems for work in the community, are obvious.

When professionals who work in mental health services talk of an 'integrated, comprehensive, seamless service' they mean a service where acute hospital beds, hostels, group homes, community teams, and services for people in their own homes are all managed as one service with one team of people who have total responsibility. In practice this is rarely achieved by health services and local authorities and almost never includes private and voluntary sectors. Nevertheless, most professionals aspire to a flexible, easily accessible service where 'users' can move rapidly between home, day care and hospital when the need arises. One of the major anxieties about the new NHS and Community Care Act is the further fragmentation of services with health services even more isolated and hospital-bound, yet still consuming massive resources. One radical but simple solution to this problem is joint contracting and joint buying consortia.

Buying consortia and joint contracting

Under this system the two statutory authorities would create a new joint mechanism for purchasing services in which health-service resources for mental health services and the local-authority social services resources for domiciliary, residential, and day-care services would be pooled. A new organisation, or consortium, might usefully be developed to create joint contracts with provider organisations. The joint consortium could have powers delegated to it to design and buy services across an area coterminous with the local-authority boundary. Indeed, the local authority *must* be the key agency around which services are designed if we are to make the best use not only of social services but also of housing, education and leisure facilities.

Apart from the clear advantages of having a joint strategic plan for mental health services, a joint buying consortium would have much enhanced buying power and could lead, too, to considerable economies in developing information systems and a pooling of skills in service development and the maintenance of standards of care. Figure 7.2 shows diagrammatically how the new community care proposals by the government are currently planned. Figure 7.3 shows how a Joint Purchasing Consortium would work.

There are, of course, drawbacks to this proposal. It may, for example, be politically 'undeliverable' in many areas at present – both authorities

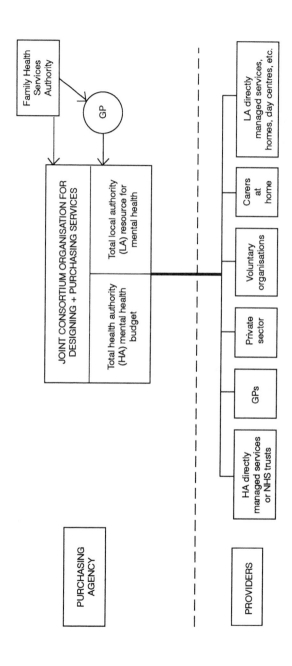

Fig. 7.3. The seamless service: a buying consortium for mental health services

would lose some sovereignty over their current funds and may find this unacceptable. There would inevitably also be a fear among some health service professionals that their hard-won services would be dissipated into a 'support-only' service and that accurate diagnosis and treatment would be sacrificed in favour of providing a better living environment. There will be an equally potent fear that new, less appropriate priorities may take precedence in planning, for example the large numbers of people with minor disorders who pose a burden to social-services departments and GPs. Social services council members may fear they will be left with nothing very much to do if they delegate their decision-making to an independent body. Nevertheless, some authorities are already exploring, albeit gingerly, the possibilities of 'joint purchasing'.

Maintaining flexibility and responsiveness

Health-care planning is often carried out assuming that the planning systems will remain stable and that the characteristics of the population to be served will remain steady. But in the real world, we cannot assure political or economic stability; health-service personnel often complain that 'the goal posts keep moving'. Public-sector services operate in a permanent climate of upheaval and change imposed both from above as a result of political change and from pressure upwards from the changing nature of populations and disorders. For example in south-east London, the inner-city area has witnessed in the past 10 years the influx of a large refugee population, the Vietnamese boat people, a dramatic rise in the population of those aged over 85 and a sharply increased incidence of acquired immune deficiency syndrome (AIDS). Within one decade very significant changes can derail a 10-year strategic plan. Because of the changing needs of mental health services, it is important to have plans that are sufficiently flexible for facilities and services to be used by future generations. This must be kept in mind when planning for the resettlement outside hospital for the old 'long-stay' population.

Flexibility is improved by:

(a) developing services which do not depend on specific purpose-designed capital building development, but by using, whenever possible, ordinary housing and small-scale developments which can be turned to alternative purposes over a timescale of a year or two

(b) maintaining a workforce which possesses core skills common to serving a wide range of disabilities, not so highly specialised that it cannot turn its skills to people with related disorders.

There is a tendency to develop specific and quite separate 'community teams' for rehabilitation of adults with long-term mental disorders, people with mental handicap, elderly people with mental disorder and so on, all of which develop operational policies exclusively focused on one care group. Since the members of those teams may be performing very similar work, a service can retain future flexibility by enhancing the cross-training and exchange by rotational staff training and by ensuring that senior champions of specific services do not create a separatist ethos of service development which tends to set the existing services in concrete until the 'champion' retires.

Priorities will change as the years pass and no plan should remain static. Setting priorities is part of a cyclical process of current-service analysis, joint planning, analysis of options, implementation, review of progress, reanalysis of service and new priority setting. What must not change is the vision and aspirations of the individuals who lead the priority-setting process.

References

GOLDBERG, D. & HUXLEY, P. (1980) *Mental Illness in the Community*. London: Tavistock.

GRIFFITHS, R. (1988) *Community Care. Agenda for Action*. London: HMSO.

HOUSE OF COMMONS (1990) *National Health Service and Community Care Act*. London: HMSO.

NICHOL, D. K. (1986) Action research and development in strategic planning. In *Managers as Strategists* (ed. G. Parston). London: King's Fund.

STEIN, L. I. & TEST, M. A. (1980) Alternatives to hospital treatment. 1. Conceptual model, treatment program and clinical evaluation. *Archives of General Psychiatry*, **37**, 392–397.

8 Community sectors for needs-led mental health services

GERALDINE STRATHDEE & and GRAHAM THORNICROFT

This chapter is written from the perspective of clinicians involved in the development of community-based mental health services. We shall consider here how needs assessment relates to the planning, implementation and evaluation of routine clinical services. We shall focus on the stages required to establish services which are locality, rather than hospital, orientated. We seek to see in place services which reflect those principles for the development of community mental health services which now have such a wide measure of agreement (MIND, 1983; National Institute of Mental Health, 1987; Royal College of Psychiatrists, 1990).

(a) Services should meet the range of special needs of psychiatric patients with particular attention being paid to those with physical disabilities, mental retardation, the homeless or imprisoned.

(b) Services should be local and accessible and to the greatest extent possible delivered in the individual's usual environment.

(c) Services should be comprehensive and address a wide range of needs.

(d) Services should be flexible by being available whenever and for whatever duration needed. There should be a range of complementary models which provide individuals with choice.

(e) Services should be consumer-orientated, that is, based on the needs of the user rather than those of providers.

(f) Services should empower clients by using and adapting treatment techniques which enable clients to enhance their self-help skills and retain the fullest possible control over their own lives.

(g) Services should be racially and culturally appropriate and include use of culturally appropriate needs-assessment tools, representation on planning groups, cross-cultural training for staff, use of ethnically appropriate workers and bilingual staff, identification and provision of alternative basic facilities.

(h) Services should focus on strengths, and should be built on the skills and strengths of clients to help them maintain a sense of identity, dignity and self-esteem. Patients should be discouraged from developing an identity organised around permanent illness with lowered expectations.

(i) Services should incorporate natural supports by being in the least restrictive, most natural setting possible. The usual work, education, leisure and support facilities in the community should be used in preference to specialised developments.

(j) Services should be accountable to the consumers and informal carers and evaluated to ensure their continuing appropriateness, acceptability, and effectiveness on agreed parameters.

We have framed our discussion in terms of the geographical sector, as we consider this to be the most useful local level of organisation for service needs assessment, and the most manageable level of analysis for mental health service evaluation.

The policy background

Two basic themes have underpinned Government policies for the practice of community care for the past three decades. These are that policies should be needs-led, rather than service-led, and that this objective can best be met by replacing the large psychiatric institutions with a more balanced and flexible range of local alternative services (Hunter & Wistow, 1987). However, with the exception of the White Paper, *Better Services for the Mentally Ill* (Department of Health and Social Security, 1975), the plethora of government policy documents (House of Commons, 1985, 1990; Audit Commission, 1986; Griffiths, 1988; Secretaries of State for Health, 1989, 1990) have provided little specific guidance on what should constitute the components of comprehensive local psychiatric services. Nor has any central coordinating or consultancy agency assisted districts in the task of developing the organisational and management framework necessary for such services. Still less has there been any expert guidance from academics on the application of standardised assessment techniques suitable for use by hard-pressed clinicians in the rigours of busy clinical practice. Indeed, the tendency for otherwise excellent texts (Talbott, 1983; National Institute of Mental Health, 1987; Torrey *et al*, 1990) to focus on qualitative, rather than quantitative descriptions of the needs in community psychiatric services has drawn criticism from Andrews (1990) in his own vigorous attempt to redress their deficiencies.

With a similar lack of focus, clinicians, while accustomed to making *ad hoc* assessments of an individual's need before prescribing treatment, have been slow to incorporate this approach into planning terms (Stevens &

Gabbay, 1991; and Chapter 4). Although there has been a qualified consensus that closure of the large psychiatric hospitals is a preferred option (Jones, 1972; Thornicroft & Bebbington, 1988), little agreement has been reached on how best to structure the services which replace them. The traditional path of service developments in medicine owes as much to serendipity and opportunism as to rational strategic planning (Todd, 1984). In current practice, community developments are frequently determined by financial expediency, lacking any theoretical basis, and focus more on buildings than on the flexible recruitment and deployment of personnel (Holloway, 1988).

Mental health service developments in Great Britain have tended to be based on replications (often uncritical) of models in America or Europe, rather than as a product of a well considered local strategy. As Kingdon (1989) found, in his study of 192 English Districts, only three-fifths had an up-to-date mental health strategic plan. Nevertheless, there are indications that at the level of grass-roots clinicians, locally relevant developments do occur, either in response to crisis management or based on accumulated knowledge of local needs and resources (Strathdee & Williams, 1984).

Setting the scale of local mental health services

Establishing sector boundaries

The early proponents of community care concentrated less on specifying the components of care than on developing the organisational framework within which such services could be effectively delivered. Philippe Paumelle, working in Paris, formulated three essential principles: that services should provide continuity of care, coordination of care and integration of care (Walsh, 1987). In order to fulfil these requirements, it was his view that the planning and operation of services should take place at a defined local level. Thus the concept of a 'sector' as the denominator in local planning evolved and has subsequently gained wide support. The term sector now generally refers to a delineated geographical area, with a defined catchment population.

Internationally, the concept of the sector permeates community-service development. Following the emergence of the first sectors in France in 1947, by 1961 over 300 had been established. In the USA, the Community Mental Health Centers Act (Levine, 1981) introduced the principle of a catchment area for each CMHC, and by 1975, 40% of the population had sectorised services. In Europe, throughout the 1970s, sector development grew but sizes varied between countries (Lindholm, 1983) . Germany has sector sizes in the range of 250 000, the Netherlands around 300 000, while the areas for the Scandinavian countries are smaller with Denmark averaging 60–120 000,

Finland 100 000, Norway 40 000, and Sweden 25–50 000. Of all countries, however, Italy has most comprehensively adopted the concept by virtue of Law 178, passed in 1978, which established sectors in the range of 50–200 000 population. Tansella (1989), in recognition of the vital role of such an infrastructure reiterates that "what is important in community care is not only the number and characteristics of various services but the way in which they are arranged and integrated".

In Great Britain, as in many other European countries, sectorisation is regarded by many as an essential prerequisite for the development of effective community psychiatric services (Strathdee & Thornicroft, 1993). A recent study in England and Wales (Johnson & Thornicroft, 1993) indicates that 81% of districts nationally have divided their catchment areas into sectors. Many of the claimed advantages for the sector as the basic unit of planning, organisation and service delivery are shown below, although there has been little rigorous evaluation for most of these claims.

(a) Planning advantages
    (i) high identification rates of patients
    (ii) feasible scale for clinical and social assessments
    (iii) appropriate and planned development of services
    (iv) assists development of a wide range of local service components
    (v) improved knowledge and use of community resources
    (vi) greater budgetary clarity
(b) Service delivery advantages
    (i) minimise patients lost to follow up
    (ii) individually tailored inter-agency patient programmes
    (iii) facilitates home treatment
    (iv) improved identity of staff with locality
    (v) clarity of functions of district teams
    (vi) facilitates inter-agency liaison, training and working
    (vii) allows comparative research and evaluation
(c) Quality of service advantages
    (i) less use of crisis and in-patient facilities
    (ii) improved patient education and intervention
    (iii) greater support of relatives and carers
    (iv) defined responsibility for each patient
    (v) improved communication for staff, patients and carers
    (vi) improved primary–secondary service communication.

Research has concentrated almost exclusively on establishing whether sectorisation facilitates the development of community alternatives to in-patient hospital treatment. In Nottingham, for example, Tyrer *et al* (1989) found the following reductions after sectorisation: number of admissions (5%), duration of admissions (4%), and use of in-patient beds (38%).

One Swedish study (Hansson, 1989) found a decrease in the number of admissions (20%), bed days used (40%), and compulsory admissions (25%). Another (Lindholm, 1983) found similar, but non-significant trends.

Factors influencing sector size

The division of a district into sectors is influenced by many considerations. In practice, the need to be coterminous with either social-services boundaries or general-practice locations is often the primary rationale for defining the area within the sector. However, equally important issues are the rural or urban nature of the area, and the presence of a river, main road, or other significant natural local geographical structures which impair access. Factors which influence sector size and location are outlined below.

    (a) Factors in the population
            (i) sociodemographic composition
          (ii) social deprivation indices
        (iii) ethnic composition
        (iv) age and sex structure
         (v) knowledge of identified psychiatric morbidity
        (vi) knowledge of existing service-utilisation patterns
      (vii) assessment of model of service needed
    (b) Factors in the organisation of services
            (i) social-services boundaries
          (ii) primary-care organisation
        (iii) extent of sheltered housing
        (iv) number of old/new long-stay
         (v) presence of a large institution
        (vi) presence of a district general hospital
      (vii) manpower and other resource parameters
    (c) Factors in the locality
            (i) significant geographical structures
          (ii) inherent community cultures
        (iii) presence of sites for development.

There is strong evidence that such social and demographic factors are closely associated with the measured rates of psychiatric disorder (Thornicroft, 1991a; Jarman *et al*, 1992). The age structure of the population also serves as a pointer for service needs. Over-representation in the 20–29 age range will predict a higher rate of population at risk of developing psychotic disorders. The association between psychiatric disorders and social class (particularly for schizophrenia and depression) is one of the most consistent findings in psychiatric epidemiology (Eaton, 1985; Jablensky, 1986). The Jarman combined index of social deprivation has been shown to be highly correlated with psychiatric admission rates for Health Districts in the South East Thames Region, and may be used to estimate the degree of excess morbidity (Jarman, 1983, 1984; Hirsch, 1988; Thornicroft, 1992; Chapter 5). It seems reasonable therefore to use a deprivation-weighted population score to estimate morbidity within psychiatric sectors.

Ethnicity also has a powerful influence on service utilisation with non-white ethnic groups having a higher risk than their white neighbours of being admitted to psychiatric hospital, an increased risk of compulsory admission, and a substantially raised risk of being diagnosed as suffering from schizophrenia (Ineichen *et al*, 1984; Moodley & Thornicroft, 1988; Harrison *et al*, 1988, 1989). A further modifier of service use is the presence within a district of a large psychiatric institution and the nature of local psychiatric resettlement facilities (Paykel, 1990).

The acceptability and appropriateness of the service model to be implemented is an important consideration. For example, in some areas, general practices are seen as the non-stigmatising facility which the local population traditionally use as the pathway into mental-health services. In other localities the pathways into care are less defined, with less use of statutory services and more presentation to voluntary organisations and ethnic-group facilities. This appears to be particularly likely in areas where the ethnic composition is not homogeneous. In such cases rational division into patches should take into account the need for development of innovative services, which reflect the likely help-seeking behaviour acceptable to the local population.

The process of determining sector service requirements

Clarifying service priorities

The range of services needs to be considered when planning for the sector is begun (Table 8.1). The scheme outlined is not intended as a comprehensive, sequential pathway to a 'sector development blueprint', but seeks to delineate the routine elements of clinical, training, organisational, and evaluation work likely to be encountered with some suggested mechanisms for action.

An issue which needs to be addressed early in planning needs-led services is: which patient groups are to be prioritised, and by implication, which will not be targeted (Patmore & Weaver, 1990). Although the broad grouping of 'the seriously mentally ill' are often set as the highest priority, this is rarely specifically defined, with notable exceptions. Operational definitions of severe mental illness used by health-service providers are outlined below.

TABLE 8.1
The range of planning and service requirements in a sector

Need	Information sources and mechanisms for action
To define philosophy and client group	Mission statement Information on morbidity Define priorities
An information database	Office of Population Censuses and Surveys Jarman indices Public health report Psychiatric case-register Regional Körner data Family Health Service Authority lists Social services Mental Health Authority data
Organisational structure	Establish inter-agency structures Define agency working roles Delineation of responsibilities Budgetary definitions Sector management control of resources Planning expertise
Multidisciplinary team and its base	Development of operational policy Knowledge of local structures and facilities for statutory planning departments Joint commissioning mechanisms
Routine quantitative & qualitative assessments	Inherent clinical knowledge Development of standardised routine clinical assessments
Flexible service models	Appropriate community service journals Literature searches of international models Local planners modification and application User involvement in planning Development of customised good practice protocols with GPs and other primary agencies
Training	Joint Community Care Planning Group inter-agency training group Integrated service models Team-building courses Continuing training programme
Evaluation	Multidisciplinary inter-agency audit Regional research funds Partnership with academic centres

(a) Goldman (1981)
    (i) Diagnosis   diagnosis (DSM–III–R) of:

	schizophrenia and schizoaffective disorder	295.x
	bipolar disorders and major depression	296.x
	delusional (paranoid) disorder	297.x

    (ii) Duration   at least one year since onset of disorder
    (iii) Disability   sufficiently severe disability to seriously impair functioning or role performance in at least one of the following areas:
        occupation
        family responsibilities
        accommodation

(b) McLean & Liebowitz (1989)
    At least one of the following must be present:
    (i) two or more years contact with services
    (ii) depot prescribed
    (iii) ICD 295.x or 297.x
    (iv) three or more in-patient admissions in last two years
    (v) three or more day-patient episodes in last two years
    (vi) DSM–III highest level of adaptive functioning in the past year rates 5 or more

(c) Tyrer *et al* (1985)
    Patients with chronic psychosis
    Two or more in-patient admissions in the past year
    Contact with two or more psychiatric agencies in past year
    Frequent consultations
    Risk of being homeless/imprisoned

These are all health-service-only definitions, but it could be argued, that in order to implement the current legislation on community care which has an inherent assumption that agencies will form closer working links, there is a need to identify a common language to define service priorities. Table 8.2, which is derived from a problem-orientated, rather than a diagnostic approach, goes some way to meet this need (Falloon, 1988).

The philosophy of the service

The next step is the creation of a mission statement and establishment of a defined philosophy and objectives on which the service will be based. The involvement of users, staff and other major stakeholders at this stage presents an opportunity for joint working and forms the basis of a partnership in the future planning of the service. Below are two examples of mission statements. The first is that defined in the National Institute of Mental

TABLE 8.2
A framework for inter-agency definition of severely mentally ill

Impairments	Disabilities	Handicaps
	Cognitive:	
Difficulties in thinking	Inefficient problem solving	Lack of friends
Interference with thought processes	Slowed learning	Unemployment
Distressing experiences of sight, sound or touch		
	Affective:	
Unusual, strange beliefs	Severe anxiety and fear	Limited leisure
Difficulty in movements and actions	Feelings of inadequacy	activities
Decreased concentration		Poor housing and self-care
	Behavioural:	
Loss of energy and drive	Low rate of constructive	Carers burden
Reduced ability to solve problems	actions	

Health's policy document on planning a comprehensive client-centred mental health service. The second, and influenced by the former, was developed by the mental health unit in Greenwich in South London in 1989.

Examples of mission statements

"To implement programmes and services that assist adults with severe, disabling mental illness to control the symptoms of the illness; to develop the skills and acquire the supports and resources they need to succeed where they chose to live, learn and work; and to maintain responsibility, to the greatest extent possible, for setting their own goals, directing their own lives, and acting responsibly as members of the community." (National Institute of Mental Health, 1987)

"To provide services to meet the individual needs of people in Greenwich who are disabled by mental health problems, giving priority to those people whose lives and well-being, or that of others, is most threatened by mental illness. Our services will aim to:

(a) provide an accessible 24-hour assessment and management facility with a coordinated multidisciplinary framework
(b) enable people to take responsibility for their own lives
(c) develop and acquire the skills to make choices over where they live, work and form social relationships
(d) give recognition to peoples' needs for care as well as for independence
(e) be sensitive to racial and cultural needs
(f) maximise the effective use of resources in an environment of audit and evaluation with staff support and training." (Greenwich Mental Health Unit, 1989)

The information infrastructure

To set up and monitor locally-based mental health services, it is necessary to estimate the numbers of patients who fall within the priority group. One approach to this issue is to conduct a case-identification exercise, drawing upon contacts by people with severely disabling mental illness with a wide range of services as outlined below.

(a) Service-user care
    Peer group support, advocacy, education, relapse prevention, coping strategies.
(b) Primary-health care
    Physical care and education, dental care, chiropody, opticians, family planning, identification, crisis intervention, education.
(c) Social care
    Occupation, rehabilitation, day care, education/leisure, respite, continuing care and outreach, income support and entitlements, housing.
(d) Mental health care
    Identification, continuing care and outreach, crisis intervention, family support, education, occupation, sheltered work, rehabilitation.

A clear, systematic and continuing method of collecting clinical and social-need and service-usage data is required to inform the planning of the most appropriate service model for the local situation. As Shapiro *et al* (1985) conclude, there are limitations in each of the three methods most commonly used for this assessment. Firstly, there are the broad estimates and projections derived from utilisation rates of services by defined patients (Goldberg *et al*, 1980; Goldman *et al*, 1981). Secondly, there are calculations based on the relationships of mental health disorders to age, sex, race, marital status, economic status, and other social variables (Rosen & Goldsmith, 1981). Finally, needs are often defined by a focus on the seriously impaired chronically mentally ill (US Department of Health, 1980; Thornicroft & Strathdee, 1991).

The most comprehensive method to elicit, code and store the data listed above is the case register (Wing, 1989). Although such systems were formerly labour intensive and tended to be used primarily as research and epidemiological tools, the recent availability of on-site microcomputers and minicomputers has made their widespread use for clinical-service delivery a practical option in many areas. A rapidly growing number of general practices now have such systems and there is increasing evidence that the establishment of the health promotion or disease registers such as those for asthma and diabetes improve the quality of patient care. Kendrick *et al* (1991) present convincing evidence that this method is equally applicable to the care of individuals with mental health disorders.

Establishing the organisational framework

Inter-agency planning and organisation

Between sectors and districts there are wide variations in the functions served by different agencies. In general, health authorities have provided the bulk of in-patient and acute care, with day care being administered by a combination of the statutory agencies. In the case of sheltered housing and work facilities the situation is more variable and in some areas it is social services or the voluntary sector which provide the majority of facilities. Likewise, those with psychological and social distress can present initially to housing, policy, and social services, as well as to mental health facilities. General practitioners, too, in Britain play a major role in the care of those with both acute and chronic psychological disorders (Murray Parkes *et al*, 1962; Shepherd *et al*, 1966; Goldberg & Blackwell, 1970; Johnstone *et al*, 1984; Brown *et al*, 1988; Strathdee, 1992*a*). In many districts they constitute the front-line for patients in crisis, whether or not they are concurrently in contact with the mental health teams.

While there is no core agency responsible for assuring the delivery and coordination of all services, informal joint working patterns are vital to meet the full range of needs, to achieve jointly owned policies and to avoid unnecessary duplication of services through parallel developments. At a strategic level, many districts have a mental illness subgroup of the Joint Community Care Planning Team (JCCPT), which negotiates joint financing and management initiatives (Jeffreys, 1979). Arguably these should be extended to formal arrangements at the operational level (Department of Health and Social Security, 1978), for example by the creation of multidisciplinary, interagency teams. These, by integration of personnel such as occupational therapists, community psychiatric nurses and social workers, might work productively on crisis intervention, home-based continuing care, treatment and rehabilitation teams. Work with social services at the ground level has been improved by the development of community mental health centres, which allow joint crisis and assessment initiatives to flourish (Sayce *et al*, 1991). In addition, the development of case management (House of Commons, 1990; Thornicroft, 1991*b*), and care coordination fora (Strathdee, 1992*a*) appear likely to facilitate the development of joint assessment instruments and the organisation of joint training.

The effective delivery of community care

However, some fundamental questions remain. What constitutes the most effective form of organisation between patients, relatives, and statutory and non-statutory agencies, in the assessment of need? What is the best way to form an active partnership to provide a comprehensive range of services? As mentioned earlier, Philippe Paumelle, one of the first proponents of community care, provides some guidance for the theoretical resolution of this dilemma. He considered that effective services were those which offered continuity of care, coordination of care, and integration of care. *Continuity of care*, he believed, could best be achieved by ensuring that persons and families were dealt with at all stages and at all levels of illness by the same team who had their own associated structures such as beds and clinics. Given the range of needs of individuals with mental health problems, *coordination of care* required the introduction of multidisciplinary and interagency teams to ensure that the range of treatments necessary to overcome the impairment and disability of the mentally ill be delivered. The need for *integration of care* is underpinned by the premise (World Health Organization, 1983) that in any community, first contact for individuals in distress is often not with the psychiatric specialist team, but rather persons in key positions of responsibility in the community such as teachers, police, public-health nurses, community nurses, social workers, and general practitioners. Any specialist team must therefore integrate its efforts with those of the non-specialists, as well as taking the lead in educating and counselling non-specialists.

Dichotomies in relation to the development of sector services

Within each agency a similar issue requires attention. What is the most appropriate configuration of services provided by any single agency? Four dichotomies arise.

The sectorisation/district-wide dichotomy: how to achieve the most appropriate balance between services which should be provided within the local sector and those which should have a district-wide remit. This applies particularly to rehabilitation services and crisis intervention services.

The specialist/generalist dichotomy: what is the optimal method of integrating specialist and generic staff both within sectors, for an entirely sectorised service, and between district and sector services for other configurations. For example, specialist rehabilitation outreach or drug and alcohol teams might primarily be a district service but have identified members who provide continuity for patients by dual membership with specific sector teams. Similar issues apply to forensic facilities and psychotherapy services.

The acute/continuing care dichotomy: what is the best distribution of workload and skill-mix within the sector teams? A one-team sector model could, for example, care for either the whole range of psychiatric morbidity within a small defined area or, alternatively, two teams might divide responsibilities – with one providing primary care and acute assessment and treatment services, including acute in-patient work, and a second team accepting responsibility for the longer-term patients including respite, rehabilitation, outreach, support, and crisis intervention.

The primary care/mental health specialist dichotomy: How should integration and clear definition of responsibilities between primary and secondary care teams be developed? First contact for patients presenting in crisis or in the early signs of relapse are often the primary-care agencies (Strathdee, 1992*b*) including GPs and primary-health teams, social workers, or housing offices. Therefore, to what extent should mental health team personnel be attached to, or integrated within, the primary-care framework? How can they ensure their commitments to the priority patient group against competing demands? Traditionally, this dilemma has confronted community psychiatric nurse (CPN) services.

The resolution of the final dichotomy is likely to be facilitated in future by the presence of large health centres and group practices which provide the critical number of incumbent GPs, referring an adequate number of patients and providing adequate space for these 'attached' specialist clinicians. These forms of integration are taking place insidiously with the move of psychologists (Broadhurst, 1972; Earll & Kincey, 1979), nurse therapists (Paykel *et al*, 1982; Marks, 1985), community psychiatric nurses (Robertson & Scott, 1985; Oyebode *et al*, 1990), social workers (Corney & Bowen, 1981) and counsellors (Marsh & Barr, 1975; Martin & Mitchell, 1983) into primary-care teams. Furthermore, there has been a relocation of psychiatric out-patient clinics to health centres (Strathdee & Williams, 1984; Tyrer, 1985; Pullen & Yellowlees, 1988).

Commissioning clinical teams and their bases

Fundamental to the success of a sectorised service is the nature and functioning of its multidisciplinary team(s). Although the various disciplines were established to perform specific tasks, discussion about multidisciplinary teams has taken place in the absence of close analysis. Ambelas (1991) proposes two approaches for determining skill and discipline mix within any team: to focus on the needs for treatment, or to focus on the coordination of treatment and management. But there is disagreement on this point: Horder (1990), for example, dismisses the role of job descriptions, separate training, and professional boundaries and suggests that what counts are the personality, understanding, and behaviour of the individual worker. Ovretweit *et al* (1989) have suggested that these and other relevant issues such as responsibility, degree of autonomy, accountability, leadership, and management are best determined by the creation of an operational policy which includes such practical issues as aims, criteria for referral and discharge, nature and format of meetings and agendas, case allocation and management, reporting of workload, and development, support and training.

The siting of the team-base is a fundamental decision which often reflects the philosophy of the model of service being developed, but is influenced by many variables. First, there is the need for efficient resource allocation. Central, highly resourced facilities, for example hospital-based units, may appear more efficient and effective in terms of easy movement of staff between wards, training, information gathering, and reduction in staff isolation, but be inflexible in addressing patient's needs. Secondly, the degree to which local statutory and non-statutory agencies inter-relate is vital, and thirdly, the availability of suitable sites for the chosen model may be a decisive and pragmatic local factor. From a consideration of these issues, clinicians may choose between versions or hybrids of the following four service models.

Model 1. The Hospital Core Model is exemplified by Tyrer's (1985) Hive model which advocates that the hospital base should form the core of a system with closely coordinated sub-units of care such as day hospitals, community clinics, or mental health centres located in areas of greatest morbidity.

Model 2. The Community Mental Health Centre Model which involves the development of a community base for both acute and continuing-care services within each sector, providing both a location for services and acting as a base for a range of outreach services with links to a range of dispersed local social services and voluntary facilities (Bowas *et al*, 1986).

Model 3. The Integrated Primary Care Model which focuses on first contact sites as the location for the majority of assessments and treatments. Members of both acute or crisis intervention and continuing-care elements of the sector team would have specific liaison with general practice, social service, and other agencies. While a range of in-patient facilities for both the acute and chronic patients would remain on the hospital site, all assessment, crisis intervention and out-patient work would take place at the health centre (Strathdee, 1992*a*). This would then form the base for a case-register and case-management system for a sector.

Model 4. The Assertive Outreach or Home-Based Treatment Model. This model may be the most suitable for a core of patients who are either unable or unwilling to attend the mental health services. Stein, for example, has concluded that it applies to those 10% of patients in a service. In areas where, as indicated above, the tradition of help-seeking behaviour of the population is with local community agencies rather than the statutory services, the model can be adapted to integration with these agencies.

Assessing the needs of patients in clinical practice

In an ideal planning framework, a comprehensive needs assessment would be undertaken on all patients and the aggregated data would be used to plan

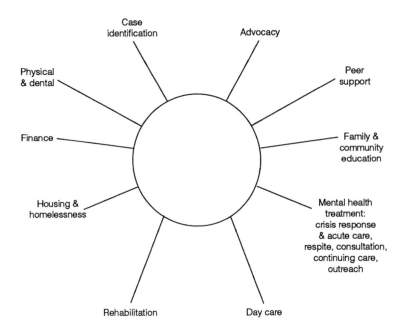

Fig. 8.1. The range of needs of individuals with mental health disorders

the services. In practice this is seldom possible, but systematic assessment, review, and evaluation over months and years of contact should allow teams to work with their users to evolve services more appropriate to their needs. Patients who suffer from severe mental illness have a range of needs which goes far beyond the purely medical. The list below identifies many of these and is adapted from the National Institute of Mental Health's document *Towards a Model Plan for a Comprehensive Community-Based Mental Health System* (1987). The distinction between need, demand, and supply is clearly defined (Holland, 1983). In this section Stevens & Gabbay's (1991) working definition of need will be used, that is ''the ability to benefit in some way from health (and social) care''.

The issue of how best to make such an assessment has taxed both researchers and clinicians, not least because their requirements differ. An ideal assessment tool for use in a routine clinic setting would be one which is brief, takes little time to administer, does not require the use of personnel additional to the usual clinical team, is valid and reliable in different settings and across gender and cultures, and above all, which can be used as an integral part of routine clinical work, rather than as a time-consuming extra. Macdonald (1991) suggests that in addition they should be sensitive to change, their potential inter-rater and test-rater reliability should be high, and they should logically inform clinical management (Hillier *et al* 1990).

In practice, the reality is far from this ideal. The commonest problems are that the same information is collected by a wide variety of disciplines and agencies in a number of settings; much of the information gathered is based on subjective judgements by individual clinicians, which although enormously valuable, can make transfer of vital knowledge impossible; a proportion of it is documented illegibly; and some recorders lack expert knowledge (such as the assessment of housing needs by health professionals, rather than housing-department experts). For example, even the collection of basic sociodemographic information suffers from a lack of reliability. These data are collected on several occasions and by several disciplines in the course of a patient's career through the morass of an episode of care. In any in-patient episode, for example, the same information is frequently sought on registration by admission staff, nursing and ward staff, the admitting doctor, the psychologist and occupational therapist involved in care, the night-staff returns, the Mental Health Act administrator, CPNs, and social workers if involved. The problem is compounded by the fact that most of these groups keep their own set of notes, resulting in waste of scarce clinical time. In one district, the inter-rater reliability on many of the variables was as low as 30% (Lelliot, personal communication). In response to the lack of uniformity nationally in the information gathered, Turk *et al* (1988) suggest a format for the routine collection of summary data based on a training instrument used by a high proportion of British psychiatrists. Regarding more structured approaches, there are many rating scales which may be used for routine clinical practice, and these are reviewed elsewhere (Thornicroft & Bebbington, 1993). The decision of which to use will depend on whether the approach is to focus on particular diagnostic or care groups, and on the balance to be struck between economy of time and inclusiveness of the ratings.

Needs for training

In an interesting review, Sturt & Waters (1985) advocated that for work in community-based settings, clinicians are required to develop skills beyond the purely clinical. In particular, they advocated the development of the ability to "recognise alternative resources to those found in hospital settings, obtain the skills of networking and the ability to administrate and manage". Cooper (1991) suggests that it is ignorance of each other's training background that leads to difficulties in resolving issues of authority and responsibility within multidisciplinary teams. He advocates that a regular activity within each team should be explanatory sessions when each discipline explains the rationale behind their thinking and formulates their concept of discipline-specific skills. The Royal College of Psychiatrists has suggested a valuable range of training experiences in psychiatry, and both the theoretical and practical elements are as follows. However, there is a clear hiatus in the provision of practical training in service planning, development, implementation, and evaluation.

Need for clinical audit

Until the recent introduction of audit, the majority of service evaluations have been the activity of researchers, rather than clinicians in routine settings. However, as Glover (1989) points out, audit offers the opportunity for clinicians to develop methods which will inform the planning process better and place arguments for resources on a more reasoned path. Four categories of audit have been defined for use in routine clinical settings:

(a) *Medical audit*, which refers to matters related exclusively to medical personnel and responsibilities, e.g. quality of medical case-notes, prescribing patterns, etc.

(b) *Clinical audit*, which refers to the activities of the multidisciplinary team in the assessment and treatment of patients, e.g. evaluation of care coordination systems.

(c) *Service planning audit* which involves assessment of current usage of services and implications for future service developments, e.g. use of current in-patient and emergency facilities.

(d) *Needs-related groups (NRGs)*. While in psychiatry diagnostic-related groups (DRGs) have been demonstrated to be inadequate measures of the resource implications of treating patients, with the availability of information technology and thus the facility for accurate information gathering, a more rational basis for the development NRGs which will predict financial and service resource needs more accurately can be developed. Examples of audit which can be carried out at the sector or district level are outlined below.

Medical audit

(a) An analysis of the content of case-notes and identification of existing patient information pathways in relation to duplication of information, areas of information gathered, internal consistency, consultation details, and outcomes.

(b) The determination of an agreed minimum data set for all patients having contact with the service including pertinent historical and mental-state details, agencies involved in care, medication and legal status.

(c) Medication chart review both by clinicians and pharmacy departments.

Clinical audit

(a) Discharge planning. An assessment of the effectiveness of discharge planning in relation to the care programme approach and the level of communication and joint working between sector agencies.
(b) The development of good practice clinical treatment profiles, in terms of assessment, management and treatment profiles of major psychiatric conditions.
(c) A review of the patients admitted under the Mental Health Act to determine numbers admitted under section, nature of sections, ethnic mix of patients on section, efficiency of tribunal procedures, efficiency of administration in ensuring consent to treatment and renewal of treatment orders.

Service planning audit

(a) Analysis of the use of in-patient facilities, such as that of Bebbington *et al*, Chapter 15.
(b) Audit of the utilisation of crisis intervention services including domiciliary consultations and casualty attenders.
(c) A census of all patient contacts with the service in a defined period.

Conclusions

We have argued that the geographical sector, with a defined population of about 50 000, forms a workable unit for the planning, provision and evaluation of community-orientated mental health services. As yet there is a dearth of information on the quantitative effects of such an approach to organising services. We would emphasise the importance of empirical research to test whether the claims set out on p. 143 operate in practice. In our view these questions are central to the proper implementation of community care for people with severe mental health problems, and to ensure that the spirit guiding the 1990 NHS and Community Care Act is enacted. It is clear to us that many different service models can deliver the essential functions required of an, at least adequate, mental health service, as indicated in Table 8.3.

Pending fuller evaluation of the claims of community facilities, and given our current limited knowledge of the exact effectiveness of many mental health interventions, we have worked with Dr Rachel Jenkins and consulted with many expert colleagues in Britain to come to a view about what combination of services should be considered in each health district, and our consensual views are shown in Table 8.4. Three points need to be kept

TABLE 8.3

The relationship between service functions and service models

Service functions	Service models
Crisis intervention	Domiciliary visits
	Casualty department
	Crisis-intervention teams
	Drop-in services at community mental health centres
	Community crisis beds
	CPN crisis-response service
	General practitioners
	Approved social worker day/night service
	24-hour telephone help line
Acute care/asylum	Local/district intensive care
	Local/regional medium-secure facilities
Assessment	Hospital out-patient clinics
	Primary-care/health-centre liaison clinics
	Community mental health centre clinics
	Sessional input to social services, housing, voluntary sector

TABLE 8.4

Proposed range of district acute and continuing care general adult psychiatric places for a 250 000 population

Type of provision	Range of places
24-hour staffed residences	40–150
Day-staffed residences	30–120
Acute psychiatric care	50–150
Unstaffed group homes	48–80
Adult-placement schemes	0–15
Local secure places	5–10
Respite facilities	0–5
Regional secure unit	1–10

in mind in interpreting these proposed service levels. First, we have deliberately indicated the number of places potentially required in each category, rather than the number of beds. In future we expect that a greater degree of flexibility will be required of mental health purchasers and providers in moving staffing resources across sites according to the needs of patients, and we shall see staff decreasingly fixed to beds. Secondly, we have given a range of places for each category, as we now find strong evidence for variations in local service requirements primarily according to local social and demographic characteristics. In this way the normative view taken in Better Services for the Mentally Ill (Department of Health and Social Security, 1975) was, we believe, misleading. Finally, a truly comprehensive service could be expected to have provisions in most or all of the categories, although this is currently far from the case, and indeed many districts have places in only two or three of the categories. There is a clear interdependence between these types of provision, and where whole groups of services are absent, this will produce a greater demand upon, and use of, those services which do exist. In our view, a necessary mechanism to realise such plans is to set clear, realistic and ambitious service-development targets (Department of Health, 1991; Thornicroft & Strathdee, 1991). We expect that among the prime challenge to mental health services for the 1990s will be: extending the variety of services offered, diversifying working relationships with voluntary, user, informal carer and statutory services, and carefully measuring the outcomes of these interventions.

References

AMBELAS, A. (1991) The task of treatment and the multidisciplinary team. *Psychiatric Bulletin*, **15**, 77–79.

ANDREWS, G. (1990) *The Tolkien Report. A Description of a Model Mental Health Service.* Sydney: University of New South Wales.

AUDIT COMMISSION (1986) *Making a Reality of Community Care.* London: HMSO.

BOURAS, N., TUFNELL, G., BROUGH, D., *et al* (1986) Model for the integration of community psychiatry and primary care. *Journal of the Royal College of General Practitioners*, **36**, 62–66.

BROADHURST, A. (1972) Clinical psychology and the general practitioner. *British Medical Journal*, *i*, 793–795.

BROWN, R., STRATHDEE, G., CHRISTIE-BROWN, J., *et al* (1988) A comparison of referrals to primary care and hospital out-patient clinics. *British Journal of Psychiatry*, **153**, 168–173.

CORNEY, R. H. & BOWEN, B. A. (1980) Referrals to social workers: a comparative study of a local authority intake team with a general practice attachment team. *Journal of the Royal College of General Practitioners*, **309**, 139–147.

DEPARTMENT OF HEALTH AND SOCIAL SECURITY (1975) *Better Services for the Mentally Ill*, Cmnd 6233. London: HMSO.

—— (1978) *Collaboration in Community Care.* Central Health Services Council, London: HMSO.

DEPARTMENT OF HEALTH (1991) *The Health of the Nation.* London: HMSO.

EARLL, L. & KINCEY, J. (1979) Clinical psychology in general practice: a controlled trial evaluation. *Journal of the Royal College of General Practitioners*, **32**, 32–37.

EATON, W. W. (1985) Epidemiology of schizophrenia. *Epidemiologic Reviews*, **7**, 105–126.

FALLOON, I. (1988) The prevention of morbidity in schizophrenia. In *Handbook of Behavioural Family Therapy* (ed. I. Falloon). London: Hutchinson.

GLOVER, G. R. (1989) Private sector psychiatric services. *Psychiatric Bulletin*, **13**, 198–199.

GOLDBERG, D. P. & BLACKWELL, B. (1970) Psychiatric illness in general practice: a detailed study using a new method of case identification. *British Medical Journal*, *ii*, 439–443.

——, REGIER, D. & BURNS, B. (1980) *Use of Health and Mental Health Outpatient Services in four Organised Health Care Settings.* Mental Health Services System Reports, Series DN No. 1 Washington DC: US Government Printing Office.

GOLDMAN, H., GATTOZZI, A. & TAUBE, C. (1981) Defining and counting the chronically mentally ill. *Community Psychiatry*, **31**, 21.

GRIFFITHS, R. (1988) *Community Care: an Agenda for Action.* London: HMSO.

HANSSON, L. (1989) Utilisation of psychiatric in-patient care. *Acta Psychiatrica Scandinavica*, **79**, 571–578.

HARRISON, G., OWENS, D., HOLTON, A., *et al* (1988) A prospective study of severe mental disorder in Afro-Caribbean patients. *Psychological Medicine*, **18**, 643–657.

——, HOLTON, A., NEILSON, D., *et al* (1989) Severe mental disorder in Afro-Caribbean patients: some social demographic and service factors. *Psychological Medicine*, **19**, 683–696.

HILLIER, W., ZAUDIG, M. & MOBOUR, W. (1991) Development of diagnostic checklists for use in routine clinical care. *Archives of General Psychiatry*, **47**, 782–784.

HIRSCH, S. (1988) *Psychiatric Beds and Resources: Factors Influencing Bed Use and Service Planning.* London: Gaskell.

HOLLOWAY, F. (1988) Day care and community support. In *Community Care in Practice* (eds A. Lavender & F. Holloway). Chichester: Wiley.

HORDER, E. (1990) *Medical Care in Three Psychiatric Hostels.* London: Hampstead and Bloomsbury District Health Authority, Hampstead and South Barnet GP Forum, and the Hampstead Department of Community Medicine.

HOUSE OF COMMONS (1985) *Second Report from the Social Services Committee, Session 1984–85, Community Care.* London: HMSO.

—— (1990) *National Health Service and Community Care Act.* London: HMSO.

HUNTER, D. & WISTOW, G. (1987) Mapping the organisational context. 1 Central departments, boundaries and responsibilities. In *Community Care in Britain: Variations on a Theme* (eds D. Hunter & G. Wistow). London: King Edward's Hospital Fund for London.

INEICHEN, B., HARRISON, G. & MORGAN, H. (1984) Psychiatric hospital admissions in Bristol. 1. Geographic and ethnic factors. *British Journal of Psychiatry*, **145**, 600–604.

JABLENSKY, A. (1986) Epidemiology of schizophrenia: a European perspective. *Schizophrenia Bulletin*, **12**, 52–73.

JARMAN, B. (1983) Identification of underprivileged areas. *British Medical Journal*, **286**, 1705–1709.

—— (1984) Underprivileged areas: validation and distribution of scores. *British Medical Journal*, **289**, 1587–1592.

——, HIRSCH, S. & WHITE, P. (1992) Predicting psychiatric admission rates. *British Medical Journal*, **304**, 1146–1150.

JEFFREYS, P. (1979) Joint approaches to community care. In *New Methods of Mental Health Care* (ed. M. Meacher). London: Mental Health Foundation.

JOHNSON, S. & THORNICROFT, G. (1993) The sectorisation of psychiatric services in England and Wales. *Social Psychiatry and Psychiatric Epidemiology* (in press).

JOHNSTONE, E. C., OWENS, D. G. C., GOLD, A., et al (1984) Schizophrenic patients discharged from hospital – a follow-up study. *British Journal of Psychiatry*, **145**, 586–590.

JONES, K. (1972) *A History of the Mental Health Services.* London: Routledge and Kegan Paul.

KENDRICK, A., SIBBALD, B., BURNS, T., et al (1991) Role of general practitioners in care of long term mentally ill patients. *British Medical Journal*, **302**, 508–511.

KINGDON, D. (1989) Mental health services: results of a survey of English district plans. *Psychiatric Bulletin*, **13**, 77–78.

LEVINE, M. (1981) *The History and Politics of Community Mental Health.* Oxford: Oxford University Press.

LINDHOLM, H. (1983) Sectorised psychiatry. *Acta Psychiatrica Scandinavica*, **67** (suppl. 304).

MACDONALD, A. (1991) How can we measure mental health? In *Indicators for Mental Health in the Population* (eds R. Jenkins & S. Griffiths). London: HMSO.

MCLEAN, E. & LIEBOWITZ, J. (1989) Towards a working definition of the long-term mentally ill. *Psychiatric Bulletin*, **13**, 251–252.

MARKS, I. (1985) Controlled trial of psychiatric nurse therapists in primary care. *British Medical Journal*, **240**, 1181–1184.

MARKS, J. N., GOLDBERG, D. P. & HILLIER, V. F. (1979) Determinants of the ability of general practitioners to detect psychiatric illness. *Psychological Medicine*, **9**, 337–353.

MARSH, G. N. & BARR, J. (1975) Marriage guidance counselling in a group practice. *Journal of the Royal College of General Practitioners*, **25**, 73–75.

MARTIN, E. & MITCHELL, H. (1983) A counsellor in general practice: a one year survey. *Journal of the Royal College of General Practitioners*, **33**, 366–367.

MIND (1983) *Common Concern.* London: MIND Publications.

MOODLEY, P. & THORNICROFT, G. (1988) Ethnic group and compulsory detention. *Medicine, Science and the Law*, **28**, 325–328.

MUIJEN, M., MARKS, I., CONNOLLY, J., et al (1992) Home based care versus standard hospital care for patients with severe mental illness: a randomised controlled trial. *British Medical Journal*, **304**, 749–754.

——, ——, ——, et al (1992) The Daily Living Programme: a preliminary comparison of community versus hospital bed treatment for the seriously mentally ill facing emergency admission. *British Journal of Psychiatry*, **160**, 379–384.

MURRAY PARKES, C., BROWN, G. W. & MONCK, E. M. (1962) The general practitioner and the schizophrenic patient. *British Medical Journal, i,* 972–976.

NATIONAL INSTITUTE OF MENTAL HEALTH (1987) *Towards a Model for a Comprehensive Community-Based Mental Health System.* Washington DC: NIMH.

OVRETWEIT, J. (1986) *Case Responsibility in Multi-disciplinary Teams (BIOSS).* London: Good Practices in Mental Health.

OYEBODE, F., CUMELLA, S., GARDEN, G., *et al* (1990) Diagnosis-related groups: implications for psychiatry. *Psychiatric Bulletin,* **14,** 1–3.

PATMORE, C. & WEAVER, J. (1990) *A Survey of Community Mental Health Centres.* London: Good Practices in Mental Health.

PAYKEL, E. (1990) Innovations in mental health in the primary care system. In *Mental Health Service Evaluation* (eds I. Marks & R. Scott). Cambridge: Cambridge University Press.

——, MANGEN, S., GRIFFITH, J., *et al* (1982) Community psychiatric nursing for neurotic patients: a controlled trial. *British Journal of Psychiatry,* **140,** 573–581.

PULLEN, I. & YELLOWLEES, A. (1988) Scottish psychiatrists in primary health care settings: a silent majority. *British Journal of Psychiatry,* **153,** 633–636.

ROBERTSON, H. & SCOTT, D. J. (1985) Community psychiatric nursing: a survey of patients and problems. *Journal of the Royal College of General Practitioners,* **35,** 130–132.

ROSEN, B. & GOLDSMITH, H. (1981) *Evaluation and Program Planning Vol 4. the Health Demographic Profile System.* Elmsford, NY: Pergamon Press Ltd.

ROYAL COLLEGE OF PSYCHIATRISTS (1990) *Caring for a Community: 1. The Model Mental Health Service.* London: Royal College of Psychiatrists.

SAYCE, L., CRAIG, T. K. J. & BOARDMAN, A. P. (1991) The development of Community Mental Health Centres in the United Kingdom. *Social Psychiatry and Psychiatric Epidemiology,* **26,** 14–20.

SECRETARIES OF STATE FOR HEALTH, WALES, NORTHERN IRELAND AND SCOTLAND (1989) *Working for Patients.* London: HMSO.

—— MEDICAL AUDIT (1990) *Caring for People.* London: HMSO.

SHAPIRO, S., SKINNER, E., KRAMER, M., *et al* (1985) Measuring need for mental health services in a general population medical care. *Medical Care,* **23,** 1033–1043.

SHEPHERD, M., COOPER, B., BROWN, A., *et al* (1966) *Psychiatric Illness in General Practice.* London: Oxford University Press.

STEVENS, A. & GABBAY, J. (1991) Needs assessment, needs assessment. *Health Trends,* **23,** 20–23.

STRATHDEE, G. (1990) The delivery of psychiatric care. *Journal of the Royal Society of Medicine,* **83,** 222–225.

—— (1992*a*) The interface between psychiatry and primary care in the management of schizophrenic patients in the community. In *The Primary Care of Schizophrenia* (eds R. Jenkins, V. Field & R. Young). London: HMSO.

—— (1992*b*) Liaison between general practice and secondary care teams towards the prevention and treatment of neural disorders. In *The Prevention of Depression and Anxiety in Primary Care* (eds R. Jenkins & J. Newton), pp. 113–124. London: HMSO.

—— & THORNICROFT, G. (1993) Setting up services in the community. In *Principles of Social Psychiatry* (eds D. Bhugra & J. Leff). Oxford: Blackwell Scientific (in press).

—— & WILLIAMS, P. (1984) A survey of psychiatrists in primary care: the silent growth of a new service. *Journal of the Royal College of General Practitioners,* **34,** 615–618.

STURT, J. & WATERS, H. (1985) Role of the psychiatrist in community-based mental health care. *Lancet,* March 2nd, 507–508.

TALBOT, J. (1983) *Unified Mental Health Systems: Utopia Unrealised.* Washington, DC: Jossey-Bass Inc.

TANSELLA, M. (1989) Evaluating community psychiatric services. In *Scientific Approaches in Epidemiological & Social Psychiatry. Essays in Honour of Michael Shepherd* (eds P. Williams, G. Wilkinson & K. Rawnsley), pp. 386–403. London: Routledge.

THORNICROFT, G. (1991*a*) Social deprivation and rates of treated mental disorder: developing statistical models to predict psychiatric service utilisation. *British Journal of Psychiatry,* **158,** 475–484.

—— (1991b) The concept of case management for long-term mental illness. *International Review of Psychiatry*, **3**, 125–132.

—— (1992) The TAPS Project (6): new long stay psychiatric patients and social deprivation. *British Journal of Psychiatry*, **161**, 621–624.

—— & BEBBINGTON, P. (1988) Deinstitutionalisation: from hospital closure to service development. *British Journal of Psychiatry*, **155**, 739–753.

—— & —— (1993) Quantitative method in the evaluation of community mental health services. In *Modern Community Psychiatry* (ed. W. Breakey) (in press).

—— & STRATHDEE, G. (1991) The health of the nation: mental health. *British Medical Journal*, **303**, 410–412.

TODD, J. W. (1984) Wasted resources. Referral to hospital. *Lancet*, *ii*, 1089.

TORREY, E., ERDMAN, K. & WOLFE, S. (1990) *Care of the Seriously Mentally Ill. A Rating of Scale Programs* (3rd ed). Washington, DC: Public Citizen Health Research Group and National Alliance for the Mentally Ill.

TURK, J., LOZA, N., KASINSKI, J., *et al* (1988) The Bethlem Royal and Maudsley Hospital Item Sheets – the development and reliability of an instrument for routine collection of summary clinical data. *Psychiatric Bulletin*, **12**, 422–426.

TYRER, P. (1985) The 'hive' system: a model for a psychiatric service. *British Journal of Psychiatry*, **146**, 571–575.

——, TURNER, R. & JOHNSON, A. (1989) Integrated hospital and community psychiatric services and use of in-patient beds. *British Medical Journal*, **299**, 298–300.

US DEPARTMENT OF HEALTH AND HUMAN SERVICES STEERING COMMITTEE ON THE CHRONICALLY MENTALLY ILL (1980) *Towards a National Plan for the Chronically Mentally Ill*. Washington, DC: US Government Printing Office.

WALSH, D. (1987) Mental health service models in Europe. In *Mental Health Services in Pilot Study Areas: Report on a European Study*. Copenhagen: WHO.

WING, J. (1989) *Health Services Planning and Research. Contributions from Psychiatric Case Registers*. London: Gaskell.

WORLD HEALTH ORGANIZATION (1983) *First Contact Mental Health Care*. Copenhagen: WHO Regional Office for Europe.

9 Costing psychiatric interventions

JENI BEECHAM and MARTIN KNAPP

> "When we mean to build,
> We first survey the plot, then draw the model;
> And when we see the figure of the house,
> Then must we rate the cost of the erection;
> Which, if we find outweighs ability,
> What do we then but draw anew the model
> In fewer offices, or at least desist
> To build at all?" (Shakespeare, *King Henry IV, Part 2*)

The demands and needs for cost information in psychiatric contexts have multiplied considerably in recent years, but have often been frustrated by inadequate data. The typical costs data available to the policy maker, manager, clinical professional, or researcher have been dominated until recently by age-old accounting practices and line-management arrangements, and constrained by fragmentation of responsibility. Most limiting of all, costs data have rarely been used in taking decisions about individual cases. In considering the demands and needs for costs in psychiatry, this chapter describes a research instrument – the Client Service Receipt Interview (CSRI) – which has been developed and extensively applied in order to meet some of these needs. The chapter includes illustrations of applications of the CSRI.

Scarcity and costs

There have been few occasions in recent British history when policies for health or social care have not been constrained by lack of funds, and often financial pressures have forced the complete redrawing or abandonment of promising plans and laudable aspirations. An obvious current example is the policy to develop community care services for long-stay hospital residents. In many regions and districts, the needs-led intentions of the mid-1980s have

163

given way to supply-led services, often dominated by whatever is the latest administrative or legal ruling on eligibility for social security benefits. Of course, we should not be surprised by this and other examples of policy fettered by resources, not for the cynical reason that there is often an enormous gulf between political rhetoric and actual delivery, but because of the fundamental fact that resources are always scarce relative to needs or wants. To indulge in a second literary quote, it was Robert Browning who wrote that ''a man's reach should exceed his grasp, or what's a heaven for?'' Aspiration will and must always run ahead of ability in this as in other areas of public and social policy.

It is the recognition that there will always be insufficient resources to meet society's demands that signals the need for a careful examination of how those resources are being used. Almost every debate in and about Britain's health and social care services boils down to a disagreement about how resources should be used, and whether they can be employed more productively or more fairly. These are the efficiency and equity questions, and almost any answer to them must range across the needs for health or social interventions, the outcomes for service users and the costs.

The demands for cost information thus stem from a variety of policy, practice and research needs. There is, for example, long-standing interest in the financial implications of particular treatment or care procedures, manifested most visibly in cost evaluations such as cost-effectiveness and cost–benefit studies. The demand for information on the costs of social or public expenditure on mental illness is another long-standing feature of psychiatric debate and research. What has been different about the last few years has been the greater emphasis on the place of costs in management and clinical decision-making. Costs also underpin pricing or charging decisions, feeding into the calculus of contracting and preparation for the marketing of services. Costs data are needed by the 'value for money auditor' checking on efficiency, and the elected or appointed member monitoring progress towards local goals. The introduction of case or care management would signal another demand if case managers are charged with putting together packages of care with given budgets.

These and other demands could hardly contrast more vividly with the supply of available costs information. This information is usually dominated by age-old line management arrangements: within a local authority, for instance, there will usually be separate budgets for field social work and residential care. Different agencies will have separate financial recording mechanisms, an obviously necessary requirement for the purposes of probity and budget-making, but the accounting and reporting procedures may also be so different as to make it impossible to pull them together for the purposes of comparison or aggregation. How often, for example, are local district health authority and family health service authority expenditures looked at together? The inclusions and exclusions may also pose difficulties for the researcher or manager trying to determine the costs of alternative care strategies. Capital expenditures may bear no relation to the 'real' cost to society of using the durable resources such as buildings to which they relate. Costs to service users and the indirect financial effects on the public at large are inevitably omitted. Worst of all is the lack of financial information systems to allow clinicians, managers or others to easily and regularly monitor levels of spending against available income.

In none of these respects have health departments or local-authority finance departments acted improperly or inappropriately; indeed, many of the problems posed by today's available cost information derive from the diligence and watchfulness of accountants and finance departments. The accounting and reporting procedures carefully built up over a number of years are no longer equal to the task of responding to such a diversity or bombardment of demands as is currently to be witnessed.

We are neither inclined nor qualified to discuss how cost-information systems could be constructed to meet the many demands set out earlier, nor, we suspect, would most readers of this book be particularly interested in those particular details. Instead we will describe a *research* tool which has been developed and successfully employed in the collection of information on costs, service utilisation, income, and related matters. We then illustrate its use from some of our own research. Like the plans for the new health and social care systems being set in place in Britain in the early 1990s, the aim of this research method (and its accompanying tools) has been to produce costs data which are client-focused rather than agency-centred, and consolidated rather than fragmented, and which are constructed and employed with consistency. Our costing method has not, however, been designed as an information system, although it shares some common features.

In this chapter we first describe the method and its accompanying instrumentation, and then illustrate its employment in practice by examining some of the demands for cost information.

A costing method for research in psychiatry

The basic cost rules

In an earlier paper we recommended four general rules when costing health and social care services (Knapp & Beecham, 1990). The first rule recommends that it must be possible for costs to be comprehensively measured. They should therefore range over as many service components of care programmes or 'packages' as is relevant in any particular circumstance.

"Unless costs are defined and measured comprehensively, one treatment mode may appear to be less costly than another when in reality that mode merely shifts costs into forms that have not been measured". (Weisbrod *et al*, 1980, p. 403)

The calculation of comprehensive costs is most usefully effected at the individual level, partly because this is the level at which clinical data are collected, and partly because this preserves inter-client variability in the research domain – an essential feature of any needs-based service system. The second costing rule then urges that these variations between clients, facilities or areas of the country should not be overlooked. Handled properly, these cost variations can produce useful policy and practice insights, for costs will usually be linked to differences in individual characteristics, needs, and outcomes.

When an examination of differences in cost tempts one into drawing conclusions about comparative performance, the third rule should come into play: such comparisons must be made on a like-with-like basis. It is of little value, for example, to report how community care costs less than hospital if clients in the community have fewer behavioural or health problems than those in hospital. Finally, cost information is far more useful if it does not stand in isolation from other relevant evidence, particularly outcome data. Reliance on cost information alone could be dangerous, just as it is inadvisable to *neglect* costs in policy and practice discussions and decisions. As Griffiths wrote,

"To talk of policy in matters of care except in the context of available resources and timescales for action owes more to theology than to the purposeful delivery of a caring service". (Griffiths, 1988, para. 9)

For example, underpinning most evaluations is the hoary old question: for whom and under what circumstances is one intervention preferable to another? But to define the criterion 'preferable' solely in clinical outcome terms without regard to cost is to invite unnecessary (that is, avoidable) difficulties of implementation.

These cost rules embody two sets of principles: they are consistent with the demands of economic theory as applied to health and social care (Drummond, 1980; Knapp, 1984), and they are also essentially the costing counterparts to the usual principles of any evaluation. This congruence and the economic theoretical grounding help considerably in the design and interpretation of empirical research. With these four rules in mind we will describe the instrumentation developed for collecting data on service utilisation and for calculating comprehensive costs. Although the potential undoubtedly exists within a case management system with devolved budgets, it is not yet possible to ask any one individual about the full cost implications of a client's care package. The process of costing can be broken down into three connected tasks:

(a) the collection of service receipt or utilisation data by individual clients or patients over a consistently defined period

(b) the costing or pricing of each of the services used

(c) the combination of these two sets of information in order to cost full care packages.

Each of these tasks is described below. For simplicity the method has been described by reference to a single research project, although the flexibility of the approach and instrument should be stressed and is evidenced by a variety of other applications.

Collecting data on service utilisation – the CSRI schedule

In order to calculate the costs of community care for people moving from long-stay hospital residence, we developed and employed a new instrument, the Client Service Receipt Interview (CSRI). Although the instrument needed to be tailor-made to fit the research context, an early requirement was easy adaptability, for the CSRI was to be employed in the Personal Social Services Research Unit's (PSSRU's) evaluation of the Department of Health's Care in the Community demonstration programme of 1984–88, which concerned all the main adult client groups, and also in the evaluation of the psychiatric reprovision services being established under the closure programmes for Friern and Claybury hospitals in North East Thames Regional Health Authority. The CSRI was built on previous research in the PSSRU, particularly on services for child care and young offenders (see Knapp & Robertson, 1989, for partial reviews), and incorporated relevant parts of previously developed instruments in the mental health field, particularly the Economic Questionnaire of Weisbrod *et al* (1980).

The CSRI was piloted in the summer of 1986 in the Maidstone Care in the Community project for people with learning difficulties where a wide range of services had been developed, affording the chance to test the instrument under different conditions. A second round of instrument refinement was based on use of the CSRI in another three care in the community projects. Since its introduction the CSRI has been used in more than a dozen evaluation studies, some of which are listed below:

(a) the Care in the Community programme, under which more than 800 people left hospital (Renshaw *et al*, 1988; Knapp *et al*, 1992*b*)

(b) the North East Thames Regional Health Authority (NETRHA) psychiatric reprovision study of what will eventually be as many as 1000 former residents of Friern and Claybury hospitals (see, for example, Knapp *et al*, 1990; Beecham *et al*, 1991)

(c) the Maudsley Hospital Daily Living Programme (Marks *et al*, 1988), where costs research is due to be completed in early 1992

(d) a study of people with schizophrenia living in the community in two London districts (Melzer *et al*, 1991)

(e) the evaluation of the rundown of psychiatric and mental-handicap hospitals and developments in community care in Northern Ireland, results from which will be published from mid-1992 onwards

(f) an ongoing follow-up study of more than 250 people with learning difficulties who moved from hospital under the Care in the Community programme, looking now at outcomes and costs after four and a half years in the community, to be reported in 1992

(g) an evaluation of community psychiatric nursing in Greenwich which compares an experimental service orientated towards case management with a more traditional model (McCrone *et al*, 1992).

In describing the CSRI we will concentrate on its development for the NETRHA study of people with a history of long-stay hospital residence who are moving to the community under a planned and well funded reprovision programme. In this and the Care in the Community evaluations we could be certain that most clients would have a key carer or case manager, or that the client would be living in a group home where a diary would be kept of residents' activities (especially contacts with health, social care and related services, and with peripatetic professionals). The questionnaire was therefore originally designed for administration by an interviewer from the research team to the principal carer of the person with mental health problems. Very often the carer was a member of staff at the residential unit. Where it was impossible to identify a carer, for example when a client was living in an independent flat, the questionnaire was often successfully completed in an interview with the client. It has also been completed by staff without need for an interview, although it is not specifically intended for that mode of use. In some research projects, the key questions of the CSRI have been incorporated into other schedules. However, experience has confirmed our initial expectations that a trained interviewer is needed to tease out accurate and comprehensive information.

The questionnaire is printed on ten A4 pages and takes approximately 40 minutes to complete. The questions are largely structured, some with a multiple-choice answer format and some open-ended but, given the complexity of community care arrangements, it is not surprising that a few narrative answers are required. The questionnaire design also incorporates blank spaces to write additional comments or interpret the occasionally confused responses of the interviewee. A series of 'prompt cards' supplements the CSRI. These contain indicative lists of accommodation types, different services, and social security benefits.

The CSRI collects retrospective information on service use, service-related issues, and income. The retrospective period (up until the date of the interview) is a compromise between the accuracy that comes from not asking respondents to cast their minds back too far and the comprehensiveness which can only come by allowing sufficient time to elapse for some rarely used but potentially expensive services to be used. We have generally found it helpful to divide the interview about service use into two parts, one covering the previous month – in the NETRHA case this is the 12th month after discharge from hospital – and the other asking about less-regularly received services (such as dentist or general practitioner (GP) visits) over the past 12 months. These durations are not fixed, and we have ourselves varied them to fit particular uses. For example, repeated use of the CSRI – as in the Daily Living Programme evaluation, when interviews were conducted at 3, 6, and 18 months after entry to the study – allows one to ask only about the period between interviews. For this longitudinal study, information gathered at all interviews has been recorded on the same schedule. This had the important advantage that the interviewer could use data from the previous interview to prompt or guide questions.

The first section of the CSRI covers *background and client information*, for example recording client code number, gender, and date of birth. Depending on the availability of information from other instruments, the interviewer could then ask for details of past admissions and discharges from hospital, participation in a special programme, registration with a GP, and medication. The opening section also records the date and place of interview and identifies the interviewer. The second section concentrates on *accommodation* and the living situation generally. Accommodation is usually a major component in both provision and cost. The CSRI thus covers: address, partly for the purposes of identifying facility type and budget, and partly because location influences cost (London is more expensive than the rest of the country, for example) and some adjustment may be needed; tenure of accommodation (council or private rent, residential home, owner-occupier); a simple description of the size of the unit (the number of different types of rooms and the number of other residents); the amount paid by the client or household in rent or other payments; and receipt of housing benefit, if any.

Most clients leaving long-stay hospital care do not live in domestic accommodation but in specialised facilities such as residential or nursing homes, hostels, or group homes. The interviewee is asked for *their* classification of the facility, although later we would impose a standardised categorisation using other information on tenure, staffing arrangements, and managing agency. (Where several clients live in the same unit some of these questions need be completed only once and can be separated from the main questionnaire.) Unfortunately, many people with mental health problems (although generally not the former long-stay in-patients moving to planned community care schemes) quite frequently move from one address to another, and the CSRI records such changes of address, including hospital readmissions. Instability of accommodation obviously complicates cost calculation; for clients it can have dire consequences for ability to work, entitlements to social security or indeed mental health itself. In some other applications of the CSRI in projects where clients are more likely to live in domestic accommodation with other members of their families, the accommodation questions have been more comprehensive, asking about the composition of the household and whether the clients themselves have any care responsibilities. More attention is also paid to how household expenses are covered.

Research has shown that concerns about money can have an adverse effect on some mental health conditions (Brugha *et al*, 1985; Granzini *et al*, 1990). Many people in this client group have low incomes, due in part to their heavy reliance on social security benefits and also to problems associated with under-claiming of benefits, low wages if work is found, and unstable work patterns. Information on *employment history, earnings and other personal resources* is therefore collected. Questions on employment are not usually relevant to clients with a history of long-term hospital residence, and it is more important to clarify receipt of social-security benefits. (In strict economic terms these should be considered as transfer payments, not representing an aggregate cost to society, but they are also good proxies for living expenses, since clients usually rely on these benefits as their only source of income. For example, in the NETRHA study we found that few people had any other sources of income at their disposal.) Details of regular outgoings are also collected in this section; we have found that only very rarely have clients had the opportunity to accumulate any savings. Data on *changes* in benefit status over the past year are also collected. In some of the accommodation units managed by voluntary organisations or by private individuals, carers receive benefits on behalf of the clients.

Former long-stay hospital residents rarely find (open) employment, but for many other groups of people with mental health problems, employment and its loss are important facets of both service effectiveness and cost. More questions are therefore sometimes needed on employment history, and a number of questions may be needed on current employment activities. The costs of lost employment resulting from mental ill health or in-patient treatment will fall to clients (lower income) and to society (lost production), the actual values to be attached depending on a variety of labour market and individual circumstances.

The *service receipt* section is at the core of the CSRI, and can take up most of the interview time. Community care is delivered and received in a 'fragmented' system, many agencies providing a variety of services. There is certainly no standard package of care handed out as people are referred to psychiatric care, and so there will be much variation between clients' packages of care. At this point the questionnaire identifies receipt of services which are not funded within the accommodation budget; these could be either services for health or social care available to everybody or specialist mental health services. Information is collected on services which the client leaves the accommodation to attend, such as day-centre activities, hospital-based services, appointments at the GP surgery, or leisure activities. Some professional support or services are provided for the client at home. Examples here would be home help, community psychiatric nurse or field social-worker domiciliary visits. These service utilisation fields are both divided into two parts, firstly to enable collection of information pertaining to the 12th month since discharge from hospital (representing some form of 'steady state', for to record service use since the first day after discharge will pick up the high transition costs which were not our concern in this study), and secondly to allow adjustment of this picture to account for regularly but infrequently used services such as out-patient appointments. For each service outside the place of residence, information is collected on: type of service, such as day care or out-patient appointment; name of providing establishment, for example the name of a day centre or hospital attended; providing agency, such as MIND or Hampstead Health Authority; professionals involved, such as psychiatrist; frequency of attendance or receipt per week; duration of attendance, such as one day or one hour; mode of clients' travel to and from the service; time spent travelling; and any charges made for the service. For domiciliary services, the interviewer asks for a similar range of data, but in addition a question on the total number of clients sharing the service is included. This is important where a professional visiting an establishment will see several clients for a group session (as with occupational therapy) or will see them sequentially (as with GP visits) and the allocation of cost to individuals must take the scope of the visit into account.

Two further questions complete this section. One asks about use of aids or adaptations to property. Although more relevant for other client groups, these are used quite frequently by older people with mental health problems. The other question asks for details of time spent by the *principal carer* both on direct care activities (face-to-face contact) and indirect care activities (telephone calls, record keeping, contacting other agencies to arrange services, etc), and whether there has been above-average administrative or managerial involvement in the client. Interestingly, we have found virtually no input from personnel at this level once the client has been living in the community for a year, except where a serious threat is posed to other residents or the wider community.

The importance of clients' *informal care* networks has been highlighted in recent policy documents such as the White Paper on community care (Cm 849, 1989), but the availability of such care arrangements for people leaving long-stay psychiatric hospitals appears to be limited (Knapp *et al*, 1992*b*, chapter 14). The CSRI includes questions on the input of informal carers in terms of time spent (frequency and duration of visit) and tasks undertaken (personal care, shopping, domestic tasks, and social visits).

If a number of clients are known to be living in domestic accommodation with other members of their families, more weight will need to be given to informal care in the interview.

Two aspects of *satisfaction with services* are covered in the interview, and gaps in service availability are identified. Because the interview refers to a single client, the same GP or day-care facility may be considered appropriate or satisfactory for one client but not for another. Service availability is assessed very broadly on a four-point scale: usually sufficient, sometimes insufficient, usually inadequate, or service not required. Quality of contact is similarly measured: usually helpful, sometimes unhelpful, generally unhelpful, or not applicable (where the service is not used). The final question on the CSRI schedule on gaps in service availability fulfils two functions. It draws the interview to an end by providing a discussion point for the interviewee and, when completed, it obviously provides information on 'service gaps' in the client's total care package, thus supplementing the data on satisfaction. Where this question was completed, inadequacy and inappropriateness of day-care activities and lack of personal resources were frequently noted responses. Aggregated data from these responses can point to gaps in service provision within a particular district or locale.

Costing individual health and social care services

The second major task in measuring the costs of mental health services is the costing or pricing of the various services used by clients. Economic theory advocates basing cost measures on *long-run marginal opportunity cost*. In practice, by *long-run* we mean to move beyond the small scale and immediate development of community care which could probably be achieved by using present services more intensively at very low marginal cost. Since national policy intentions are to substitute community services for most long-term hospital beds, it would hardly be credible to measure only short-run cost implications. By *marginal* we mean the addition to total cost attributable to the inclusion of one more client (the production of one more unit of output in general economic parlance). By *opportunity cost* we mean that the resource implications should reflect opportunities forgone rather than amounts spent. The opportunity cost measures the true private or social value of a resource or service, based on its value in the best alternative use. In a perfectly informed and frictionless market economy, this 'best alternative use value' would be identical to the price paid in the market. Not everything is marketed, not every market works smoothly, and information is rarely complete, with the result that observed prices and opportunity costs diverge. Thus the recorded depreciation payments on capital equipment or buildings will not usually reflect the opportunity costs of using these durable resources, nor will the (zero) payments to volunteers and informal carers usually indicate their social value.

In application of these principles, it happens that today's (short run) average revenue cost, plus appropriate capital and overhead elements, is probably close to the long-run marginal cost for most services we would encounter. In making this assumption we are following a precedent (see, for example, Jones *et al*, 1980; Mangen *et al*, 1983). In this chapter we will say no more about the calculation of these average revenue costs or their capital add-ons, for once we open the description we will need more space than can presently be made available. Moreover, the details are not everyone's cup of tea. We have written about them elsewhere, briefly (Knapp & Beecham, 1990), in more detail in relation to our evaluation of the Care in the Community demonstration programme (Allen *et al*, 1990), and in much greater depth with various health and social care examples (Netten & Beecham, 1993).

Three types of information are used to calculate the costs of services: facility-specific accounts, national data on pay and working conditions, and similar local data. Facility-specific costs information are most relevant for services which show a wide variation in scale, purpose, and location, such as accommodation or day activity services. Here, financial accounts compiled by the providing agency within their normal processes are the starting point, although to enable comprehensive costing these data require careful scrutiny. For other services, national costs (with regional weighting) are more appropriate. For example, some professional groups have nationally applicable pay and working conditions from which costs can be calculated. Although some variation in client-level costs would be accounted for by different grades of staff it is often not feasible to collect salary data for specific members of staff, and anyway a greater source of variation will be the *amount* of the service each client receives. In calculating costs for clients who use services in one locale it would be more appropriate to use a similar method applied to local pay and working conditions for the professional groups involved.

The costs for all services should be calculated at a constant and relevant unit, the choice of which depends on the nature of the service. For accommodation or hospital stays the cost per resident week or in-patient day is the most convenient and useful. For day care, cost per attendance, session or day could be used, whereas an average appointment or per minute cost is more appropriate for peripatetic professionals.

Costing full care packages

The CSRI is a means to an end rather than an end in itself. The interview collects the data that enable packages of care to be identified. This information must then be manipulated and joined with information on the costs of those services. This data preparation stage allows service receipt to be allocated at a constant unit over a defined period of time.

The unit of calculation for service receipt should be the same as that used for the calculation of service costs. The period of time is often defined by the research: for the NETRHA study the follow-up period was one year after discharge from hospital, for the Care in the Community programme evaluation, the follow-up was nine months, and for the Daily Living Programme several follow-up periods, varying from three to nine months, are used.

These tasks employ a particular method. To facilitate the process, the Service Entry And Numeration (SEAN) form has been developed. This schedule enables the components of a client's package of care to be listed alongside the amount of that service received. We have found this information is most usefully presented as receipt per week relating, for the NETRHA study, to the month before interview with adjustments for infrequently but regularly used services over the past 12 months. The third and final task is also completed on the SEAN form, to combine each client's average weekly use of services with the unit costs for each service so as to calculate total cost of care. (A computerised version of the SEAN form is currently being developed.)

Meeting the demands for cost information

The demands for cost information are many and various, and have certainly grown rapidly over the last few years. For the traditional top-down, supply-led, single-agency, planning of public expenditure, too often with little scope for innovation, the cost information currently available is probably adequate in design and quantity to satisfy most needs. However, the systems and incentives promoted by the 1990 *National Health Service and Community Care Act* (House of Commons, 1990) require a rather different approach to service planning and delivery. Ideally, health and social care decision-making will be bottom-up, needs-led and multiple-agency, with innovations encouraged by financial and other incentives, and system implications couched in terms of social and not merely public expenditures. The cost information requirements of the 1990s will be rather different from those of previous decades.

One of the requirements to be introduced as a result of the 1990 Act is the development of community care plans, jointly drawn up by local and health authorities, agreed with central government, and published for wider consideration. Any plan which is to have a chance of succeeding must be affordable, and the context for the new community care plans will help to encourage individual public authorities to define 'affordability' less narrowly than before. One of the criticisms of the community care arrangements of the 1980s voiced by the Audit Commission (1986), Griffiths (1988), and others focused upon the perverse incentives within the system which encouraged authorities to try to minimise their own costs while simultaneously increasing everyone else's. Community care planning circa 1993 will require information on population needs and preferences, the services to meet those needs, and the costs of providing those services. With case management and similar arrangements supporting the voice of the individual client and encouraging needs-led planning, there will be a tremendous demand for comprehensive and disaggregated costs data, with the funding sources made clear. Indeed, case management itself will have its own costs needs, for the community care White Paper advises local authorities to devolve budgetary responsibilities down to case managers or case-management teams. The British evidence for other client groups suggests that such devolution can work rather well to improve client quality of life at affordable cost (Challis & Davies, 1986; Challis *et al*, 1988). Social services departments of some local authorities are therefore putting financial-information systems in place which can supply case managers with costs and other data.

Equivalent in some respects to case management is the introduction of care programmes into psychiatric services, the consultant psychiatrist being required to set out the services needed by a patient not admitted to, or no longer resident in, hospital. Such care programmes will need to take account of the agencies capable of supplying the services. Although cost-consciousness is not written into the care programme recommendations, and although consultant psychiatrists will not hold client-specific budgets, the approach has obvious costs implications. Once again, drawing up plans which are unattainable because of their expense is not going to be helpful to the client or anyone else.

From April 1991, local social services authorities could apply for funding assistance "to enable [them] to improve the social care they can provide to people with a mental illness in need of specialist psychiatric care" (Department of Health, 1990, para. 7.13). Provided it is jointly agreed by both social services and health authorities, this discretionary Mental Illness Specific Grant (MISG) can subsidise social care of any kind for people accepted for treatment by the specialist psychiatric services (hence those covered by the care programme approach), and also for those not currently in touch with those services but who would clearly benefit from them. The grant is paid as a recurrent annual contribution to social services authorities' revenue spending, initially for up to three years. A comparatively small sum of £21 million of central money was made available for England in 1991–92, provided local matching funds totalling £9 million were also committed. Any grant calculation and allocation requires detailed cost data, and in many local social services authorities the work necessary to draw up bids for MISG funds represented the first detailed costing of social care for people with mental health problems for many years.

The employment of costs information in needs-based planning, preparing community care plans, devolving budgets to case managers, examining the implications of care programmes, and bidding for specific grants, is all relatively new. Demands for costs data of greater vintage stem from the need to evaluate both the outcomes and the resource implications of different, and especially new, policies and practices; the occasional calculation of the 'social costs of mental ill health'; the pricing of services for sale, either to clients and their relatives or to public authorities embarking on a policy of contracting out; and in the perennial performance reviews required for public probity, now often built around 'value for money audits' and 'efficiency scrutinies'.

In each and every case, whether new demands of the 1990s or long-established needs, the cost data requirements are rarely met. Had there been good cost and service receipt data to hand we would not have needed to develop the CSRI, health authorities would not have such a difficult time establishing the information bases for the new internal market, value for money auditors would have had fewer disagreements with the public authorities they were auditing, and the Department of Health could have spent rather less in contracting with a variety of commercial firms for the development of computer-based information systems.

We cannot illustrate the information responses to each and every one of these demands or needs for decent costs data – some of which we have considered in a review of recent literature (Knapp & Beecham, 1991) – but we can briefly describe some of the results of using the CSRI, long-run marginal opportunity costing, and the SEAN form to gather, price, and process information on service use and costs.

Illustrations of costs research

In debates about the rundown of long-stay hospital provision and its replacement by community care, doubts about economic viability are rarely far from the surface. Is community care less or more expensive than hospital? If it is less expensive, is this because it pays insufficient attention to client well-being? Of the many variants of community care, which are the more costly, and which the more cost-effective? If, in some long-term steady state, community care costs less than hospital, how feasible is it for expenditure savings from hospital rundown to be used to finance new services in the community?

These are among the questions addressed in two studies, the first evaluating the Care in the Community demonstration programme and the second, which is still ongoing, examining psychiatric reprovision in the North East Thames Region. We concentrate here on the latter. (For details of the evaluation findings for the Care in the Community programme, see Knapp *et al*, 1992*b*).

Two of the largest psychiatric hospitals in North London, Friern and Claybury, are due to close in the next few years. The decision to close was taken in 1983, since which date the Regional Health Authority has funded research to examine the psychiatric reprovision services being established to replace them. In association with the Team for Assessment of Psychiatric Services (TAPS), the PSSRU has been studying the economics of reprovision (see Team for the Assessment of Psychiatric Services, 1990). Thus far, the research has concentrated on in-patients who have been in continuous residence for at least a year, and who, if over 65 years old, do not have a current diagnosis of dementia. Most attention is focused on people who leave hospital, for whom follow-up CSRIs are completed one year and five years after discharge. The first reprovision patients moved to the community in 1985. Community care comprises an almost bewildering variety of services and arrangements, and the costs work has therefore ranged widely across agencies and services.

Describing community care costs

By August 1988 a total of 357 people who met the study criteria had left the two hospitals under the rundown plans, and most under the reprovision arrangements which carried financial transfers. Baseline information for all patients in the hospitals was collected by the TAPS researchers, covering: mental health status, using the Present State Examination (PSE; Wing *et al*, 1974) and the Social Behaviour Schedule (SBS; Sturt & Wykes, 1986); the Physical Health Index; patient personal and historical data; patient attitudes; living skills using the Basic Everyday Living Skills schedule; information on patients' social networks using the Social Network Schedule; and an assessment of living environments. These latter schedules were developed by TAPS (1992). Altogether, including the 'new long-stay' patients who had accumulated in the two hospitals since the study began, baseline information has been assembled on 964 in-patients. The TAPS research design compares aspects of the quality of life for patients discharged from the two hospitals with similar patients who remain behind, and some of our costs work has also made comparisons between community and hospital care. Service utilisation and costs data are collected for most leavers. For example, for 254 people who had left Friern or Claybury by August 1989, we can summarise community reprovision costs as in Table 9.1. The figures are self-explanatory: they illustrate the variety of services used by psychiatric reprovision clients, the dominance of accommodation in the total package costs, and the small proportion of clients in receipt of community psychiatric nursing services.

Costs, needs and outcomes

It is more interesting and relevant, of course, to set the costs data alongside the outcomes. Costs and outcomes are obviously not measured in identical

TABLE 9.1
NETRHA psychiatric reprovision: disaggregated costs (for a sample of 254 clients)

	Clients using the service: %	Average contribution of total cost	
		Among users: %	For all clients: %
Accommodation	100	82	82
DHA hospital services			
in-patient	15	15	2
out-patient	26	3	1
day care	24	19	5
DHA community services			
psychiatry	57	1	$-^1$
psychology	13	2	–
physiotherapy	2	–	–
nursing (CPN)	28	2	–
chiropody	34	–	–
drugs	12	3	–
FHSA services			
general practitioner	81	1	1
dentist	22	–	–
optician	15	–	–
pharmacy	5	–	–
LA social services			
day care	26	10	3
social club	4	1	–
field social work	34	6	2
occupational therapy	12	3	–
travel	30	1	–
miscellaneous	11	2	–
Voluntary sector services			
voluntary organisation day care	18	9	2
volunteers	4	4	–
Education classes	6	10	1
Police	2	2	–

1. – indicates less than 0.5%.

units, so we cannot say that the costs of community care are greater or less than the outcomes, but we *can* compare the costs of achieving given levels of outcome in different types of community provision or placements. In short, we can conduct cost-effectiveness but not cost–benefit analyses (Knapp & Beecham, 1992). In this way we can ask *for whom* and *under what circumstances* was community care more cost-effective than hospital, or was one community care arrangement more cost-effective than another. We have not yet examined the links between costs and outcomes for the 254 clients whose care services are summarised in Table 9.1, but for a subsample of 132 people (who had left hospital up until August 1988 and for whom we had the necessary data), we explored the relationships between costs, outcomes, needs and certain other individual and facility characteristics. Half (49%) of the subsample included in the analysis of cost variations were female, and 22% were of non-white ethnic origin; 69% had never married, and 92% were single, divorced, separated, or widowed. Mean age was 56 years. Mean length of stay in hospital since the most recent admission (at the time of the hospital assessments, not at the time of discharge) was 13 years, and sample members had spent another 5 years on average in previous hospital in-patient stays. The mean number of previous in-patient admissions was 4.4. The most common primary diagnosis (made at first presentation to psychiatric services, coded as per the ICD–9, but collapsed into groups), was schizophrenia (72% of these 132 people). A further 11% had a diagnosis of affective disorder, diagnoses of neurosis and personality disorder were made for 11% and organic disorders for 7%.

Using a cost–function approach, ordinary least-squares regression was employed to explore the causal links between cost and its hypothesised determinants. The method, full results and implications are considered at greater length in another paper (Beecham *et al*, 1991). Four particular hypotheses were addressed, reflecting some current issues in psychiatric practice and community care policy.

Firstly, is there an association between the cost of mental health care and patient or client outcomes? Defining outcomes as changes in the scores on each of the measures of individual health, welfare, and quality of life (such as the PSE and the SBS), it was found that more costly care packages appear to result in better outcomes. For example, a higher score on the various component scales of the PSE indicates worse symptoms of mental illness, so that a negative difference (absolute or relative) between the community and hospital assessments indicates an improvement in health. The analyses show improvements on the PSE measures of negative symptoms, and delusions and hallucinations are associated with higher costs; more costly community care packages have brought about reductions in symptoms. A general broadening of social networks is also associated with greater cost. The overall conclusion was that higher community care costs are linked with better outcomes. This is obviously an encouraging finding at a time when some people are having doubts about running down long-stay hospital provision. The results suggest that spending more on community care will bring about desirable improvements in clients' health and welfare.

The second research question asked whether client needs or problems are related to cost? Do people with greater needs or problems get more support? We use the term *problem* to describe those psychosocial character-istics of clients upon which psychiatric and associated support services are expected to have an impact. If costs summarise, albeit imperfectly, the resources expended or services delivered to clients, how well are services tailored to address these problems? The estimated cost functions indicated that community care costs are sensitive to a variety of client characteristics, including incontinence, mobility, affect, and the absence of certain community-living skills. In each case, greater need, as indicated by the presence of these problems, was associated with higher cost. A second encouraging finding, therefore, was that more is expended through community care services on clients who have more severe problems (but this does not necessarily mean that all their needs are actually being met).

Thirdly, we were interested in intersectoral cost differences. Are public-sector services more costly or less efficient than non-public? Does the high cost of care in health authority facilities, in contrast to facilities run by social services departments, voluntary (non-profit) or private (for-profit) agencies, reflect the creation of environments which encourage client dependency, or at least do not encourage independence? Or, alternatively, is high cost the logical corollary of the tendency for the facilities of health authorities to accommodate those former residents with greater needs? The answer suggested by the cost–outcome analyses is that health authority facilities are more costly than would be expected, and that private and voluntary accommodation placements are less costly than expected. After standardisation for differences in client characteristics, outcomes and needs, costs are still significantly different between the sectors. In fact, we have something approaching an inter-sectoral *efficiency* difference, although more work is needed to explore why this is happening as well as the policy implications.

The fourth and last hypothesis concerned the link between cost and type of accommodation. Once again, cost differences were explored having held constant the effects of outcomes and needs. It was found that residential homes, nursing homes, and hostels (all fairly highly staffed) are more costly than predicted by the cost function, and other facility types less costly.

Predicting the full costs of hospital closure

A third illustration of the use of the CSRI and the costs information it generates in the NETRHA study is the prediction of community reprovision costs for people who have not yet left hospital. We examined statistically the association between community costs and the characteristics of the former in-patients when they were still in hospital. The prediction equation, estimated from multiple regression analysis, was used to extrapolate costs for the full population of Friern and Claybury hospital in-patients, and subsequently for all residents of English psychiatric hospitals (in both cases excluding those who had been in-patients for less than one year or had a diagnosis of dementia). For Friern and Claybury, we concluded that the full costs of community care were marginally *less* than hospital, not just for the first cohorts of leavers, but for the full populations of the two hospitals (Knapp *et al*, 1990). The parallel TAPS research concluded from the client outcomes' analyses that people generally do no worse and possibly slightly better in the community than in hospital (TAPS, 1990). Thus, if the short-term and eventual savings from running down hospitals can be fully or mainly transferred to psychiatric reprovision, and with the added assistance of social security funding, future community care for people with long-term needs should be no worse, and probably marginally better, than hospital.

At the national level, our interest was slightly different. What would be the cost of supporting in the community every long-stay resident in England's psychiatric hospitals? Excluding people with dementia, we estimated that the cost for the approximately 24 000 psychiatric hospital residents would be £271 per person per week (Knapp *et al*, 1992a). This is equivalent to a need for annual community care expenditure of £341 million. From data on the community care packages for the sample of leavers we also calculated the proportion of total community care cost which is allocated to social care, so as to be able to comment on the size of the Mental Illness Specific Grant. Mean social care revenue cost accounted for 12.3% of total community care cost, with social care playing a proportionately larger role in the support of those people with fewer social-behaviour problems and fewer negative psychiatric symptoms. The total revenue cost of social care was calculated to be approximately £33 per person per week, equivalent to a total cost for social care of £42 million per annum. This estimated annual revenue cost covers only one group of clients with mental health problems identified as needing support from agencies providing social care (such as, local authority SSDs) – long-stay hospital residents without a diagnosis of dementia – and so the funding needs of community social care provision are actually considerably greater.

Conclusion

In 1980, in the Foreword to Drummond (1980), Alan Williams suggested that:

> "One cannot but help sympathise with clinicians and other health service professionals who feel that with so many pressures upon them they might at least be spared the distasteful task of having to think about efficiency, and the husbanding of scarce resources, on top of all their other problems". (p. vii)

More than a decade later, the pressure to economise has increased markedly. The cost-effectiveness imperative is stronger than ever. The demands for cost information have grown, and requirements for cost information now permeate all levels of decision-making. Terms and practices such as quality assurance, clinical or management budgeting, value for money audit, devolved case-level budgeting, and purchase of service are not only more common, but serve to emphasise the changed context within which mental health services are planned, delivered and received. As we have argued, the supply of (decent) cost information has not kept pace with the demands which these terminological and practical changes have created. Yet, methods have been developed and banks of data and experience are being constructed to bolster the supply response and to aid cost-sensitive decision-making. There will never be answers to each and every cost question, and there has been comparatively little costs work in psychiatry in the UK, but the distance between what is demanded and what can be supplied appears to be narrowing.

Acknowledgements

Research described in various parts of this chapter has been funded over a number of years by the Department of Health and North East Thames Regional Health Authority, and some has been conducted in collaboration with PSSRU colleagues Caroline Allen and Andrew Fenyo, and with the Team for the Assessment of Psychiatric Services, Friern Hospital, led by Julian Leff. We record our considerable gratitude for this support and assistance, but we bear the sole responsibility for the chapter.

References

ALLEN, C., BEECHAM, J. & KNAPP, M. R. J. (1990) *The Methodology for Costing Community and Hospital Services used by Clients of the Care in the Community Demonstration Programme*, Discussion Paper 647, Personal Social Services Research Unit, University of Kent at Canterbury.
AUDIT COMMISSION (1986) *Making a Reality of Community Care*. London: HMSO.
BEECHAM, J., KNAPP, M. R. J. & FENYO, A. (1991) Costs, needs and outcomes: community care for people with long-term mental health problems. *Schizophrenia Bulletin*, **17**, 188–208.
BRUGHA, T., BEBBINGTON, P., TENNANT, C., *et al* (1985) The list of threatening experiences: a sublist of twelve life event categories with considerable long-term contextual threat. *Psychological Medicine*, **15**, 189–194.
CHALLIS, D. J. & DAVIES, B. P. (1986) *Case Management in Community Care*. Aldershot: Gower.
——— , CHESSUM, R., CHESTERMAN, J., *et al* (1988) Community care for the frail elderly: an urban experiment. *British Journal of Social Work*, **18** (suppl.), 13–42.
CM 849 (1989) *Caring for People: Community Care in the Next Decade and Beyond*. London: HMSO.
DEPARTMENT OF HEALTH (1990) *Caring for People: Community Care in the Next Decade and Beyond*, Policy Guidance. London: HMSO.
DRUMMOND, M. F. (1980) *Principles of Economic Analysis in Health Care*. Oxford: Oxford University Press.
GRANZINI, L., MCFARLAND, B. H. & CUTLER, D. (1990) Prevalence of mental disorders after catastrophic financial loss. *Journal of Nervous and Mental Disease*, **178**, 680–685.
GRIFFITHS, R. (1988) *Community Care: Agenda for Action*. London: HMSO.
HOUSE OF COMMONS (1990) *National Health Service and Community Care Act*. London: HMSO.

JONES, R., GOLDBERG, D. & HUGHES, B. (1980) A comparison of two different services treating schizophrenia: a cost-benefit approach. *Psychological Medicine*, **10**, 493–505.

KNAPP, M. R. J. (1984) *The Economics of Social Care*. London: Macmillan.

—— & ROBERTSON, E. (1989) The costs of child care services: implications for research and policy. In *Child Care Research, Policy and Practice* (ed. B. Kahan). Milton Keynes: Open University Press.

—— & BEECHAM, J. K. (1990) Costing mental health services. *Psychological Medicine*, **20**, 893–908.

—— & —— (1991) Mental health service costs. *Current Opinion in Psychiatry*, **4**, 275–282.

—— & —— (1992) Health economics and psychiatry: the pursuit of efficiency. In *Principles of Social Psychiatry* (eds J. Leff & D. Bhugra). Oxford: Blackwell Scientific Publications.

——, ——, ANDERSON, J., *et al* (1990) The TAPS project. 3: Predicting the community costs of closing psychiatric hospitals. *British Journal of Psychiatry*, **157**, 661–670.

——, ——, GORDON, K., *et al* (1992a) Predicting the community costs of closing psychiatric hospitals. *Journal of Mental Health* (in press).

——, CAMBRIDGE, P., THOMASON, C., *et al* (1992b) *Care in the Community: Challenge and Demonstration*. Aldershot: Avebury.

MANGEN, S. P., PAYKEL, E. S., GRIFFITH, J. H., *et al* (1983) Cost-effectiveness of community psychiatric nurse or out-patient psychiatrist care of neurotic patients. *Psychological Medicine*, **13**, 407–416.

MARKS, I., CONNOLLY, J. & MUIJEN, M. (1988) The Maudsley Daily Living Programme: a controlled cost-effectiveness study of community based versus standard in-patient care of serious mental illness. *Bulletin of the Royal College of Psychiatrists*, **12**, 22–23.

MCCRONE, P., BEECHAM, J. & KNAPP, M. (1992) *Community Psychiatric Nursing in a Community Support Team: A Cost Evaluation of the Greenwich Innovation, Discussion Paper 794* (October). Canterbury: University of Kent at Canterbury, Personal Social Services Research Unit.

MELZER, D., HALE, A. S., MALIK, S. J., *et al* (1991) Community care and schizophrenia: one year after hospital discharge. *British Medical Journal*, **303**, 1023–1026.

NETTEN, A. & BEECHAM, J. (eds) (1992) *Costing Community Care: Theory and Practice*, (working title). Aldershot: Avebury.

RENSHAW, J., HAMPSON, R., THOMASON, C., *et al* (1988) *Care in the Community: The First Steps*. Aldershot: Gower.

STURT, E. & WYKES, T. (1986) Assessment schedules for chronic psychiatric patients. *Psychological Medicine*, **17**, 485–493.

TEAM FOR ASSESSMENT OF PSYCHIATRIC SERVICES (1990) *Better out than in?* London: NETRHA.

—— (1992) The TAPS project: evaluation of community placement of long-stay psychiatric patients. *British Journal of Psychiatry* (in press).

WEISBROD, B. A., STEIN, M. & TEST, L. I. (1980) Alternatives to mental hospital treatment. II. Economic benefit–cost analysis. *Archives of General Psychiatry*, **37**, 400–405.

WING, J. K., COOPER, J. E. & SARTORIUS, N. (1974) *The Measurement and Classification of Psychiatric Symptoms*. Cambridge: Cambridge University Press.

IV. Evaluating the ability of psychiatric services to meet needs

10   Identifying unmet needs: the NHS Health Advisory Service

PHILIP SEAGER

". . . because the two most important things I achieved in my two years here were firstly the setting up of the Hospital Advisory Service. . . . It should be an independent group of people inspecting and reporting to me."
The Diaries of a Cabinet Minister, Volume 3 (Crossman, 1979)

Scandal and outrage have been two words in common usage, particularly by the media, when referring to unfortunate episodes of the mishandling of disabled, sometimes frail, people who are dependent on the support of staff in various institutions. A series of disquieting reports in the 1960s culminated in an inquiry by Sir Geoffrey Howe into practices at Ely Hospital, Cardiff. Richard Crossman, in his Diaries, describes how he had been unaware of this and other worrying episodes, even though the officials in the Department of Health had known of what had been described.

He therefore decided to set up a multidisciplinary inspectorate which would visit each long-stay hospital and report to him directly about the state of clinical practice. Thus was born the Hospital Advisory Service, and it was agreed that there were major disadvantages in developing an inspectorate, resulting in the decision to give the new body an advisory role. It was felt that this would have a much greater ability to influence professional colleagues and carry them along in discussing and evaluating all aspects of clinical work, not only with their separate professions but as a multidisciplinary team working together to achieve the best possible outcome for patients and their care (Freeman, 1990).

Three teams were established, and in 1970 commenced visits to hospitals for the elderly, the mentally ill, and the mentally handicapped in England and Wales. A proportion of hospitals in each region was visited consecutively, enabling a broad overview of services to be described to each Regional Board. Within about four years, all hospitals in the three specialities had been visited, but the service has continued for two decades. Similar hospital advisory services were established for Scotland and for Northern Ireland.

The remit of the Hospital Advisory Service was to examine the range of clinical and hotel services supplied to patients in the relevant hospital, to talk to the various professionals involved, and to be satisfied that the best available use was made of resources. It soon became clear that services for these three groups of individuals should not cease at the hospital gate, and much was to be learned by visits to day hospitals, day centres and other community activities.

By 1976, a new organisation was set up with the Social Services Inspectorate (SSI) (formerly the Social Work Services) of the Department of Health, renamed the Health Advisory Service (HAS). The new body no longer visited services for mentally handicapped individuals, since this was now catered for by the National Development Team for the Mentally Handicapped (NDT) (except in Wales, where the HAS retained these visits for some years). The new HAS/SSI visits continued the model with a team of five or six people – a consultant in the relevant field, administrator, nurse manager, clinical nurse, occupational therapist or physiotherapist, and Social Services Inspector, with, on occasions, a clinical psychologist.

Since 1985 all reports are published jointly by the Health Authority and Local Authority, and it has been possible for a number of studies on the findings of HAS teams to be reported on and critiques of the work of the organisation have appeared (Horrocks, 1987; Day *et al*, 1989; Henkel *et al*, 1989; Denham & Lubel, 1990; Seager, 1991).

Since the inception of the HAS, the practice has been for the Director to be medically qualified with an alternation between psychiatrist and physician in geriatric medicine seconded from their work for a period of three to four years. The principle underlying the selection of teams and Director is that these are professionals in active clinical practice or recently retired, of senior status and considerable experience, with a broad knowledge of current clinical issues, bringing their own experience and expertise to membership of the team. There are no specific HAS policies, despite popular belief to the contrary.

Aims and objectives

The middle word of the title is *advisory*, and the responsibility for deciding priorities must lie with the authorities locally. The HAS will draw attention to deficiencies in the particular services with which it is concerned, but it would be impossible to take over the responsibility for deciding priorities without knowing the full range of issues confronting the district. Cries for 'teeth' for the HAS always seem to me to fly in the face of this important consideration. The HAS does not avoid pointing out that adequate health services for elderly and mentally ill people include the provision of the full range of hospital services for acute admissions and an extensive rehabilitation service for the majority of people after assessment.

An important feature of the visit is the assessment of the interaction between various components of the total service. Any complex organisation dealing with the provision of health and personal care for extensive populations cannot avoid splitting into divisions, sectors, segments, localities, buildings, units, wards, and homes. Many advantages lie with such subdivisions, allowing a small group of people to provide a service for a discrete population. Difficulties arise when people refuse to fit neatly into one pigeonhole or another. Beautiful drawings of management charts are effectively reduced to a tangle of wool in the hands of a small child when that child has learning difficulties, the mother is schizophrenic, the father an out-of-work alcoholic living apart from the family but returning periodically to beat the mother and abuse the child, while the demented grandfather sits rocking in the corner, or setting the place on fire in attempting to make a cup of tea.

The HAS establishes that there are clear lines of communication between managers and clinicians, the Health Authority and the Social Services Department, professional staff and volunteers, the hospital and the community service, and the many other components of the complex of services that such a family may need. It is not sufficient to say, "We have a policy"; the policy must work all day and every day.

Observations of the HAS teams

One of the more striking conclusions is that it is almost impossible to find, or even to define, a standard psychiatric service. Districts vary in size from 100 000 population to nearly one million, many largely rural or largely urban, but with the majority having a mixture of both. Some populations are cohesive with well marked local characteristics, while others are multiracial, multicultural and multireligious. Some services are almost entirely mental-hospital based, others have psychiatric units in district general hospitals, while a growing number are developing community mental health centres for each locality. Some newly created districts have taken the opportunity to shake off dependence on a distant mental hospital and have developed local services for new patients and accepted responsibility for the long-term care of former residents of the district in a distant mental hospital; a proportion of these large mental hospitals are scheduled to close within five years.

The majority of psychiatrists still see hospital beds as an important component of any district or locality service, but an increasing number, together with a much larger proportion of nurses, believe that highly staffed local community services, possibly with a few crisis beds, can cope with all the problems a district is likely to offer. Various patterns of service are developing, sometimes in a random fashion throughout the country.

The complexity of district services may arise as a result of the drive and enthusiasm of particular individuals, new ideas forced on a district by closure of an out-of-district mental hospital, financial and property-led constraints, or some combination of all of these. A balance has to be struck between two differing theories about relevant psychiatric services. On the one hand there is the localised community mental health service dealing with a population of perhaps 30 000, usually urban and closely linked with the primary health-care teams of the locality, reliant on the provision of a general service to the majority of people and expecting to deal with virtually all the problems within the community mental health team. The alternative pattern of care is a more centralised, specialised, often hospital-based, secondary psychiatric service composed of a number of sector teams, each taking on in addition a district-wide specialist service – rehabilitation, alcohol and drug abuse, etc.

The role of age-related psychiatry, both child and adolescent which tends to link more with paediatric than with general psychiatry, and psychiatry of the elderly which, while it has some links with the medical geriatricians, usually retains its base within the psychiatric services, may pose particular problems to both of these models. In many districts, general psychiatrists see all or some of the older patients. Occasionally, one sees the pattern of general psychiatrists with specific sessions defined for care of the elderly. More commonly, the development of an age-related policy, when one or more consultants take on clinical responsibility for all patients with organic psychiatric conditions, including some under the age of 65, and have their own assessment and treatment unit for functional illness in the elderly, is becoming much more commonplace. The clinical team takes on responsibility for planning services, organising their developing needs and reinforcing links with appropriate professional groups such as the geriatricians, the district nurses, the home care and other social-services' staff, and the general practitioners and the primary health-care team.

While all these changes in organisation and management have been developing over recent years, the quality and style of services has been improving only gradually. Mental hospitals have been closing, and with the loss of large, grim, impersonal wards has also gone the loss of pleasant gardens, open spaces, regular meals, and opportunities to behave bizarrely without too much comment. Many former mental-hospital residents who have been questioned about the loss of these 'homes' in which they lived for several years, have usually preferred the alternative of a share in a small house with acceptance of personal responsibility for their own ways of living. It is not easy to get a detailed balance sheet of the advantages of differing ways of living and their effects on the different people living in them. Probably the most important issue is to ensure the level of support and encouragement which may or may not have been present in the large institutions is available for the more isolated individuals living 'in the community'.

Two decades ago, psychiatry was on its way back to rejoining the medical profession, assisted by the presence of psychiatric units in the general hospitals. For many years there had been out-patient clinics, but often there was little or no contact between the visiting psychiatrists and the other clinic users except as a useful disposal service responding to the Department of Health recommendation that all patients who had taken drug overdoses and carried out other forms of self-harm should have a psychiatric assessment. As psychiatric wards appeared, so some psychiatrists attended clinical seminars in the postgraduate medical centre, and appeared at lunch in the staff dining room. Opportunities became available to ask advice from these psychiatrists about the management of someone who had been thoroughly investigated for chest pain and no abnormality found; general nurses could discuss with their psychiatric nursing colleagues the problem of the painfully thin girl who had been investigated for weight loss and seemed to eat well on the ward but still did not put on weight. Such patients could be casualties of the move to the community, where the psychiatric team is now developing links with the primary health-care team in health centres, and offering a range of management programmes for the people disparagingly referred to as the 'worried well'.

Because of the large number of individuals involved, whether in the field of liaison psychiatry in the general hospital or in treatment of individuals with disturbing, if not disabling, psychiatric symptoms in the community, in the end the solution to the problem must lie with the Colleges of Medicine and of Nursing. Too much emphasis has been placed on the need to make a physical diagnosis in the first instance and to be sure that such a diagnosis is excluded before considering the possibility of 'a psychological overlay'. Before one can consider a doctor, a nurse, a social worker, or an occupational therapist adequately trained, it should be incumbent that they can each in their different ways identify the physical, psychological, and social components of their patient's condition. Several professions claim a unique attitude of holistic care of each individual; they decry the 'medical model', a vague but pejorative description of a narrow focus of inappropriate treatment. All need to bring into effect a range of treatment possibilities depending on the identification of the different components of the problem, either dealing with all aspects themselves or calling in colleagues to deal with the identified elements.

Standards of care

A continuing argument during the existence of the HAS has been the advisability of setting out defined criteria for appropriate clinical care and environmental conditions. Such norms and standards have formed the basis of accreditation of hospitals in the United States of America, in Canada, Australia (World Health Organization, 1991), and more recently in the organisational audit carried out by the King's Fund in Britain. The idea of a minimum standard has been resisted for a number of reasons. Defined criteria are often difficult to specify in terms of the particular circumstances obtaining in the ward, the unit, or the hostel visited. Variation may be found between different shifts, between day and night, and dependent more on the quality of staff than on numbers. Five poor-quality staff may or may not be better than two excellent ones. Perhaps in psychiatry more than in other specialities there is much more exchangeability between different professions and different levels of qualification. An experienced assistant nurse may be more effective at making relationships than a neophyte staff nurse; a community psychiatric nurse may offer the necessary expertise in a particular setting, albeit not replacing the different contributions of a social worker. These issues may be compounded by recruitment problems for one profession compared with another, resulting in the rise and fall in the work of one therapeutic field compared with another.

In extreme situations, problems are apparent. No-one would be satisfied with overcrowded dormitories without personal space and room for personal possessions; no-one would accept as appropriate the absence of any form of therapeutic care other than dispensing of medication three times a day. It is less easy to define the other end of the continuum, and even more difficult to pinpoint the transition from unacceptable to acceptable in terms of a specific criterion.

The change in the pattern of care can itself produce deficiencies in the appropriate level of support. Because of the complex nature of arrangements for continuing personal and health care, the change from hospital to community services has not always been able to carry along with it the necessary altered patterns of provision of the different service requirements. A more rapid assessment and acute treatment in hospital of elderly people with mental illness has resulted in a greater demand for specialist community psychiatric nurses, social workers, home care staff, day centres, lunch clubs, transport, and help and advice for carers than may be readily available. Furthermore, with the division of services into a hospital unit, possibly a self-governing trust, and social services and voluntary provision in the community, as well as the primary health-care team, communication between the various components in terms of immediate needs and, in some ways more importantly, in planning and projecting the demands for necessary staff and other resources, often falls behind the immediate decision of the therapeutic team to discharge a particular individual. The solution of this problem by recourse to private institutional care of one kind or another may firstly be unsuitable for the particular individual, and, secondly, may be an unacceptable decision once proper assessment is to be made under the terms of the community-care provisions.

Conclusions

At the time of major changes in the National Health Service, brought about by the *NHS and Community Care Act* 1990, the HAS is also undergoing a change. It is constructive to examine what has gone before in order to improve what is to come next. The Secretary of State has taken the decision to continue the work of the Health Advisory Service, with its responsibility for monitoring services for the elderly and mentally ill people in hospital and in the community. It will be available to advise purchasers of the relevant services and will also be used by the Secretary of State in those instances where services may be suspect. It may be asked to concentrate on specific aspects of a service, or on particular client groups.

A review of two decades of the HAS brings the inevitable question, one that is asked by many team members, staff, and perhaps, not least, by professional colleagues and families of those team members who disappear for a month at a time to unfamiliar parts of the country. What has the HAS achieved? What does the HAS achieve now? To answer 'nothing' would be entirely incorrect; to suggest that the HAS has been responsible for the major changes in psychiatric practice over the past 20 years would be foolish and untrue. Evidence for the value of the HAS can be found from local discussions, during which information is given on the changes brought about by earlier visits and the welcome for a further opportunity of sharing ideas. Suspicion and mistrust did occur in the early days of the Hospital Advisory Service, but a more mature attitude towards discussion of problems and issues, and an acceptance of fellow professionals specifically selected from more distant regions, is a welcome improvement in the ethos of the visit and therefore its value to the district.

The HAS team may find its support is canvassed for the development of particular services which have been held in abeyance, often for financial reasons, in competition with other demands. It is the responsibility of the Authority to make the final decision, but the fact that this team has supported the need for an enhanced community psychiatric nursing service or the development of a locality base for a community mental health group may be sufficient added pressure for a priority service to be given priority.

Almost without exception, team members comment on the valuable educational experience participation in the HAS has been for the particular individual. This is an aggregation of discussion with a wide range of colleagues, patients, carers and volunteers in a confidential context and an opportunity to exchange ideas with team colleagues at a much more intensive level than is usually available. Alex Baker, the first Director, mentioned it (Freeman, 1990), and the same message is still received.

Major changes in the National Health Service, with the development of clinical audit, quality assurance specialists, and with the purchasers having responsibility for ensuring that the needs of the community are being met by the providers, suggest that all the issues on which the HAS concentrated will now be assured at a local level. Ultimately, this should be so, but experience has indicated that, while many people may be aware of problems, a series of anxieties, of vested interests, of apathy and of carelessness militate against the best interests of those people whose condition may inhibit their opportunities for comment and complaint.

To work effectively, there may well be changes. Advantage could be derived from enhanced training in the assessment of services within a district, interaction with the staff providing that service, and the formulation of clear, concise and well presented advice. Such activities cost money and, perhaps more importantly, take up the time of busy people, whether team members or HAS permanent staff. At the moment, the HAS uses the expertise and authority of senior people already in demand for membership of the other 'Inspection Industries', such as the Royal College accreditation teams, nursing validation visits for the English and Welsh National Boards, and the Mental Health Act Commission. The value of the work of teams and the reports they produce will stand or fall by the recognition that membership of a team has educational value for those participating and is therefore worthwhile to the releasing Authorities, as well as an important, constructive and effective review of services for a particular Health District. It is in the interests of all concerned, and not least the patients and their carers, that standards are frequently and effectively reviewed by a group whose opinion is appreciated and respected.

References

CROSSMAN, R. (1977) *The Diaries of a Cabinet Minister. Vol 3: Secretary of State for Social Services*. London: Hamish Hamilton Ltd. (With kind permission of the publishers, Hamish Hamilton Ltd.)

DAY, P., KLEIN, R. & TIPPING, S. (1988) *Inspecting for Quality*. Bath: University of Bath Centre for the Analysis of Social Policy.

DENHAM, M. & LUBEL, D. (1990) Peer review and services for elderly patients. *British Medical Journal*, **300**, 1635–1636.

FREEMAN, H. (1990) Interview: in conversation with A. Baker. *Psychiatric Bulletin*, **14**, 386–394.

HENKEL, M., KOGAN, M., PARKWOOD, T., *et al* (1989) *The Health Advisory Service: an Evaluation*. London: King Edward's Hospital Fund.

HORROCKS, P. (1987) *Health Advisory Service Annual Report*. Sutton: NHS Health Advisory Service.

SEAGER, P. (1991) General consideration regarding external independent reviews with a description of the health advisory services of England and Wales. In *National Perspectives on Quality Assurance in Mental Health Care* (ed. J. Orley). Geneva: WHO Division of Mental Health.

WORLD HEALTH ORGANIZATION (1991) *National Perspectives on Quality Assurance in Mental Health Care*. Geneva: Division of Mental Health.

11 Assessing systems of care for the long-term mentally ill in urban settings

M. SUSAN RIDGELY, HOWARD H. GOLDMAN and JOSEPH P. MORRISSEY

Measuring the perceived needs of a community for mental health services can serve as a valuable complement to a direct assessment of the needs of individuals. Often it is too difficult or too expensive to assess the needs of a population directly, and an indirect survey of the opinion of key informants about the need for services in the community may usefully substitute for a direct assessment. Several indirect approaches are being employed to assess systems of care for the long-term mentally ill in the evaluation of a service demonstration sponsored by The Robert Wood Johnson Foundation in nine large cities in the United States. This chapter describes this demonstration programme and its evaluation, focusing in particular on a key-informant survey used to assess changes in the system of care. In the process, we attempt to explain its relevance to mental health services assessment and planning in the United States and the United Kingdom.

Background

The organisation and financing of mental health care in the United States is complex, especially when contrasted with the centralised UK National Health Service. In the United States, public mental health care is provided by an array of public and private mental health facilities, financed by an equally perplexing array of funding sources, including federal, state, and local-government categorical funds and public (Medicaid and Medicare) and private health insurance.

A nationwide system of state mental hospitals, first built in the second decade of the 19th century, dominated public mental health care for many years. By the early 20th century the US had become the locus of public responsibility for mental health care. Following World War II, with the community mental health centre movement of the 1960s, and the subsequent community-support movement of the late 1970s and early 1980s, responsibility for mental health care became more diffuse as the focus broadened from state mental hospitals to community general hospitals and other community-based facilities, and from the treatment needs to the social welfare needs of severely mentally ill persons in the community. Alarmed by the release of thousands of patients from state mental hospitals to alternative community settings, critics of the policy of deinstitutionalisation pointed to the widespread neglect of the needs of severely mentally ill persons. Patients were faced with obtaining care in a highly differentiated system where many critical supportive services were either non-existent or fragmented and poorly funded. Increasingly, then, since the 1980s, the focus in the development of mental health policy has been on the need to coordinate fragmented systems of care in local communities. The focus has been on pushing the locus of public responsibility for mental health care to the most local of geopolitical entities, in the case of the United States, city and county government.

The Robert Wood Johnson Foundation Program

In the autumn of 1985, The Robert Wood Johnson Foundation, the largest private health-care philanthropy in the United States, announced the Program on Chronic Mental Illness, one of the foundation's largest health-care initiatives and its first initiative in mental health care (Shore & Cohen, 1990). The Program, funded in 1987 for five years, has been contributing $29 million in grants and low interest loans to nine demonstration sites[1]. The demonstration is designed as a test of comprehensive systemic changes in the organisation, financing, and delivery of mental health and other supportive services to individuals with severe mental illness. Nine cities were chosen to participate in the five-year demonstration: three on the east coast (Baltimore, Maryland; Philadelphia, Pennsylvania; and Charlotte, North Carolina); three in the midwest (Columbus, Cincinnati, and Toledo, Ohio); and three in the west (Denver, Colorado; Austin, Texas; and Honolulu, Hawaii).

Earlier reforms of public mental health systems focused on the need to address the individual's social welfare needs as well as their mental health needs by including housing, income support, and vocational programmes explicitly. The Robert Wood Johnson Foundation Program on Chronic Mental Illness went beyond advocating for a more inclusive view of the mental health system of care by proposing that major organisational and financing changes may be necessary to ensure the delivery of that care. In

---

1. A 'site' of the demonstration is the city or county recipient of the grant from The Robert Wood Johnson Foundation, the specified benefits from the federal government, and ongoing technical assistance from the Program Office (Miles Shore, MD and Martin Cohen, MSW of the Massachusetts Mental Health Center in Boston).

the 20 years before the demonstration, state, federal, and local funding sources had allowed localities to develop services, many of which were outside the bounds of the public mental health system. These 'systems' of services included a variety of providers, none of whom bore ultimate responsibility for meeting the needs of severely mentally ill persons. The Robert Wood Johnson Foundation Program focused on the need for coordination and integration of services and each city in the demonstration was expected to create a local mental health authority, which would constitute an organisational locus of responsibility for the care of severely mentally ill adults in the geographical area. (The approach to managing mental health care proposed by RWJ is built loosely on the experience of public authorities. See Walsh & Leigland (1986). For a more complete discussion of the concept of a local mental health authority within the RWJ Program on Chronic Mental Illness see Shore & Cohen (1990) and Goldman *et al* (1990).) According to the application guidelines and subsequent documents, the authority was described as:

> "An entity combining public accountability with the flexibility of the private sector (public accountability to ensure continuation of the public funding that pays for the greatest part of services and private-sector flexibility to solve the problems created by the civil service, legislative and political constraints on public operation of services)." (Shore & Cohen, 1990)

Thus, the intervention in this demonstration goes beyond the development of a specialised programme, but, instead, includes governmental and organisational changes in each city/county site, integrating both decision-making and service delivery for severely mentally ill persons, including housing, disability, rehabilitation, financing, and crisis management 'interventions'. The local mental health authorities were intended to assume fiscal, clinical, and administrative responsibility for meeting the treatment, housing and supportive-care needs of these persons. Specifically:

> "As a single point of administrative, clinical and fiscal responsibility, the authority is fully accountable for all aspects of the organization and functioning of the system of care: which services are provided, including which are purchased versus which are provided directly by the authority; which consumers are served and by which providers; how consumers are served; and finally, how the available resources, including finances, are allocated to serve consumers." (Shore & Cohen, 1990)

Once in place, the local mental health authority was expected to plan and implement a series of system-improvement strategies or activities directed at improving service delivery to severely mentally ill persons. The development of affordable housing for severely mentally ill persons is a particular focus of the demonstration. The US Department of Housing and

Urban Development (HUD) is a co-sponsor of the demonstration and is contributing approximately $85 million in federal rental subsidies (Section 8 housing vouchers).

The development of a local mental health authority is central to the demonstration. The Robert Wood Johnson Foundation identified the lack of such an authority as one of the main problems in the delivery of mental health care in urban areas. During the 1960s, under the Community Mental Health Centers (CMHC) programme, *catchment areas* divided jurisdictions across large cities, and often represented barriers to access for severely mentally ill people. Some clients simply were not fortunate enough to live in a catchment area equipped with the particular service they needed. Others were mobile across catchment area boundaries with no CMHC or speciality mental health agency taking responsibility for their care. Issues of availability and accessibility dominated the discussion of the shortfalls of this and other federal programmes delivering health and social services to the poor.

The Robert Wood Johnson Foundation Program represents an important social reform on behalf of individuals with severe mental illness. It builds on experimental evidence that cost-effective treatments can be developed and administered in community settings (Weisbrod *et al*, 1980; Hoult & Reynolds, 1984) and on quasi-experimental evidence that governmental intervention can put community support systems into place in states and local communities (Tessler & Goldman, 1982). There is considerable evidence, however, that large metropolitan areas are failing to care for persons with severe mental illness adequately. The reasons for these historic and current failures have been enumerated elsewhere (Goldman & Morrissey, 1985; Mechanic, 1991) and, in the particular case of large cities, focus on the effects of bureaucracy, entrenched interests and 'perverse financial incentives' over a more reasonable approach to delivering services. This demonstration of services not only provides a test of a remedy to this problem in large urban areas but also provides an opportunity for a programme of research to be conducted by a large number of investigators at multiple sites, integrated into a national evaluation.

Relevance of RWJ model to the UK situation

The specifics of the national evaluation will be discussed below. First, however, it seems germane briefly to address the relevance of the RWJ Program model to the current situation in the UK. Recent changes in National Health Service (NHS) policy, as a result of the government White Papers, are stimulating variations in the organisation and financing of public health care. With the advent of self-governing trusts, health authorities are now in the position of contracting for, as well as providing, health services. As some health authorities move to a more decentralised system of care, involving multiple providers, including voluntary organisations, the issues of coordination of care will arise.

In addition, the Audit Commission Report (1986) makes reference to the need for better coordination of services across district health authority and local authority social-services boundaries. While much recent discussion has focused on the use of 'key workers', analogous to case managers in the US systems, undoubtedly some attempt will be made to cope with the larger structural and financing barriers that result from the lack of one authority responsible for the community mental health and social-welfare needs of severely mentally ill persons. (For a discussion of the origins and uses of case management in a variety of human services, see Willenbring *et al* (1991).) The development of 'community support systems' (CSS) for severely mentally ill persons may have been an American concept, but it seems clear that District Health Authorities will need to address the social welfare, housing, and vocational, as well as mental health treatment, needs of the mentally ill in their local communities. Joint planning has not been a successful mechanism for many communities, raising the possibility that alterations in the organisation of care may be deemed necessary to make the most efficient use of health and welfare dollars. It is precisely the need for one authority for mental health and social-services support that produced the RWJ model, although each of the demonstration sites implemented the concept of a centralised mental health authority in their own way, based on local conditions and opportunities.

The design of the national evaluation

The principal objective of the national evaluation is to assess the impact of interventions associated with the development of a local mental health authority in each of the demonstration cities. The evaluation assesses whether organisational and financing changes at the city level result in improved systems of care for those with severe mental illness, and whether mature systems (later in the demonstration) are able to produce greater continuity of care. The evaluation is an agenda of research more than it is an 'evaluation' in the narrowest sense of the word. The national evaluation comprises five inter-related components: a site-level study, a community-care study, housing studies, financing studies, and disability studies. Table 11.1 outlines the five components and Table 11.2 lists data sources and instruments used in these studies.

It is not possible to discuss each of these studies at length. Therefore we will focus on the study most germane to the issue of measurement of needs, the key-informant survey within the site-level study, and will explain the method and the relationship of this aspect of the site-level findings to client outcomes.

TABLE 11.1

Research components of the national evaluation of the Robert Wood Johnson Foundation Program on Chronic Mental Illness

Component	Features
1 Study of the mental health authority and the systems of care	political and administrative changes implementation of innovative services inter-organisational coordination
2 Community care	individual client assessment of symptoms, functioning, and quality of life quasi-experimental, pre-post design needs, service use, and continuity of care
3 Housing studies	site-level assessment of housing development (finance and acquisition) effect of housing arrangements and residential supportive services on individual outcomes in terms of functioning and quality of life use of special rental subsidies
4 Financing studies	effect of mix of revenue sources and financial incentives on services patterns of utilisation and costs
5 Disability and vocational studies	acquisition of benefits for disabled individuals effect of vocational rehabilitation on employment

Developing the key-informant survey

As the view of providing for the needs of chronically mentally ill persons has broadened, beyond 'treatment' to ensuring that basic life needs (such as those for food and shelter) are met, the view of what constitutes the system of mental health service has also broadened. Rather than the traditional delivery system for mental health services, the concept of a 'community support system' (CSS) is central to current programme development efforts (Turner & TenHoor, 1978; Tessler & Goldman, 1982). This concept encompasses a much more complex reality because of the sheer number and types of providers (e.g. mental health, social welfare, employment, housing, rehabilitation, and criminal justice) operating in the system of care.

Systems concepts for describing service delivery (such as availability, accessibility, accountability, adequacy, quality, continuity, comprehensiveness, and viability) have become well-accepted in the health and mental health service arenas. These key service variables, taken together, define a 'good' service-delivery system, as opposed to simply a set of 'good' services. Despite widespread acceptance of these concepts of good system performance, survey methods for assessing the capacity and performance of service systems for severely mentally ill persons are not well developed. After looking for an established instrument without success, a 'key informant survey' was developed to obtain performance ratings of the local service system from knowledgeable persons in each of the demonstration sites. (The idea for this

TABLE 11.2

Data sources and instruments for the national evaluation of the Robert Wood Johnson Foundation Program on Chronic Mental Illness

Study component	Data sources	Instruments
Site-level study	Documents	
	Site visits	
	Key-informant survey	Assessing local service systems for chronically mentally ill persons
Community-care study	Management information system	
	Client interviews	Community-care client questionnaire (baseline and follow-up)[1]
	Case-manager interviews	Case-manager questionnaire[2]
Housing studies		
site level	Documents	
	Site visits	
	Housing management information system	
client level		
community care	Client interviews	Community-care client questionnaire[1]
Section 8	Client interviews	Section 8 questionnaire (identical to community-care client questionnaire follow-up)
Financing studies		
site level	Site visits	
	Financial reports	
	Budgets	
	Management information system	
Medicaid	State Medicaid plan	
	State Medicaid files	
Disability and vocational rehabilitation studies		
site level	Site visits	
client level	Social Security Administration pilot study	

1. Derived from the Quality of Life (Lehman, 1988), Denver CMI Consumer Questionnaire (Demmler *et al*, 1988), Uniform Client Data Instrument (Goldstrom & Manderscheid, 1984), Continuity of Care Provider Questionnaire (Tessler, 1987), Symptom Checklist (SCL-90) (Derogatis & Cleary, 1977), and American Housing Survey (US Department of Commerce, 1989).
2. Derived from the Uniform Client Data Instrument (Goldstrom & Manderscheid, 1984) and Continuity of Care Provider Questionnaire (Tessler, 1987).

type of survey came from earlier research on CSS programmes in New York State (Morrissey *et al*, 1986). In that study, respondents were asked to rate the extent of service-delivery problems, but the range of items was quite limited.)

We recognised that these surveys would yield only relatively 'soft' measures of system capacity and performance. Short of a large-scale epidemiological survey in each demonstration community, however, there is no easy and reliable way of measuring service needs. Nor is there any straightforward way of assessing the adequacy of a service system in meeting such needs. A survey of key informants (participants and stakeholders) in each site provides a broad base of informed judgements about the service system's performance. We reasoned that, by obtaining these judgements at two points in time (mid-1989 and mid-1991), we could assess the extent to which system performance is perceived to have changed during the course of the demonstration. Then, by combining these ratings with information from other components of the evaluation, we could develop a reasonably comprehensive assessment of the demonstration projects.

In addition to the key-informant survey, the site-level evaluation team is employing three other methods to collect data pertinent to organisational and service-system changes. These include periodic interviews with local RWJ Program staff to obtain updates on the status of the local mental health authority and other system improvements; site visits to obtain assessments of mid-course corrections; and an inter-organisational network study to obtain quantitative measures of the centrality of the local mental health authority and system coordination in five of the nine cities. (This separate study, funded by the National Institute for Mental Health, is being conducted by Robert Paulson (University of Cincinnati) and Joseph Morrissey (University of North Carolina at Chapel Hill), Co-Principal Investigators. RO1 MH 44839.) A variety of contextual information is also available through secondary sources.

Our approach to the development of the key-informant survey was informed by a number of sources. First, the goals of the RWJ Program on Chronic Mental Illness, as reflected in application materials (Program for the Chronically Mentally Ill, 1985), and associated published reports (Aiken *et al*, 1986), were reviewed to identify the relevant domains and dimensions of the interventions. Next, on the basis of this analysis, we developed a template for conducting site visits to each of the nine cities. These visits, in turn, provided an initial view of the systems of care through the eyes of local stakeholders and a range of ideas about the ingredients and criteria for service-system performance. We then looked at the available literature for instruments to measure service-system capacity and performance and for characterisations of well-developed service 'systems' that would help us construct items for inclusion in the questionnaire. (Two such instruments deserve mention. First, the Denver CMI Initiative Attitude Survey (Wilson *et al*, 1988) influenced our thinking on how to ask about specific service-delivery problems. We used some of these questions, added others and rearranged the questions along specific categories of service. Second, the work of Grusky & Tierney (1988) influenced the development of our section on service-system performance. (See, for example, Walsh & Leigland, 1986; Dickey & Goldman, 1986; Mechanic & Aiken, 1987.)) From these reviews we developed an extensive list of items which were then revised, grouped under the various system concepts, and organised as indicated below.

Construction of the survey

The key-informant survey, Assessing Local Service Delivery Systems for Chronically Mentally Ill Persons, was constructed to have five discrete parts. The basic building blocks of the instrument allow us to tap the respondents' informed judgements about three key areas: client needs, service-system performance, and the specific performance of the local mental health authority.

The questionnaire yielded both quantitative and qualitative data. The quantitative data are derived from a series of Likert-type scale items that relate to several distinct constructs. The first section was designed to provide an indication of client needs or the extent to which persons with a severe mental illness were experiencing service-delivery problems. This section probes the types of problems encountered with regard to the eleven CSS elements. The eleven CSS service elements include the basic services believed to be essential to maintain severely mentally ill persons in the community, and they include: outreach services, emergency services, mental health treatment services, psychosocial rehabilitation services, case management, assistance with basic human needs, vocational and prevocational services, shelter/housing, medical/dental care, substance-abuse services, and supportive services (peer and family support). Respondents are asked to indicate whether certain situations are occurring in their community and, if so, their judgement of the severity of the problem. The following examples of items are illustrative.

To what extent are the following problems occurring for chronically mentally ill (CMI) persons in City A:

(a) not having access to in-patient services because there are too few public in-patient beds
(b) not having access to adequate amounts of food and clean clothing
(c) lacking opportunities for vocational training or sheltered work.

In the next section, the respondent is asked specifically to rate the adequacy and quality of existing services within each of the 11 service categories. Adequacy is examined by asking how many of those who need each service are getting it (all, most, some, few, none) and quality is measured by asking respondents to consider the technical and interpersonal aspects of care and the physical setting. Respondents are not rating the care given by particular facilities, but rather making global judgements about care in these categories across the city. The next section of the questionnaire is devoted to measuring current service-system performance, in terms of availability and accessibility, as well as the level of coordination of services and information. Respondents are asked to assess how well the current service system performs on a number of dimensions. Some examples of items include:

> How well does the current service system for CMI persons in City A perform on these activities?
>> avoiding excessive waiting lists or long delays in scheduling
>> providing services at reasonable cost to CMI persons
>> training staff to work caringly and comfortably with CMI persons
>> developing agreements between agencies at the level of direct-service delivery to avoid needless duplication of effort.

The final section focuses on the performance of the mental health authority, with regard to its structure and administrative effectiveness, its role in articulating a clinical plan for services to the target population, and its success in securing and coordinating the flow of fiscal resources to individual service providers.

Qualitative data are obtained in the last section of the questionnaire in the form of several open-ended questions about the major accomplishments and shortcomings of the local RWJ Program. These data are a rich source of detail and observations that are complementary to the numerical data provided in the main body of the questionnaire.

The respondents

The respondent pool was developed in consultation with the RWJ Program staff at each of the nine sites. The process was iterative. We relied upon the concept of a community support system and its associated functions to ascertain the sectors from which knowledgeable respondents could be identified. For most agencies the key informant was to be the chief executive officer (CEO), but for some more centrally involved agencies, multiple points of view were sought. (One of the reasons to seek multiple points of view within an agency is the prevailing view that issues may be differentially perceived depending on one's place in the agency (i.e., the 'front lines' versus the 'top floor').) We reviewed the lists created by the Program staff, adding and substituting agencies and informants where appropriate. We sought to apply the same selection criteria and sampling strategy in each city (regardless of the boundaries of the service system as viewed by local participants) so that cross-site comparisons would be meaningful.

Finally, the key-informant survey was pretested in Rochester, New York, in collaboration with the Monroe-Livingston Demonstration Project. This site was chosen because a capitation financing project, being operated by Integrated Mental Health, Inc., is a demonstration of systems reorganisation in the mental health field, similar to, but not a part of, the RWJ Program.

While the focus of the reorganisation in Rochester is a particular financing mechanism, Integrated Mental Health acts as a local mental health authority, managing and coordinating services much as the authorities in the RWJ sites are doing. The pretest indicated that the key-informant instrument had face validity to participants in the various sectors and could be administered as a mailed questionnaire with an acceptable response rate after two follow-ups.

Findings from the key-informant survey

Information concerning analysis of the data from the key-informant survey, as well as the specific findings from the first wave of data collection (mid-1989), have been reported elsewhere (Morrissey *et al*, 1990). Briefly, the findings indicate that key goals of the Robert Wood Johnson Foundation Program were being addressed in the sites. While respondents indicated that dramatic improvements had occurred in specific services (e.g. outreach, housing, and case management), their ratings of service-system performance also indicated that there continued to be significant problems in service coordination across the demonstration cities. Clearly respondents felt that much more work was needed. Respondents in most cities gave high marks to the mental health authorities created under the RWJ Program. These ratings may have reflected enthusiasm for the Program and optimism about the prospect of change early in the demonstration. Of course there were significant differences between sites, reflecting the differences in service-system development between the nine cities.

We are currently collecting a second wave of data (mid-1991) to obtain another set of service-system performance ratings at the end of the demonstration. This will provide us a way of comparing 'early' with 'late' ratings of key informants, providing an assessment of the extent to which service-system performance changed over the course of the demonstration. This, when taken together with findings from the other components of the national evaluation, will provide guidance for improving systems of care for people with severe mental illnesses.

Other methods for assessing needs

The key-informant survey is not the only tool used in the evaluation to measure the need for services, and several of the component studies examine the extent to which the identified needs of individual clients are met. Furthermore, the key-informant survey is only one element in the assessment of changes in the system of care in each city. Each element is designed to characterise the implementation of innovation and to predict (or explain) the impact of changes in the system of care on individual client outcomes.

First, each administration of the key-informant survey was preceded by a three-day site visit to each city. The visit was conducted by two or three members of the site-level evaluation team who spoke with stakeholders (e.g. providers, consumers, government officials, etc.) serving analogous roles in each site. Additional visits were made to study special aspects of the demonstration, including the mechanisms for financing services or developing new housing units. The site visits provided more detail than could be gained from a questionnaire and more comprehensive observations of actual services and interactions among individuals. The key-informant surveys confirmed a great many observations made during the more subjective site visits. They also suggested aspects of the demonstration that we had not seen, or raised questions that required further inquiry. While believing in the strength of site visiting as an evaluation tool (Silverman *et al*, 1990), we have noted some problems. For example, the data from the key-informant survey in one site indicated that the larger group of respondents in that site were more positive about the demonstration than was evident at the site visit. This discrepancy suggests limits of these data-collection strategies. While civic pride in this community may have artificially inflated responses, site visits can reach only a limited number of informants. Consequently, we feel strongly that site visiting and key-informant surveys are complementary, rather than alternative, methods for collecting qualitative data on programme implementation.

Second, data from the key-informant surveys and site visits are supplemented by documentary evidence (e.g. annual reports, planning reports, government documents, newspaper accounts) used in further assessment of programme implementation. Third, a study of inter-organisational networks and how they may have changed over the course of the demonstration completes our assessment of the development of a system of services.

Our design then calls for us to describe and assess these changes at the system (or site) level and predict what kind of impact these changes might have on individual client outcomes (in terms of symptoms, functioning, and quality of life). Client outcomes are assessed using self-reports in structured interviews. Clients are asked about their needs (what needs they have identified for themselves and what needs have been identified by others), what services they have received to meet these needs, and how they felt about the services they received. Service utilisation data (e.g. patterns of use) will be analysed to describe *continuity* in episodes of care. The relationships between client outcomes, continuity of care, exposure to particular services and service agencies, and the nature of system coordination (based on data from the site-visits, the key-informant survey, and the inter-organisational analysis) will be studied. Taken together, these analyses constitute an integrated evaluation of the RWJ Program on Chronic Mental Illness.

The results of these assessments may be used to guide the planning of future mental health services, as well as making mid-course corrections in the current system of services. The key-informant survey was constructed to capture information about the eleven elements of a community-support system. Data about client needs and system performance in each of these 11 areas can be translated into recommendations for the enhancement of specific service domains. For example, if the needs for housing are being met and the system of residential services is viewed as performing well, then a planner for a local mental health authority might conclude that the current strategy has been working and the approach and level of effort should be maintained. Conversely, if the rehabilitation needs of the population are not being met because of poor performance by the service system in this area, remedial activity would be indicated. This survey would not identify particular agencies where remedial action might be taken but would highlight areas of need according to the 11 service elements.

Overall, the key-informant survey provides feedback on the performance of the local mental health authority, providing guidance as to changes in the structure or process of governance and administration of mental health and support services in the community. It is hoped that such assessments will encourage a process of ongoing evaluation and quality assurance for planning of mental health services.

As this chapter has indicated, the evaluation of the RWJ demonstration has focused on the development of *systems of care*. What this emphasis has overshadowed is the assessment of the *quality* of services at the level of individual service programmes. The demonstration *assumes* that there is an effective technology for treating, rehabilitating, and caring for individuals with severe mental illnesses; the evaluation assumes that these demonstration sites will implement the proper technology, *if* they can implement a system to deliver the services. Although these may not be completely reasonable assumptions, they are embedded in the conceptualisation of the demonstration and its evaluation. The primary focus of the demonstration is on system creation, service integration, and continuity of care.

If we set aside the conceptual reasons for avoiding the assessment of quality of care, there are two other reasons for skirting the issue of quality: there is little consensus on operational measures of quality, and it is very difficult to make the observations necessary to evaluate quality. Such observations often require intimate access to the interactions between client and provider – and the very act of observing the interaction probably distorts that interaction. Proxy measures of quality often are not satisfactory substitutes. Because of limitations in evaluation methods and restricted access to observe clinical interactions, we continue to focus on structural and process measures. We assess individual outcomes without being able to connect these dependent measures to specific service interventions. It is a bit like looking for one's watch beneath the street lamp, even though the watch was lost at the other end of the street, just because the light is better at this end. At some point we need to bring the light to the assessment of the quality of services and programmes.

Acknowledgements

While this chapter bears the names of three investigators participating in the national evaluation of The Robert Wood Johnson Foundation Program on Chronic Mental Illness, it reflects the work of the larger group. The authors thank Anthony Lehman and Catherine Jackson at the University of Maryland; Clara Muschkin and Deborah Franks at the University of North Carolina; Sandra Newman, Richard Frank, Don Steinwachs, and E. Ann Skinner, at The Johns Hopkins University and Dee Roth at the Ohio Department of Mental Health.

The national evaluation is supported by grants from The Robert Wood Johnson Foundation, the National Institute of Mental Health, several other federal agencies, and the Ohio Department of Mental Health to the Mental Health Policy Studies Program, Department of Psychiatry, University of Maryland, 645 W. Redwood Street, Baltimore, Maryland 21201 USA.

References

AIKEN, L., SOMERS, S. & SHORE, M. (1986) Private foundations in health affairs: a case study of the development of a national initiative for the chronically mentally ill. *American Psychologist*, **41**, 1290–1295.

AUDIT COMMISSION (1986) *Making a Reality of Community Care*. London: HMSO.

DEMMLER, J., SHERN, D. L., COEN, A. S., *et al* (1988) *Denver CMI Initiative Study 3: Client Needs, Life Situation and Satisfaction and Initiative Program: Client and Collateral Survey*. Colorado: Division of Mental Health.

DEROGATIS, L. R. & CLEARY, P. A. (1977) Confirmation of the dimensional structure of the SCL-90: a study in construct validation. *Journal of Clinical Psychology*, **33**, 981–989.

DICKEY, B. & GOLDMAN, H. (1986) Public care for the chronically mentally ill: financing operating costs, issues and options for local leadership. *Administration in Mental Health*, **14**, 63–77.

GOLDMAN, H., MORRISSEY, J. & RIDGELY, M. S. (1990) Form and function of mental health authorities at RWJ Foundation program sites: preliminary observations. *Hospital and Community Psychiatry*, **41**, 1222–1230.

—— & —— (1985) The alchemy of mental health policy: homelessness and the fourth cycle of reform. *American Journal of Public Health*, **75**, 727–731.

GOLDSTROM, I. D. & MANDERSCHEID, R. W. (1984) The chronically mentally ill: a descriptive analysis from the Uniform Client Data Instrument. *Community Support Service Journal*, **2**, 4–9.

GRUSKY, I. & TIERNEY, K. (1988) *Evaluating the Effectiveness of Countywide Mental Health Care Systems*. Working Paper Number 5. Los Angeles: University of California.

HOULT, J. & REYNOLDS, I. (1984) Schizophrenia: a comprehensive trial of community oriented and hospital oriented care. *Acta Psychiatrica Scandanavica*, **69**, 359–372.

LEHMAN, A. F. (1988) A quality of life interview for the chronically mentally ill. *Evaluation and Program Planning*, **11**, 51–62.

MECHANIC, D. (1991) Strategies for integrating public mental health services. *Hospital and Community Psychiatry*, **42**, 797–801.

—— & AIKEN, L. (1987) Improving the care of patients with chronic mental illness. *New England Journal of Medicine*, **317**, 1634–1638.

MORRISSEY, J., TAUSIG, M. & LINDSEY, M. (1986) Interorganizational networks in mental health systems: assessing community support systems for the chronically mentally ill. In *The Organization of Mental Health Services: Social and Community Systems* (eds W. Scott & B. Black). Beverly Hills, CA: Sage.

―――― , MUSCHKIN, C., FRANKS, D., *et al* (1990) *Client Needs, Service System Characteristics, and Mental Health Authority Performance: An Interim Report from the Site-Level Evaluation of the Robert Wood Johnson Foundation Program on Chronic Mental Illness.* Chapel Hill, NC: University of North Carolina, Sheps Center for Health Services Research.

PROGRAM FOR THE CHRONICALLY MENTALLY ILL (1985) *Program Announcement.* Princeton: The Robert Wood Johnson Foundation.

SHORE, M. & COHEN, M. (1990) Creating new systems of care: The Robert Wood Johnson Foundation program on chronic mental illness. *Hospital and Community Psychiatry*, **41**, 1212–1216.

SILVERMAN, M., RICCI, E. & GUNTER, M. (1990) Strategies for increasing the rigor of qualitative methods in evaluation of health care programs. *Evaluation Review*, **14**, 57–74.

TESSLER, R. C. (1987) Continuity of care and client outcome. *Psychosocial Rehabilitation Journal*, **10**, 39–53.

―――― & GOLDMAN, H. (eds) (1982) *The Chronically Mentally Ill: Assessing Community Support Programs.* Cambridge: Ballinger.

TURNER, J. & TENHOOR, W. (1978) The NIMH community support program: pilot approach to a needed social reform. *Schizophrenia Bulletin*, **4**, 319–408.

US DEPARTMENT OF COMMERCE, US BUREAU OF THE CENSUS (1989) *Current Housing Reports, Series H-150. General Housing Characteristics for the US and Regions: 1987. Annual Housing Survey.* Washington, DC: US Government Printing Office.

WALSH, A. & LEIGLAND, J. (1986) *Public Authorities and Mental Health Programs.* New York: Institute for Public Administration.

WEISBROD, B., TEST, M. & STEIN, L. (1980) Alternatives to mental hospital treatment II: economic benefit–cost analysis. *Archives of General Psychiatry*, **37**, 400–498.

WILLENBRING, M., RIDGELY, M. S., STINCHFIELD, R., *et al* (1991) *Application of Case Management in Alcohol and Drug Dependence: Matching Techniques and Populations.* Rockville, MD: National Institute on Alcohol Abuse and Alcoholism.

WILSON, N., DAVIS, E., SHERN, D., *et al* (1988) *The Denver CMI Initiative: Evaluation, Study 1: The Key Informant and Attitude Survey.* Denver: Colorado Division of Mental Health.

12 Auditing the use of psychiatric beds

PAUL BEBBINGTON, SEAN FEENEY and CLAIRE FLANNIGAN

Audit is ideally part of a process of feedback that encourages action to remedy perceived deficiencies, the so-called 'audit cycle' (Royal College of Physicians of London, 1989). The proper basis of audit is outcome, but in practice most audit is of *process*, on the assumption that good processes will result in good outcomes. In many cases, the processes chosen for audit are selected precisely because they are readily accessible; so, for example, a major focus of current medical audit procedures is the quality of casenotes. Clearly, documentation is essential to a well-run service, but the corollary, that good documentation indicates good overall practice, is a dubious inference.

In finance, audit measures a firm's financial procedures against accepted good practice. In psychiatry the term is clearly metaphorical. Good practice in psychiatry is less well defined than in commerce, and because of this the process of audit should accommodate the possibility that practice should be changed. Otherwise there is a danger of fossilising practices that are unlikely to have been adequately established on an empirical basis and are in any case at risk of being superseded. In some cases there are not even agreed standards, and it is the job of professional bodies to formulate the basis for a consensus concerning both appropriate practice and the requisite service provisions. This has been done by the Royal College of Psychiatrists of Australia and New Zealand, and the British Royal College of Psychiatrists is currently following suit.

Clinical audit shades into evaluation research when it uses structured designs and comparisons. These may entail reference to epidemiologically defined populations. They may also involve a follow-up element. Audit and evaluative research have a common reliance on information. Since audit is envisaged as a relatively routine process, it must be based on routinely gathered information. This does not mean that information must be obtained as it always has been, and it is clear that introducing relatively formal procedures of audit has already changed the quality of information collected.

Nevertheless, while the methods of registering data must be relevant, they must also be convenient, so there is a fair chance that they will be used. Evaluative research is likely to be based on a more structured approach to information gathering, perhaps with the use of specially designed schedules. Nevertheless, audit and evaluative research cannot be precisely distinguished in terms of the quality and procedures associated with their information base.

They likewise share their reliance on concepts that are clearly value-laden, namely the acceptance that health services have certain aims worth pursuing. Some of these aims are fairly uncontentious, for instance, relieving the distress occasioned by severe mental illness. Other issues are more arguable: for example, whether mental health services should treat the 'worried well' at the expense of those with long-standing severe mental illness, or whether they should look after social needs in addition to medical ones (assuming these are separable in severe psychiatric disorder).

Among the many procedures covered by the term medical audit, one of the most crucial is the systematic and critical analysis of the use of medical resources, with the object of improving the quality of the care provided for patients. Quality of care itself is not a succinct concept, but rather operates as a catch-all phrase, encompassing all the aspects of care thought to have a bearing on the wellbeing of patients and their relatives. As such it serves as a mnemonic for the features of a service that need to be considered in any attempt to improve care. Ideally, these elements should be identified through formal research, but this is not always feasible. We are then left to fall back on expert opinion. While all evaluative research necessarily involves an interplay between observation and ideology, the canvassing of expert opinion allows little prospect of controlling the ideological component by rendering it explicit. However, it is often all that is available.

In this chapter we shall focus on the evaluation of the use of one particular element of psychiatric services, that is, of psychiatric beds. Over the last 40 years or so there has been a major change in psychiatric bed use. At the beginning of this period, patients were admitted for relatively long stays, as they always had been, and the admission rate was relatively low. The peak psychiatric bed occupancy in England occurred in 1954. The subsequent well-documented decline (Salokangas *et al*, 1985; Thornicroft & Bebbington, 1989) followed a resurgence of therapeutic optimism, vigorous policies of rehabilitation back into the community, and the introduction of neuroleptic medication. It was primarily the result of individual clinical action and a change in psychiatric attitudes. However, once the trend was noted (Tooth & Brooke, 1961) it appeared to offer financial savings, and the trend was rapidly adopted as a governmental policy. So it has remained ever since, although the resulting unholy alliance between therapeutic radicalism and economic conservation has often looked very odd. Moreover, in recent years, the engine of the move towards community care has seemed to be the economic rather than the therapeutic imperative.

One way or another, we are using fewer psychiatric beds in Britain than 40 years ago, and we are using them in a different way. It has become an article of faith that fewer beds means a better and more modern service. Indeed, services with large numbers of beds are viewed as backward to the point of being primitive. However, if we are serious about audit, this in particular is an assumption that must be subject to scrutiny. How far can the process of bed reduction go? Has it gone too far already? Can it go further by the deployment of existing alternatives to admission? If not, what level of facilities is required to accommodate, in a feasible, humane and therapeutic manner, those people for whom admission to a psychiatric bed might be avoided?

There are several ways in which information could be obtained that bears on these questions. So, for instance, controlled trials have been carried out of alternatives to hospital care for psychiatric patients (e.g. Stein & Test, 1980; Test & Stein, 1980; Weisbrod *et al*, 1980; Hoult & Reynolds, 1984; Creed *et al*, 1990). These certainly provide information relevant to the possibility of managing psychiatrically ill patients in other settings, and give an idea of the alternative facilities required to do this. In so far as they have been successful, they also add fuel to the ideological debate.

However, such studies do not indicate in practical terms what the opportunities are for modifying services in other locations. This requires an evaluation of the existing practice in these services, and in particular of current bed usage. The easiest situation in which it is possible to query the use of beds is where occupancy is low. If, over the course of a year, occupancy varies between 70% and 80%, a good argument can be made for a 10% – 15% cut in available beds. However, such situations are becoming rarer in psychiatric practice in the UK. Most services in the authors' experience have occupancies around 90% or higher. When they approach 100% the service is in danger of grinding to a halt. In this chapter we have deliberately chosen to concentrate on the problems of auditing high-occupancy bed usage, since it is in such situations that service developers may feel constrained. We propose to explore the methodological considerations that must be dealt with before bed usage can be audited, and then describe the conduct of our own study of this type, undertaken in the Bethlem/ Maudsley Joint Hospital where high bed occupancy is the rule.

Methodological issues in bed use audit

In epidemiology, studies based on incidence and prevalence answer different sorts of questions. A similar distinction can be made about the evaluation of bed usage. One strategy would be to examine the appropriateness of admission in a series of patients admitted to hospital beds over a given period. From this it should be possible to reach conclusions about the numbers of admissions that might have been avoided over the period of study. Such a study would also permit general statements about the sorts of alternative facility that seem to be indicated. Moreover, some types of workload are related to admission rates rather than to bed occupancy, for example, the work of clerking patients and performing standard investigations. Everyone working in a hospital knows that admissions mean work, and they have a natural impulse to keep patients in hospital rather than to release beds for possible new admissions.

However, avoidable admissions will relate to a range of patients with different characteristics and circumstances. In most cases, avoidable periods of in-patient care will be fairly brief. Nevertheless, they will vary in duration. Studies of admissions give information about the feasibility of changing admission rates, given the availability of alternative resources. They should also give an indication of the characteristics of patients requiring particular placements and facilities, and are thus an aid to clinical decision-making. However, they provide relatively poor information about the potential for reducing the numbers of hospital beds and about the necessary extent of the replacement facilities.

This situation can be improved by recording the duration of admission. This necessarily involves a follow-up of the selected patients. It permits the calculation of avoidable days of stay in the period over which the admissions were collected. Provided the period of collection is reasonably long in relation to the mean duration of stay, this will give a fairly accurate indication of the potential for bed closures arising from the prevention of admission, and of the requirements for alternative facilities.

An alternative approach is not to collect patients as they are admitted, but to conduct a census on a given day of all current in-patients. A small minority of these patients may have been admitted on that day, but most will already have been in-patients for varying periods of time. The probability of inclusion will be proportional to the length of stay. There will thus be a natural correction for the varying duration of admissions, and potential savings of beds can be calculated directly from the number occupied by people who in principle could have been accommodated by other services.

However, the validity of this calculation is based on the assumption that the census day adequately represents the remaining days of the year. Only in a very large (these days unimaginably large) institution could this be guaranteed. It is therefore better to go, not for a single census day, but for a much longer sampling period. In our own study we opted for three months. This means that information about the suitability of bed use must be integrated throughout the whole period. It is then inadequate just to evaluate the number of admissions for which alternatives might have been available, since it now becomes necessary to make a direct correction for the duration of admissions.

Imagine that over a three-month period there were 100 admissions, and it was felt that 40% of these were potentially avoidable. It would be improper to infer that the bed numbers could thus be reduced by 40%, because it might be that all the avoidable admissions were of very brief duration. The way to correct for this is to begin with a census of all subjects in hospital on the start date and to monitor the duration of admissions for these subjects and for all patients admitted during the subsequent three months. For each patient admitted, the period of admission lying within the three-month period of the evaluation should then be calculated. Periods of admission outside the three-month period would be ignored in all cases. It is then possible to weight the proportions of avoidable and unavoidable admissions by this figure, and thus obtain an estimate of the avoidable bed use in the period. This length of time is likely to be sufficient to be reasonably representative of annual bed occupancy.

However, we have only discussed the savings in bed use that can be obtained by directing potential admissions to alternative services. There is also the possibility of reducing bed occupancy by earlier discharge. This presupposes that admissions could not have been avoided, but that patients might have been accommodated in another way at some stage before their actual date of discharge.

Again, the technique that affords the most direct calculation of savings in bed numbers is some form of prevalence study. The point prevalence (census day) approach would then be supplemented by an evaluation of whether the patient would be accommodated elsewhere on that particular day and at what point of their in-patient stay. Likewise the period prevalence approach would now include both savings due to avoidable admissions and the number of days that, for each admitted patient, could have been saved by facilities permitting earlier discharge.

It is clear that the intensiveness and sophistication of the methods used to audit bed use will determine the soundness of the conclusions that can be drawn about the feasibility of changes in policy. However, the examination of the way that available beds are used in practice is only one side of the coin – it addresses only the potential for reducing bed numbers and the alternative facilities necessary to encompass this. In order to evaluate the overall appropriateness of bed use, one must also consider those people who were not admitted to hospital when they should have been. In some services this is a very serious matter indeed (Patrick *et al*, 1989). Unfortunately, it is much more straightforward to audit the use than the non-use of beds, since patients admitted to hospital are always easier to get hold of. In consequence, quantifying the potential for bed reduction is a simpler matter than arguing that bed numbers are inadequate.

The proper sampling frame for identifying patients considered for admission but managed outside hospital is unclear. Some method for identifying the category 'considered for admission' is required. Does this just mean patients who have been seen as a matter of urgency by psychiatrists in out-patients or emergency clinics or on domiciliary visits? Do we also have to include routine out-patients because a few of them occasionally deteriorate? How *seriously* must the patients have been considered for admission? In any case, will their doctors actually remember? Ought we to include other people who have not been considered for admission but should have been? If so, how might we find them? These questions make it obvious that this part of an overall evaluation of bed usage is much more difficult to investigate.

Once these difficulties are overcome, the results of bed usage evaluations will be of considerable value. At the moment, decisions about the appropriateness of bed numbers are often based on the Jarman indicators of the local community (Jarman, 1983; see also Jarman & Hirsch, this volume, pp. 62–80). However, these indicators are based merely on the average utilisation figures for communities with equivalent sociodemographic footprints. The average practice may or may not be ideal. The direct evaluation of bed usage can be related to an area's Jarman indices to provide a clearer notion of the discrepancy between average and ideal. Moreover, if the process is repeated in areas with different social characteristics, a judgement can be formed about the proper allocation of resources between communities. Finally, repeating the valuation of bed usage after an interval would permit the assessment of the changes currently being wrought within the National Health Service.

A study of bed-use audit

We have already stressed that any attempt at a study of this type must have an ideological component. While it is quite possible to conceal this for strategic purposes, scientific probity requires that it is made as explicit as possible. Our own evaluative instrument was developed on the basis that there is nothing ideologically good or bad about the mere fact of admissions to hospital for psychiatric illness. Moreover it is not inherent in our evaluation that admissions should be avoided at all cost. The choice between placements should be based, not on opportunities for cost reduction, but on a consideration of whether the needs of the patient can be met more effectively outside hospital. Cost should only be considered when needs can be met equally well in or out of hospital.

The current study, the South Southwark Bed Use Audit, is one of a series in different areas of the country. These are conducted under the auspices of the Royal College of Psychiatrists' Research Unit. The corresponding study in Hammersmith and Fulham has now also been completed.

The survey instrument: the Bed Use Audit Schedule

The audit procedure in our study is based on interviews with staff, in particular the admitting psychiatrist and the key worker. The information is recorded in a schedule divided into ten sections. The first two sections are devoted to orientation – identification of the patient in terms of socio-demographic attributes, hospital diagnosis, consultant, date of admission and discharge, circumstances of admission, previous admissions and so on. A third section records the source of any care received in the month before admission. Next, in order to supplement the diagnostic record, the symptoms and signs at admission are listed in a simple way, together with assessments of their severity.

The next two sections are concerned with the reasons for the admission. Obviously there may be several of these, and an attempt is made to distinguish between major reasons and those that are merely contributory. Overall, these sections cover five topics: the prevention of harm; the containment of incipient relapse; treatment; management; and the provision of security for the patient or for others. They are listed in detail below.

(a) Prevention of harm or incipient relapse

    (i) prevention of suicide attempt/other self-harm
    (ii) prevention of severe physical self-neglect
    (iii) prevention of harm to physical health
    (iv) removal from a stressful situation other than actual harm as above
    (v) prevention of harm to patient from others
    (vi) prevention of physical harm to relatives, including children
    (vii) prevention of psychosocial harm to family – includes when family cannot cope with bizarre or threatening behaviour
    (viii) prevention of physical harm to others
    (ix) pre-emptive prevention of violence
    (x) pre-emptive prevention of relapse
    (xi) to prevent the misuse of medication or drug; e.g. alcohol, benzodiazepines, opioids, cocaine, etc.
    (xii) other.

(b) Treatment, management, security of self or others

    (i) relief for relatives/other carers
    (ii) reinstatement of medication following termination by patient with risk of relapse
    (iii) supervision of medication following failure to respond or change in response to medication
    (iv) medical treatment of other problems not responsive to community management
    (v) social and/or occupational rehabilitation
    (vi) training or care of personal hygiene
    (vii) supervision because of wandering or other danger

(viii) supervision, observation, monitoring NOS
(ix) admission at patient's request.

The seventh section is concerned with possible alternative ways of managing the patient. Was 24-hour medical and nursing care in a hospital setting required, or did admission come about because one or a combination of alternative settings was not considered, or was unavailable? The object here is to rate whether any of a number of specified settings *could* have been used to prevent admission. The ratings are made on the basis of the best information at the time of rating, irrespective of whether it was known when it was decided to admit the patient. At the end of the section, there is provision for recording why an existing facility was not used, whether through ignorance of its existence, the lack of a place, or failure to make contact with it. The list of potential alternative settings is given below.

(a) Sheltered community for people with long-term disability
(b) Nursing home for people with dementia
(c) Nursing home for elderly, physically frail or ill
(d) High supervision hostel with good staffing levels able to cope with acute disturbance day and night
    (i) Long stay if necessary
    (ii) Short stay only
(e) Hostel with staff on call at night
    (i) Long stay if necessary
    (ii) Short stay only
(f) Group home, staffed during the day
(g) Unstaffed group home (visited)
(h) Other supervised residential, e.g. flat, lodging
(i) Home supervision at night by CPN or equivalent (on call or spending the night there)
(j) Other home care intensive enough to have prevented this admission (not simply occasional domiciliary visits)
(k) Other form of residential unit, e.g. for adolescents, 'battered wives', 'retreat', mother and baby, refuge, etc.

Admission sometimes comes about because the patient's impending breakdown was not identified early enough. The next section records the existence of premonitory signs and symptoms, and whether early recognition would have permitted alternatives to admission.

The final two sections cover information that can only be assessed at discharge or at the end of a follow-up period. The first allows interviewed staff to use their clinical judgement in estimating the degree of the patient's vulnerability – to being violent, attempting suicide, relapsing, or the dangers of self-neglect. Researchers are also required to record details of the aftercare plan and its implementation.

If at follow-up the patient has not been discharged, the final section permits possible reasons for this to be recorded.

The conduct of the survey

Until the catchment area was recently extended, the Bethlem and Maudsley Joint Hospital had responsibility for the area of South Southwark. It was decided that a one-day census of South Southwark beds would be conducted and that all patients admitted from the catchment area over the subsequent three-month period would then be logged and assessed.

The first requirement was to identify the patients who fell within the scope of the study. This was done from the hospital's computerised Patient Administration System (PAS). First, a list of all in-patients was made on the index date, the 1st of November 1990. The hospital's PAS records also gave information on patients' age, consultant, and ward. There were 136 apparently eligible patients in the hospital on the day of the census. Following this, a weekly update of new admissions was made. In the three calendar months following the census date there were 138 admissions of 122 patients resident in the South Southwark area. Thus, in the end, a total of 258 patients were evaluated.

Once details of patients had been established, the key worker for each patient was identified. One of us (SF) then interviewed the key worker or registrar on the ward and scrutinised the casenotes for information that was unclear. Supplementary details, particularly with regard to continuing vulnerability, were obtained later. In about two-thirds of cases the information was obtained from the patients' key worker, while in the remaining one-third the major informant was the registrar, although this information might be supplemented from the key worker. We formed the opinion that it was desirable to obtain information from both.

A number of difficulties were encountered in the process of obtaining information about patients. It was hard to get information from the hospital records department sufficiently quickly so that occasionally patients were discharged before information could be obtained about them. Because of constraints on the interviewer's time, much of the interviewing had to be done out of hours. This meant that the only informant available was the key worker rather than the registrar. Key workers were sometimes surprisingly hazy about the information we sought. Similar reservations applied to the casenotes. It was sometimes very difficult to find out whether a patient had been seen in out-patients in the month before admission. Finally, of the 136 patients who initially appeared to be in scope, four later turned out to be from outside the catchment area.

The Bed Use Audit Schedule offers two methods of entering data for analysis. As the Schedule is available in a lap-top computer version, it is possible to enter data directly during the interview. However, at the time

TABLE 12.1
Social isolation

Social isolation	N (%)
More or less isolated	5 (3.7)
Little support	17 (12.5)
Fair support	74 (54.4)
Good support	40 (29.4)

of our study the lap-top version was not available, and the data were recorded on paper and entered into the computer later.

Initial analyses from the study

Data have so far only been analysed for the admissions, rather than census patients. Of the 136 admissions during the three-month period , 46% were male, 71% were white and 21% were Afro-Caribbean. In total, 57% lived in their own flat or house, 25% were dependent on the care of relatives, 12.5% lived in a group home or hostel and three subjects were completely homeless, living on the streets. There were 21% who were married or living with someone, 46% were single and 23% were divorced or separated. Of the sample, 35% lived alone, but most patients received reasonable support from their social network (see Table 12.1).

Of the patients, 37% had a psychotic disorder in the schizophrenic spectrum, 9% schizoaffective disorder, 15% bipolar affective disorders and 22% unipolar depressive conditions. The patients typically had long-standing illness. The mean length of illness was nearly 12 years and only 19% of admissions were first admissions. One-third of all cases had received in-patient care of some sort in the month before admission.

Those admitted under a section of the Mental Health Act made up 23% of all patients. In 37% of cases, admission was decided upon by the registrar, in 53% by the senior registrar. Only 7% of admissions were referred by a consultant.

The major reasons for admission that were identified by the informants are listed in Table 12.2 along with reasons regarded as having a secondary contribution to the decision to admit. Subjects could have been admitted for more than one major reason. Only reasons present in more than 10% of cases are tabled. Most admissions were concerned with the effective provision of medication, with the protection of the patient, or with the relief of those providing care at home. Very few admissions were used pre-emptively to prevent anticipated relapse (6%).

Section 7 of the schedule provides for recording residential alternatives to admission, including intensive supervision at home. In fact, the only

TABLE 12.2
Major and secondary reasons for admission

Reasons for admission	N (%)
Major reasons	
Relief of relatives/carers	69 (50.7)
Suicide/self-harm	38 (27.9)
Misuse of medication/drug	22 (16.2)
Reinstatement of medication	20 (14.7)
Supervision of medication	16 (11.8)
Other supervision/observation	83 (61.0)
Secondary reasons	
Removal from stressful situation	27 (19.9)
Relief of relatives/carers	24 (17.6)
Prevention of severe physical neglect	15 (11.0)
Suicide/self-harm	18 (13.2)
Other supervision/observation	19 (14.0)

alternatives seen as feasible for more than a few patients looked like hospitals under a different guise – that is, a fully staffed high-supervision hostel. This was felt to be appropriate in nearly two-thirds of cases. However, this finding should be interpreted with care. The actual instruction is "Rate below, only whether any of the specified type could have been used to prevent admission". We took this to mean "Would a high supervision hostel with good staffing levels, able to cope with acute disturbance day or night, be able to house the patient?" This is obviously a broad interpretation, and in 65% of the cases it was felt that a hostel of this type would be able to manage the patient. Even so, this left a third of cases for whom admission to hospital was felt to be an absolute necessity. High supervision hostels like this are currently unavailable.

Only in three cases was it felt that intensive support at home could have prevented the admission. This obviously represents a pessimistic view of the possibilities of management of this type as demonstrated by the Daily Living Programme at the Joint Hospital, although it should be said that that dealt with first episodes only (Muijen *et al*, 1992).

Finally, it was apparent that most patients had some kind of prodrome, and in virtually all cases early intervention would have been appropriate. Only in ten cases was the appropriate action not attempted, but it is not clear from our data whether patients cooperated adequately with this. A third or so of patients did not have the means of asking directly for help.

Discussion

In this chapter we have argued for the value of structured information about the use of psychiatric services, in this instance, the use of in-patient beds. The information was not already available in the service studied and therefore required investment of time over and above that required for analysis. In fact, the Joint Hospital does conduct an annual census in which an attempt is made to judge the appropriateness of admission. This depends purely on the unstructured clinical opinions of the medical teams. The hospital's own audit is in line with the results of the current study, insofar as it reports that consultants do not see much opportunity for alternative placements. However, given the way the data are collected, it is probably easier to record the unfeasibility of alternatives than to think what might suffice. It is unlikely that the resulting data could be made as detailed as in the current study, but, in our view, worthwhile improvements could be made to this routine procedure.

The results of the South Southwark Bed Use Audit presented here are necessarily preliminary, and are indeed based only on patients actually admitted during the period of the study. They, therefore, do not comply with many of the methodological strictures outlined in the earlier part of this chapter. Nevertheless, they do give a flavour of the way in which beds are used in the Joint Hospitals.

They also give a general snapshot of the sorts of patients who are admitted to the hospitals. They mainly suffer from severe mental illness, and have done so for a long time. Despite this they retain their place in the community, living either on their own or with relatives. Marked social isolation was relatively rare. However, their community tenure is unstable in many cases: repeated admission is the rule and some patients had been discharged very recently before the index admission. In nearly a quarter of cases admission was compulsory.

Most of the patients were admitted to hospital for their own protection, because the relatives could not cope, or in order to institute effective treatment. There did not seem much scope for redirecting patients – the only feasible alternatives looked like psychiatric hospitals masquerading under another name.

South Southwark is an area of considerable social deprivation, particularly in its northern part. The overall Jarman index is a high + 40, reaching + 51 in one of the northern wards. The Camberwell Health Authority as a whole is the sixth most deprived in England. Even allowing for this, the area does have a large number of psychiatric beds per head of population (over 100 per 100 000 on the census day of the South Southwark Bed Use Audit). Our preliminary results suggest that, given the current structure of the services, these beds are largely necessary.

A service that responds *ad hoc* to crises by admitting patients repeatedly cannot be cheap. It is also doubtful if it is meeting the needs of its clientele except in a quite limited sense. The service could be changed at more than one level. Thus, assuming that crises are inevitable, it would be possible to replace admission to hospital beds with the alternatives suggested by our informants, namely, well-staffed hostels with all necessary cover. This might bring the advantage of reduced stigma and perhaps a more domestic atmosphere, without jettisoning the functions of asylum and relief for carers. It ought to be technically feasible to make such places safe for disturbed and sometimes suicidal patients. Patients are likely to prefer them, although it would not be possible to guarantee this *a priori*. However, acute hostel wards are unlikely to be cheap, particularly if equivalent cover by medical, nursing and other disciplines is to be maintained in a dispersed service.

It is possible to discern another implication of our findings. The high level of admissions in response to crisis may reflect the management of patients who have been discharged, both in our own service and in many others. In many cases, vulnerable patients with long-standing illness are managed solely through out-patient appointments, often being seen by relatively junior staff who may not know of facilities that could keep such patients well. This system is not designed to deal with those who fail to attend or to comply with treatment generally.

It is possible that a different system of out-patient management might reduce admission rates by diminishing the risk of crisis. One plausible suggestion would be a service based on outreach by the whole team responsible for the patient. This would involve home visits and the deployment of community facilities. The Daily Living Programme has demonstrated the feasibility of such techniques in the management of acute crises (Muijen *et al*, 1991): we think they would be at least as effective if they were used to prevent admissions. Only thus would it be possible to divert some of the resources tied up in the provision of beds for crisis admission.

References

CREED, F., BLACK, D., ANTHONY, P., *et al* (1990) Randomised controlled trial of day patient versus inpatient psychiatric treatment. *British Medical Journal*, **300**, 1033–1037.

HOULT, J. & REYNOLDS, I. (1984) Schizophrenia – a comparative trial of community-orientated and hospital-orientated psychiatric care. *Acta Psychiatrica Scandinavica*, **69**, 359–372.

JARMAN, B. (1983) Identification of underprivileged areas. *British Medical Journal*, **256**, 1587–1592.

MUIJEN, M., MARKS, I., CONNOLLY, J., *et al* (1992) Home based care and standard hospital care for patients with severe mental illness: a randomised controlled trial. *British Medical Journal*, **304**, 749–754.

PATRICK, M., HIGGITT, A. & HOLLOWAY, F. (1989) Changes in an inner city psychiatric in-patient service following bed losses: a follow-up of the East Lambeth 1986 Survey. *Health Trends*, **21**, 121–123.

ROYAL COLLEGE OF PHYSICIANS OF LONDON (1989) *Medical Audit. A First Report – What, Why and How?* London: Royal College of Physicians.

SALOKANGAS, R. K. R., DER, G. & WING, J. K. (1985) Community psychiatric services in England and Finland. *Social Psychiatry*, **20**, 23–29.

STEIN, L. & TEST, M. (1980) Alternatives to mental hospital treatment. *Archives of General Psychiatry*, **37**, 392–393.

TEST, M. & STEIN, L. (1980) Alternatives to mental hospitals. III. Social cost. *Archives of General Psychiatry*, **37**, 409–412.

THORNICROFT, G. & BEBBINGTON, P. E. (1989) Deinstitutionalisation – from hospital closure to service development. *British Journal of Psychiatry*, **155**, 739–753.

TOOTH, G. & BROOKE, E. (1961) Trends in mental hospital population and their effect on future planning. *Lancet*, **i**, 710–713.

WEISBROD, B., TEST, M. & STEIN, L. (1980) Alternatives to mental hospital treatment. *Archives of General Psychiatry*, **37**, 400–405.

13 Measuring individual needs for care and services

CHRIS R. BREWIN

The concept of need, currently so topical, has a long and controversial history within the social sciences. In the psychological literature, for example, needs have frequently been invoked as explanations for human behaviour. An early usage of the term was as a drive towards specific behaviour patterns (e.g. needs for achievement or dominance), but this has fallen into disfavour owing to the lack of explanatory power. Needs have also been seen as objective human requirements for physical and mental health (e.g. needs for warmth or security or self-actualisation), and as subjective expressions of want or desire (Tracy, 1986). Because of these varying meanings, subjective wants are often referred to as 'felt' or 'perceived' needs to distinguish them from needs that are considered to have a more objective basis.

Individuals lacking these objective requirements are often described as being 'in need', and hence needs are for some writers synonymous with the presence of objective lacks. Thus for Mallman & Marcus (1980) need is "an objective requirement to avoid a state of illness" (p. 165), and for Tracy (1986) "a need of a living system is a lack of a specific resource which is useful for or required by the purposes of that system" (p. 212).

Mental health professionals are not primarily interested in needs as explanations of behaviour but as grounds for professional intervention, and the concept of need as an objective lack has been interpreted in three ways. One interpretation is as a lack of health or wellbeing, and needs have been defined in terms of ameliorating symptoms, distress, behaviour problems, skills deficits, poverty, poor housing, and so on. In this usage, needs are in effect assessed failures to attain general goals of health and wellbeing (e.g. Leighton *et al*, 1963; Stein & Test, 1980). Or again, "Need is seen as a shortfall compared with a state of being which is generally acceptable" (Davies & Challis, 1986, p. 562). Some studies of needs consist largely of descriptive accounts of a set of clinical problems (e.g. Falloon & Marshall, 1983). Such failures or shortfalls must in principle fall within the domain of professional expertise although where the boundaries are drawn, e.g. between social and medical expertise, varies from study to study.

The second interpretation is as a lack of access to particular forms of institutionalised care targeted at these objective lacks. For example, Lehtinen *et al* (1990) interpret needs as reflecting an inadequate level of service for the severity of the problem. Thus patients with severe disorders receiving primary rather than specialised psychiatric care would be rated as having unmet need. Similarly, for Shapiro *et al* (1985), unmet needs are defined as the combination of definite morbidity and lack of utilisation of mental health services. A recent survey instrument, the Community Placement Questionnaire (Clifford *et al*, 1991) is designed to assess the varying types of institutionalised care required by long-stay patients resident in hospitals scheduled for closure.

The third interpretation of the term 'need' is as a lack of specific activities by (professional or lay) mental health workers. These may include both treatment-orientated activities such as medication and individual therapy, and support-orientated activities such as ensuring access to leisure facilities and arranging for a home help. Thus in the terminology developed at the MRC Social and Community Psychiatry Unit, 'needs for care' have been defined as requirements for specific activities or interventions that have the potential to ameliorate disabling symptoms or reactions. In contrast, 'needs for services' reflect institutional requirements and are defined as needs for specific agents or agencies to deliver those interventions (Brewin *et al*, 1987). Mangen & Brewin (1991) outline a procedure for deriving estimates of needs for services from individuals' needs for specific items of care.

Typically the distinction between need as a lack of health or wellbeing and need as a lack of a specific intervention is not made; to cite only one of many examples, Birchwood & Smith (1988) include among the needs of families caring for a relative with schizophrenia both the amelioration of adverse emotional reactions (an objective lack) and specific items of care such as providing information and practical advice. That the distinction is nevertheless an important one is illustrated by the existence of certain objective lacks, such as intractable treatment-resistant symptoms, for which no specific interventions are effective. Such situations, which would qualify as needs according to one usage of the term but not according to the other usage, have been explicitly described as "problems without needs" (Brewin *et al*, 1987) and as constituting "no meetable need" (Brewin & Wing, 1989). Similarly, there are examples of individuals who have unmet needs for specific items of care but no unmet need for access to agents or agencies other than those currently provided.

These three uses of the term 'need' within the psychiatric literature reflect in part the different concerns of the various investigations that have been carried out. When studying populations with inadequate provision or low contact with services, such as random community samples, the families of the mentally ill, or the mentally ill living in greatly under-resourced environments, it has generally been considered sufficient to establish lack of health or wellbeing in order to establish the presence of need. Similarly, unmet need has been equated with the combination of a lack of health or wellbeing and a lack of access to institutionalised care. This assumes a low probability that in such samples (a) all available treatment avenues would have been exhausted, so that individuals receiving services were not actually in need and (b) individuals in contact with services might still have unmet needs owing to inappropriate treatment.

However, studies of groups such as the long-term mentally ill already in high contact with services have frequently found it necessary to go further and assess the lack of the specific items of care or services that appear most appropriate to the individual's circumstances. For these groups, the equation of receiving care with having one's needs met is even more unwarranted than it is in the populations described in the previous paragraph, in part because of the lack of well-validated treatment methods and the requirement for an active and highly flexible approach to treatment. In these groups, the existence of unmet need will not only reflect the absence of any care at all but will also in some cases reflect an absence of appropriate care as measured against some ideal template.

Measuring need in low-contact groups

A number of studies, mostly community psychiatric surveys, have attempted to assess need from the presence of morbidity and/or from service utilisation. In the Stirling County study (Leighton *et al*, 1963) need for psychiatric attention was rated on a five-point scale: most abnormal; psychiatric disorder with significant impairment; probable psychiatric disorder; doubtful; probably well. Individuals considered to have a definite need for psychiatric help fell into the first two categories, these judgements being based on the presence of clear psychiatric disorder, the presence of significant impairment, and the nature of the symptoms, including conditions that needed attention for diagnostic and prognostic purposes, whether or not treatment was possible.

Shapiro *et al* (1985) presented operational definitions of need employed in the 1981 Eastern Baltimore Mental Health Survey, one of the sites participating in the NIMH Epidemiologic Catchment Area Program. In this survey the presence of a need for care or services (no distinction was made between the two) was defined in a number of ways: either (a) specialist mental health service utilisation or general health service utilisation for a mental health problem in the past six months (7.1% of the sample) or (b) the presence of two or more manifestations of a mental health problem (a further 6.4% of the sample). These manifestations consisted of either a diagnosable disorder on a standardised psychiatric interview, or a high score on a mental health screening instrument, or social-role impairment due to mental health problems for at least one entire day during the past three months. Individuals who had at least two manifestations of emotional disorder but had not used mental health services were defined as having an unmet need.

Clearly the use of multiple criteria for establishing the presence of need means that comparable data are unlikely to be obtained elsewhere unless a specific attempt at replication is made. From a purely practical point of view the criteria used have reasonable face validity, but the conflation of need, demand, and utilisation is likely to prolong the conceptual confusion already characteristic of this area. The assumptions that people who visit mental health centres have a need for treatment that is then met remain untested. It is also hard to know from this study the length of the psychiatric episodes that individuals experienced and the degree of disability: it was neither an incidence study, since current morbidity was not required, nor a prevalence study since the critical periods for the occurrence of a diagnosable disorder and for the occurrence of disability were not the same.

A different approach to measuring needs for mental health treatment was taken by Lehtinen *et al* (1990) in their epidemiological survey in Finland. This decision was primarily based on whether or not subjects reached case criteria for a recognised psychiatric disorder using the PSE-ID-CATEGO system. Subjects were rated as having a need for care at a specialist or at a primary level, depending on the severity of the disorder, and then categorised as either: (a) having an unmet need for care, by which they meant that the subject was not under care although it was needed; (b) being under inadequate care – receiving care from a general practitioner (GP) although the involvement of specialist services was warranted; (c) being under adequate care – the agent was appropriate to the severity of the disorder. Virtually all individuals reaching case criteria were judged to be in need of mental health services, half of them for specialist services, but over 50% were not receiving any treatment at all.

Although these authors referred to the measurement of needs for care, it should be noted that according to the distinction made earlier they were measuring needs for services. That is, they were mainly concerned with whether the individual was receiving treatment from an appropriate agent rather than with the appropriateness of the treatment itself. It appears that the judgement of appropriateness of services was made *a priori*, rather than reflecting any specific inadequacy or breakdown in the care being provided by the GP. Another point to note is the reliance on the Present State Examination: there were no explicit requirements concerning the duration of the illness episode or the amount of social impairment. In this respect it is interesting to note that only about a third of those who had a psychiatric diagnosis mentioned some degree of need for mental health care themselves.

In conclusion, there are problems in equating 'objective' estimates of need with perceived need, demand, or service utilisation, all of which will almost certainly result in an underestimate. Morbidity surveys are likely to yield better estimates, but specific rules must be formulated to exclude brief transient disorders that will clear up of their own accord, and to take proper account of social impairment independently of the amount of morbidity. Even these data will tend to be underestimates, because no allowance is made for the adequacy of the specific treatment being received (for further discussion of community surveys see the chapter by Bebbington in this volume, pp. 99–117).

Measuring need in high-contact groups

Citing their dissatisfaction with morbidity and service utilisation surveys, and with the method of asking consumers, who as a group are probably ill-informed about the range of potential items of care and service, to define their own needs, Levin *et al* (1978) asked intake workers in community mental health centres to rate their patients' needs for 13 types of service. They devised an instrument called SNAPOR (Services Needed, Available, Planned, Offered, and Rendered) that enquired about the need for and provision of services such as individual sessions, group sessions, family sessions, medication, hospital admission, etc. When rating services needed, workers were to ignore their actual availability. Even allowing mental health workers to define patients' needs themselves, and taking no account of the effectiveness of services actually provided, Levin *et al* found that the centres were only delivering about half the services that their own workers thought were required.

Most of the research on high-contact groups has been concerned with the long-term mentally ill. According to Stein & Test (1980), the needs of these patients can be summarised in terms of material resources, coping skills, motivation, freedom from pathologically dependent relationships, support and education of the community members who are involved with them, and a supportive system that assertively helps patients to achieve their goals. These needs, as we have seen, are a mixture of individual goals for health and wellbeing, and specific requirements for interventions and services. The original intention appears to have been to describe a treatment philosophy that would underpin intervention rather than to enumerate variables that would be specifically targeted in pre- and post-treatment assessments.

Some studies that have attempted to assess the needs of this group directly have relied on questionnaires or interviews completed by key informants. For example, Wasylenki *et al* (1981) simply asked staff members responsible for discharge planning to identify patient aftercare needs in the medical/therapeutic, housing, vocational/educational, and social/recreational areas. In the latter three areas they found strikingly low rates of referral, even in response to aftercare needs identified by staff themselves.

Solomon & Davis' (1985) study used social workers in two state receiving hospitals in Cleveland, Ohio, who completed a service-needs-assessment form for each patient. Services required were collapsed into seven categories – socialisation, individual therapy, group therapy, chemotherapy, vocational rehabilitation, residential treatment, and financial assistance – and the social workers' recommendations were compared with the records of all relevant public agencies to determine whether or not corresponding services had been delivered. Even when it is considered that the authors, like Wasylenki *et al*, took no account of the effectiveness of those services that were delivered (a serious limitation), this study too revealed high levels of unmet need, particularly for rehabilitative services. Although needs for individual counselling, chemotherapy, and financial assistance were apparently met for a high proportion of patients, the majority of the sample had either none or between a quarter and a half of their needs met. The authors note that, of the group that did receive services, 11% utilised services that did not match any of their assessed needs.

Wykes *et al* (1985) reported a similar procedure in which for each patient a member of staff was asked to assess the presence of need for 13 types of care: assessment; administration of medication; personal counselling; relative counselling; training in domestic skills; occupational therapy; industrial training or therapy; sheltered work; hotel services; behaviour modification; self-care; security; and social activities. The four possible ratings were: (a) no need, no service provided; (b) overprovision, service provided but no need; (c) need for and utilisation of service; (d) unmet need for service. These judgements were then compared with the judgements of a research team who had collected a large amount of additional information on each patient. Kappa coefficients measuring agreement on the presence or absence of need between day staff and the research team were significantly greater than chance for 10 out of the 13 items of care, but there were fewer agreements about whether particular needs were being met by services. The authors comment that "the staff's judgement of specific needs did not have a very close correspondence with the team judgements" (p. 83).

One obvious problem with having care staff assess the needs of their own patients is that their judgements may be excessively conservative, and constrained by their knowledge of current practice and the treatment resources available. It has also frequently been noted that information about any particular patient tends to be dispersed among members of a clinical team, so that no one individual is in full possession of the facts. In Mann & Cree's (1976) study of new long-stay patients they found that staff agreed with the research team about the overall proportion of patients that were suitable for discharge into the community, but that there was little agreement on specific individuals (personal communication cited in Wykes *et al*, 1985).

The alternative approach is to employ specially trained researchers. The method of team judgement used in the Wykes *et al* (1985) study and the results obtained with it have been described in more detail by Wykes *et al* (1982). The team first elicited information from patients, staff, relatives, and case records, one of their tasks being to reconcile conflicting reports. They then rated the needs for different types of care and judged whether the needs were met or unmet, or whether there was overprovision. On the whole they did not try to assess the adequacy of interventions being offered, and the need was generally regarded as being met if an identified problem was being addressed by a suitable intervention.

A similar technique has been reported by Cormier *et al* (1987), who employed trained raters to collect information from patients, staff, and medical notes. They then rated the need for 20 different items of care over the past six months, assuming an ideal system of care in which there were no constraints due to resources, staff training, etc. This proviso was made in order to avoid excessively conservative ratings that simply served to reflect the status quo. Types of care included therapeutic interventions such as medication and family therapy, and psychosocial interventions such as vocational rehabilitation and financial advice. In their study of patients with a diagnosis of schizophrenia discharged from the psychiatric units of general hospitals, Cormier *et al* reported a poor fit between needs for and utilisation of most rehabilitation and psychosocial services. Over-provision was not rated, and once again there was no explicit assessment of whether interventions were or were not effective.

Putting together the best of the needs assessments described above, one would end up with a procedure that had the following characteristics: (a) standardised assessment by trained raters; (b) measurement of over- as well as under-provision; (c) assumption of ideal conditions rather than accepting current service limitations; (d) information drawn from patients, staff, medical notes, and relatives. The importance of including relatives in assessments has been recently supported in a study by Brewin *et al* (1990). Relatives in their sample, compared with both the patients themselves and day staff, reported that patients had significantly greater numbers of problems. Interestingly, relatives' ratings did not differ from those of professional hostel staff who also knew patients in a residential setting, suggesting that relatives' perceptions reflected different opportunities for observation and were not being coloured by a more intimate relationship with the patient.

All the above methods of assessment suffer from one important limitation, namely that it is far from clear on what basis patients were rated as having needs for the various forms of care. For example, what set of clinical or social problems did raters have in mind when they made these judgements? What forms of care did they judge to be appropriate to which kinds of problem? And what did they do when patients were already in receipt of treatment or intervention aimed at a particular problem? In these respects, needs judgements have tended typically to be opaque and difficult to question.

One of the main contentions of our recent work (e.g. Brewin *et al*, 1987) is that needs cannot be properly assessed and compared between settings without an explicit model of care that states the assumptions behind the development of the instrument. Such an explicit model permits both the ideology of an instrument and the logic of individual judgements to be freely inspected. In other words, one cannot realistically measure the needs of specific groups without clear views about the therapeutic and rehabilitative process. These principles have been built into the MRC Needs for Care Assessment (Brewin *et al*, 1987; Brewin & Wing, 1989; Mangen & Brewin, 1991), which was designed for use with the mentally ill living in the community and in high contact with psychiatric services. Data on the reliability and validity of the instrument are encouraging, and are discussed in more detail by Mangen & Brewin (1991).

The MRC needs for care assessment

Model of care and definition of need

The care model on which the assessment is based attempts to reflect the clinical reality of working with individuals with chronic mental health problems. It is well-documented that this group tend to have a low tolerance for stress, difficulty in forming stable social relationships, and high levels of dependency (e. g. Stein & Test, 1980; Lamb, 1982; Shepherd, 1983). The intractable nature of their problems and consequent feelings of helplessness frequently result in demoralisation, effort withdrawal and lack of initiative in overcoming difficulties. Few treatments have demonstrable efficacy, and providing care typically involves a great deal of flexibility and persistence on the part of staff. Multiple clinical symptoms and problems in social functioning are the norm. Relatives who support patients often labour under a considerable burden and have numerous problems themselves (MacCarthy, 1988; MacCarthy *et al*, 1989).

This clinical picture leads naturally to a (much simplified) model of care. The aims of care are to reduce symptoms and distress to the maximum possible extent and to equip patients with the skills required to live independently in the community. This should have beneficial effects both on patients' self-esteem and level of dependence, and make them less vulnerable to changes in their support network, while at the same time minimising the burden on their relatives or on those who are charged with caring for them. To achieve this, a wide range of potential problems must first be assessed at regular intervals. Second, for each problem a range of possible interventions should be specified in order to ensure that all therapeutic options are considered. Third, in order to maintain an appropriately assertive approach to therapy, provision must be made for the case where interventions are initially refused or are (either wholly or partly) ineffective.

Our definition of need is therefore, as indicated above, based on the principle that some specific intervention must be identified that might reduce or ameliorate an objective lack. In this case the objective lack is social disablement, by which we mean lowered physical, psychological, and social functioning compared with societal norms (Wing, 1978, 1986). In other words, actions by care staff are not assumed to be meeting a need simply because social disablement exists, but must also satisfy additional criteria indicating whether those actions are appropriate or inappropriate. This leads to the following formal definition of need for care:

(a) need is present when (i) a patient's functioning (social disablement) falls below or threatens to fall below some minimum specified level, and (ii) this is due to a remediable, or potentially remediable, cause

(b) a need (as defined above) is met when it has attracted some at least partly effective item of care, and when no other items of care of greater potential effectiveness exist

(c) a need (as defined above) is unmet when it has attracted only partly effective or no item of care and when other items of care of greater potential effectiveness exist.

Measurement principles

These definitions are represented in Table 13.1, which specifies how assessments of social disablement and assessments of items of care are combined to yield judgements concerning need. Twenty separate areas of functioning, both clinical and social, are assessed to determine the patient's specific problems. Because of the likely dispersal of information about patients already noted, the investigator is charged with consulting a number of informants, and particularly relatives with whom the patient lives. Reliance on a single source of information is to be avoided. For each area of functioning in which there is a problem, the assessment then specifies a set of potential interventions agreed upon by a cohort of rehabilitation workers (Brewin *et al*, 1987). Each intervention is given a rating by the

TABLE 13.1
Assessment of functioning, interventions, and need status

Assessment of functioning	Assessment of interventions	Need status
No problem or mild problem	None employed	No need
Significant current or recent problem	None even partly effective	No meetable need
	Some potentially fully effective	Met need
	None fully effective: no alternatives	Met need
	None fully effective: alternatives available	Unmet need for treatment
Level of functioning not known		Unmet need for assessment

investigators that reflects whether it is appropriate, whether it has been tried, how effective it has been and, where this is known, whether it has proven acceptable to the patient. Ratings of problems in functioning and of interventions are then combined algorithmically to generate a set of 20 needs-ratings per patient. In each area of functioning the patient can be rated as having no problem and no need, a met need, a problem but no meetable need, an unmet need for intervention, or an unmet need for assessment. The rationale of our definitions of social disablement is given in more detail in Brewin *et al* (1987). The intention was to set down minimum acceptable levels of health and social functioning. Thus, health was defined in terms of the absence of various kinds of symptoms rather than in terms of the achievement of positive health goals. Similarly, acceptable social functioning was defined in terms of possession of the minimum skills required to function independently in the community, rather than in terms of higher level skills that might maximise the individual's autonomy and quality of life.

The symptoms and competencies covered in the most recent version (version Two/2) of the MRC Needs for Care Assessment (Brewin & Wing, 1989) are outlined below.

Symptoms and behaviour problems
  Positive psychotic symptoms
  Retardation (slowness and underactivity)
  Side effects of medication
  Neurotic symptoms
  Organic brain disorder
  Physical disease and disorders
  Violence or threats to self/others
  Socially embarrassing behaviour
  Distress about social circumstances

Personal and social skills
  Personal cleanliness
  Household shopping
  Cooking or buying meals
  Household chores
  Use of public transport
  Use of public amenities
  Basic literacy and arithmetic skills
  Occupational skills
  Social interaction skills
  Management of money
  Management of household affairs

Ratings reflect whether symptoms are current (i.e. were present in the past month), absent in the past month but recently present, or completely absent. The distinction between 'current' and 'recent' symptoms is necessary so that items of care offered for purely preventive purposes can be rated appropriately.

In each area of social disablement the Needs for Care Assessment specifies a list of between two and eight appropriate items of care, covering such diverse types of care as medication, counselling, behaviour programmes, remedial education, and the provision of a sheltered environment. A total of 34 different types of intervention is included. Our aim was to be over- rather than under-inclusive, and this meant including items of care not necessarily in widespread use, although we judged them to be generally acceptable to professionals. The original list of items of care was also validated against the judgements of rehabilitation care staff (Brewin *et al*, 1987), and has been slightly amended in the light of subsequent empirical work. In each area of social disablement there is the facility to add a specific item of care that seems appropriate but does not figure on the standard list.

The principle that problems can only be considered as needs if there are currently feasible or appropriate interventions deserves further comment. This principle follows logically from our definition of need as a requirement for some specifiable form of care. Hence, if all forms of care are in-appropriate, have proven to be ineffective, or have been refused by the patient, need cannot be said to exist. Instead, the individual will be rated by our methods as having a problem but no meetable need. Mangen & Brewin (1991) cite the example of a patient with terminal cancer who from the perspective of service providers does not have a meetable *need* for a cure so long as the cancer is untreatable by currently available methods. The same patient may, on the other hand, have meetable needs for pain relief and for counselling.

Problems with no associated meetable needs do occur from time to time with the long-term mentally ill, and were found to account for approximately

6% of identified problems in the Camberwell High Contact Survey (Brewin *et al*, 1988). It seems to us essential to be able to distinguish in this way those problems for which no effective care can realistically be offered *at the time of the assessment*. While recognising the limitations of current forms of care, this in no way lessens the obligation on agents to develop new and more effective interventions, or to persevere in the future with interventions that may have been unacceptable or ineffective in the past. Indeed, future repetitions of the Needs for Care Assessment would make this duty explicit, and might well result in problems without needs being reclassified as met or unmet needs. The concept of a problem with no meetable need highlights the important fact that professional knowledge and practice are sometimes inadequate to solve all our patients' problems.

In addition to the primary need status, the assessment permits three secondary judgements to be made in each area of disablement. *Overprovision* is rated whenever one or more items of care are rated as being superfluous. In some cases this will be because an item of care continues to be given even though it is not targeted at a specific problem or appears to be completely ineffective. In other cases, the rating reflects that the patient is in receipt of an item of care even though there has been no disablement for a considerable period of time, and there is no apparent danger of relapse. *Future need* can be rated when a patient is currently socially disabled but cannot receive the appropriate item of care because of incapacitating symptoms or other priorities for intervention. *Lack of performance* is rated when a patient is known to be socially competent in some area of functioning and is not receiving any care, but is not currently exercising that skill. The intention here is to draw attention to a possible area in which action might be required. In the Camberwell High Contact Survey (Brewin *et al*, 1988) instances of overprovision were found to be as common as were unmet needs for treatment, but future needs and 'lack of performance' were relatively rare.

Training and manpower requirements

The judgements required of assessors involve familiarity both with long-term patients and their characteristic problems, and with the specific items of care that are considered. Thus it is not suitable for investigators who have not had clinical experience of this patient group, unless considerable extra training is provided. The conclusion of those who have used it is that it is best completed by a clinical team or by a research team that includes members with varying professional backgrounds. Psychiatric and psychological expertise are of prime importance. All users of the instrument should first attend an authorised training programme to familiarise themselves with the instrument. At present this consists of two half-day workshops, with an intervening period in which users gain first-hand experience of carrying out assessments.

Data collection need not be lengthy if the instrument is used to shape the initial assessments conducted by a clinical team. Almost all the information is of the kind that should be routinely collected on admission, and this should be adequate for most clinical purposes. Additional manpower becomes necessary if comparability with other units or clinical teams is necessary for research purposes. This may well involve the addition of standardised assessments of functioning such as the Social Behaviour Schedule (Wykes & Sturt, 1986). Data collection will take considerably longer when the instrument is used by external investigators, as in the Camberwell High Contact Survey. Interviewing patients, day staff, relatives, and other involved persons where appropriate, summarising the medical records, and combining inconsistent information, requires substantial resources.

Applying the MRC Needs for Care Assessment to other populations

The fact that the assessment was designed for chronic but potentially remediable difficulties within a British community setting has a number of consequences for its application to other populations. While the principles of assessment may transfer with little modification to some other chronic patient groups, such as those with diabetes mellitus (Brewin *et al*, 1991), other potential applications raise important issues concerning the goals of, and the constraints on, measurement. Below, we briefly discuss some of the issues raised by applications of the instrument to acute populations, the elderly mentally ill, individuals out of contact with services, long-stay hospital in-patients, and patients from other cultures. All these examples illustrate the central theme of this chapter, namely that the design of assessment instruments is intimately bound up with the model of care being provided.

Acute psychiatric crises

The model of care on which the assessment is based assumes that the *order* in which interventions for a given problem are tried is not critical – the important thing is to persist with a range of possible options. This pragmatic approach appears acceptable for stable conditions that do not pose any immediate threat, but is less suitable for crises and other acute problems where it may be vital to intervene immediately in a particular way. At present the assessment does not include any facility for prioritising interventions, and indeed it is hard to imagine how this could be achieved without the collection of extremely detailed clinical information. Extension of the instrument in this direction would also presuppose that a reasonable degree of clinical consensus concerning crisis management existed.

The elderly mentally ill

The main issues raised by this group concern the applicability of the interventions specified in the assessment. For example, the active rehabilitative focus of Section B may not be perceived as appropriate for elderly and infirm persons permanently housed in residential units providing cooking, cleaning, leisure, and other services. Similarly, remedial education may not be perceived as appropriate for literacy problems in this group. As discussed by Brewin & Wing (1989), it is important to take age, aptitude, and residential placement into account in order not to generate unnecessary unmet needs. But equally, raters should take into account individual wishes to develop skills in a particular area, and whether such skills would lead to an increase in quality of life. Age alone is not sufficient grounds for ignoring unmet needs generated by our assessment.

Finally, adaptation of the instrument for this group might also benefit from incorporating new sections corresponding to particularly common problems, such as incontinence, and from incorporating additional interventions such as reminiscence therapy or reality orientation.

Individuals out of contact with services

Many individuals with severe psychiatric problems are out of contact with services, and sometimes homeless. Assessing their objective lacks is not without difficulty, but assessing their needs for specific items of care is considerably more problematic. The instrument is predicated on the assumption that individuals are in contact with services and that the various forms of care can simply be offered. There is therefore a major issue concerning the acceptability of items of care, individuals' willingness to visit health service or local authority facilities, and what alternative methods can be devised for delivering care in an effective way. It is likely that in many cases the goal of needs assessment should initially be simply that of establishing (a) objective lacks and (b) acceptable channels of service delivery. These might take the form of a lunch club or drop-in centre in preference to more traditional service settings.

Long-stay hospital in-patients

There is perhaps just one part of the assessment that is completely inappropriate for this group, and that is the section on management of household affairs. This section involves estimating the individual's ability to pay rent and bills, arrange repairs, and join in the running of the ordinary household. It is hard to see how information of this kind could ever be obtained for long-stay in-patients since the opportunities for observing them are most unlikely to exist. This section should therefore be rated as not applicable in long-stay samples.

Assessment problems may arise in other sections, for example those involving cooking and shopping, when hospital policy is to provide these services for all, regardless of their specific disabilities. Two choices are available here to the user of the instrument faced with a complete absence of any opportunities to observe patients' skills and abilities. The first option, which should normally be chosen when discharge from hospital is possible or inevitable, or when the patients are in an explicitly rehabilitative setting, is to rate all such examples as needs for assessment. The second option is to rate the level of functioning as unknown but the need as being met, on the pragmatic grounds that one cannot realistically train someone to develop a skill that they are then prevented from using. Once again, the model of care being employed constrains the nature of possible assessment.

Patients from other cultures

Attention must be paid to cultural constraints when using the instrument on ethnic minorities within Britain, or on patient groups outside Britain. For example, in Verona (and presumably in other parts of Italy) it appears to be inappropriate to expect men to have demonstrated competence in cooking and other household chores. These are not part of the accepted male role, and hence were not accepted as needs either by professionals using our procedure or by service users (Lesage *et al*, 1991). Once again, specific subsections of the assessment may be rated as not applicable in order to cope with this contingency.

Conclusions

Methods of assessing individual needs for care and services will depend primarily on the nature of the population to be surveyed and on whether they are in high or low contact with psychiatric services. For populations in low contact, service needs have sometimes been estimated from morbidity and existing service-utilisation rates. These data are inevitably crude, however, and do not furnish answers to important questions concerning whether individuals are in fact receiving appropriate and acceptable treatment. Such methods, although they may indicate substantial quantities of unmet need, say little about the quality of the unmet need and the factors that might improve service take-up. They also tend not to challenge the therapeutic status quo and are unlikely to result in a radical reappraisal of the adequacy of services.

For patients in high contact, brief assessments of needs for different kinds of service are sometimes made by care staff themselves. Although these methods have often demonstrated large amounts of unmet need, little is known about their validity. On the whole, what is known is not reassuring. With training, however, staff can make reasonably reliable brief assessments about needs for different kinds of day and residential placement (Clifford *et al*, 1991).

Any attempt to specify in more detail how staff should intervene is a relatively time-consuming matter. The MRC Needs for Care Assessment is at present the most comprehensive instrument available to assess the needs of the long-term mentally ill. It is also the only instrument to be based on an explicit model of patient care and, repeated at regular intervals, could form the basis of clinical management. Although this model may not find universal favour, we believe that progress in individual needs assessment is only likely to follow attempts to articulate principles of care and open up evaluation methods to public scrutiny.

References

BIRCHWOOD, M. & SMITH, J. (1988) The needs of families caring for a schizophrenic relative: developing a comprehensive service. In *Current Issues in Clinical Psychology 1986* (eds N. Eisenberg & D. Glasgow), pp. 186–200. Aldershot: Gower Press.

BREWIN, C. R., WING, J. K., MANGEN, S. P., *et al* (1987) Principles and practice of measuring need in the long-term mentally ill: the MRC Needs for Care Assessment. *Psychological Medicine*, **17**, 971–982.

——, ——, ——, *et al* (1988) Needs for care among the long-term mentally ill: a report from the Camberwell High Contact Survey. *Psychological Medicine*, **18**, 457–468.

—— & —— (1989) *MRC Needs for Care Assessment: Manual for version Two/2*. Unpublished manuscript. London: Institute of Psychiatry.

——, VELTRO, F., WING, J. K., *et al* (1990) The assessment of psychiatric disability in the community: a comparison of clinical, staff, and family interviews. *British Journal of Psychiatry*, **157**, 671–674.

——, BRADLEY, C. & HOME, P. (1991) Measuring needs in patients with diabetes. In *The Technology of Diabetes Care* (eds C. Bradley, P. Home & M. Christie), pp. 142–155. Reading: Harwood.

CLIFFORD, P., CHARMAN, A., WEBB, Y., *et al* (1991) Planning for community care: the Community Placement Questionnaire. *British Journal of Clinical Psychology*, **30**, 193–211.

CORMIER, H., BORUS, J. F., REED, R. B., *et al* (1987) Combler les besoins de service de sante mentale des personnes atteintes de schizophrenie. *Canadian Journal of Psychiatry*, **32**, 454–458.

DAVIES, B. & CHALLIS, D. (1986) *Matching Resources to Needs in Community Care*. London: Gower.

FALLOON, I. R. H. & MARSHALL, G. N. (1983) Residential care and social behaviour: a study of rehabilitation needs. *Psychological Medicine*, **13**, 341–347.

LAMB, H. R. (1982) *Treating the Long-term Mentally Ill*. San Francisco: Jossey-Bass.

LEHTINEN, V., JOUKAMAA, M., JYRKINEN, E., *et al* (1990) Need for mental health services of the adult population in Finland: results from the Mini Finland Health Survey. *Acta Psychiatrica Scandinavica*, **81**, 426–431.

LEIGHTON, D. C., HARDING, J. S., MACKLIN, D. B., *et al* (1963) Psychiatric findings of the Stirling County Study. *American Journal of Psychiatry*, **119**, 1021–1026.

LESAGE, A. D., MIGNOLLI, G., FACCINCANI, C., *et al* (1991) Standardised assessment of the needs of care in a cohort of patients with schizophrenic psychoses. In *Community-based Psychiatry: Long-term Patterns of Care in South-Verona* (ed M. Tansella), pp. 27–33. *Psychological Medicine* Monograph Supplement No. 19.

LEVIN, G., WILDER, J. F. & GILBERT, J. (1978) Identifying and meeting clients' needs in six community mental health centers. *Hospital and Community Psychiatry*, **29**, 185–188.

MACCARTHY, B. (1988) The role of relatives. In *Community Care in Practice: Services for the Continuing Care Client* (eds A. Lavender & F. Holloway), pp. 207–227. Chichester: Wiley.
——, LESAGE, A., BREWIN, C. R., *et al* (1989) Needs for care among the relatives of long-term users of day care. *Psychological Medicine*, **19**, 725–736.
MALLMAN, C. A. & MARCUS, S. (1980) Logical clarifications in the study of needs. In *Human Needs* (ed. K. Lederer), pp. 163–185. Cambridge, MA: Oelgeschlager, Gunn & Hain.
MANGEN, S. & BREWIN, C. R. (1991) The measurement of need. In *Social Psychiatry: Theory, Methodology and Practice* (ed. P. E. Bebbington). New Brunswick, NJ: Transaction Press.
MANN, S. & CREE, W. (1976) 'New' long-stay psychiatric patients: a national survey of fifteen mental hospitals in England and Wales 1972/3. *Psychological Medicine*, **6**, 603–616.
SHAPIRO, S., SKINNER, E. A., KRAMER, M., *et al* (1985) Measuring need for mental health services in a general population. *Medical Care*, **23**, 1033–1043.
SHEPHERD, G. (1983) Planning the rehabilitation of the individual. In *Theory and Practice of Psychiatric Rehabilitation* (eds F. N. Watts & D. H. Bennett), pp. 329–348. Chichester: Wiley.
SOLOMON, P. & DAVIS, J. (1985) Meeting community service needs of discharged psychiatric patients. *Psychiatric Quarterly*, **57**, 11–17.
STEIN, L. I. & TEST, M. A. (1980) Alternative to mental hospital treatment: I. Conceptual model, treatment program, and clinical evaluation. *Archives of General Psychiatry*, **37**, 392–399.
TRACY, L. (1986) Toward an improved need theory: in response to legitimate criticism. *Behavioral Science*, **31**, 205–218.
WASYLENKI, D. A., GOERING, P., LANCEE, W., *et al* (1981) Psychiatric aftercare: identified needs versus referral patterns. *American Journal of Psychiatry*, **138**, 1228–1231.
WING, J. K. (1978) Medical and social science and medical and social care. In *Social Care Research* (eds J. Barnes & N. Connelly), pp. 123–137. London: Bedford Square Press.
—— (1986) The cycle of planning and evaluation. In *The Provision of Mental Health Services in Britain: The Way Ahead* (eds G. Wilkinson & H. Freeman), pp. 35–48. London: Gaskell.
WYKES, T., CREER, C. & STURT, E. (1982) Needs and the deployment of services. In *Long-term Community Care: Experience in a London Borough* (ed. J. K. Wing), pp. 41–55. *Psychological Medicine* Monograph Supplement No. 2.
——, STURT, E. & CREER, C. (1985) The assessment of patients' needs for community care. *Social Psychiatry*, **20**, 76–85.
—— & —— (1986) The measurement of social behaviour in psychiatric patients: an assessment of the reliability and validity of the SBS schedule. *British Journal of Psychiatry*, **148**, 1–11.

14 Computerised clinical case-record systems

PETER ROHDE and JASON TAYLOR

In this chapter, the case for computerised clinical case-record systems is considered and illustrated with reference to two established systems. Needs assessment is not the primary purpose of these systems, but once a system is in use, it may be incorporated. Implementation and acceptance are major problems with clinical systems. Some of the problems involved are considered.

There is general agreement that the best data are those that come from the 'horse's mouth'. In a health-service context, the data which are collected and used by clinicians for their management of patients are the most reliable. Where information for statistical purposes is collected by a second party looking at the clinical records, it is less likely to be accurate than the clinicians' own records (Wing, 1989).

It is easy enough to persuade well motivated researchers to collect data in a standardised manner and it is also relatively easy to instruct administrative staff to collect administrative data. The problems come with clinicians. They see their primary purpose as treating patients, and their records as tools to enable them to treat the patient in the best possible way and to communicate with other professionals concerning their findings. It is notoriously difficult to get clinicians to record clinical information systematically, to complete data-entry forms or even to complete discharge summaries on time. The rewards of designing a computerised clinical system which is sufficiently attractive for clinicians to want to use it for all their patients are considerable, but the paucity of systems surviving the test of time is testimony to the difficulties.

There are many problems in establishing such a model in psychiatry and getting clinicians to use it. Hedlund (1985a,b) has reviewed the fate of clinical computer systems in the United States and shown that much of the early promise of the 1970s and early 1980s was not fulfilled, in spite of very large sums of money being spent (see also Jay & Anderson, 1982). There was a regular pattern for computer systems that involved both a clinical and an administrative element to persist in the administrative mode but for the clinical element to drop out. Recently a trend has developed towards smaller, less ambitious systems with fewer clinical data but correspondingly fewer potential clinical rewards (Hedlund, 1985*a*).

Young (1984) reviewed studies on professional acceptance of clinical computer systems and observed that it is not enough for clinicians to perceive a system as being potentially useful, it is also essential that they perceive it as not too intrusive on their personal method of practice. Anderson (1986) quoted studies of different professionals showing that computerised systems were accepted if they enhanced the professional's ability to manage patients and opposed if they infringed on the clinician's role as decision maker.

A successful computer system is likely to be one which offers real rewards for users for a minimum of effort. This chapter describes two approaches (SafetyNet and CRISP) to the problem of making a clinical computer system attractive to mental health workers so that they use it as part of their everyday work. Although the approaches differ, they share the model of a database which contains clinical data on individuals, details of their contacts with the service and an archive.

The archive enables the database to be updated and the changes to be recorded longitudinally, becoming, in effect, a self-building psychiatric register. Clinicians have a vested interest in keeping the database up-to-date as part of their clinical work, because they are using it as a clinical record. Thus the problem of updating, one of the major difficulties with such databases, is solved as part of the working process.

Figure 14.1 illustrates the concept, the initial database being gradually changed as a result of subsequent clinical contact, so that it is always up-to-date and provides a longitudinal record. A computer system incorporating such a model provides information on clinical measurements and data for research purposes as part of the regular data set. It is also an appropriate sampling frame for more detailed projects and provides a vehicle for questionnaires and enquiries. Needs assessment can be incorporated into the system by programming 'rules' into the software so that needs can be deduced from the data on problems, mental states, diagnoses and interventions. An alternative approach is to add a module such as the MRC Needs Assessment system.

SafetyNet

The background to the SafetyNet project

In preparation for the proposed closure by North East Thames Regional Health Authority of Friern Barnet mental hospital by 1993, detailed in-patient and community point-prevalence surveys were undertaken in 1985.

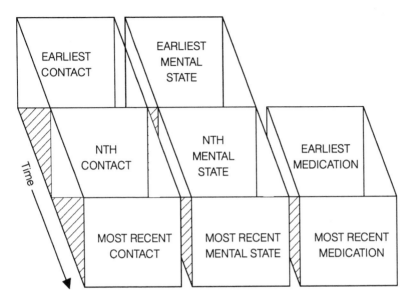

Fig. 14.1. The case-register concept represented as a card-file system

These studies focused on individuals in North and South Camden diagnosed as suffering from schizophrenia. All individuals known on a single census day to health services, social services, the probation service and to general practitioners (GPs) were included (Campbell *et al*, 1990). Data collected in these studies formed the basis for the SafetyNet information system (Taylor *et al*, 1988, 1990) which is targeted at providing clinical monitoring, case management, service evaluation, and research. SafetyNet is currently being established in around 12 sites in the UK, from Department of Health projects monitoring the homeless mentally ill to a range of in-patient and community psychiatric services.

Aims and objectives

The SafetyNet project is non-profit making and has been funded from charitable sources. The system has been programmed over the past three years and is designed to be an inexpensive and comprehensive mental health information system of the case-register type, that is highly flexible in terms of its adaptability to focus for patient management, and builds longitudinal information on each patient. Validated five-point rating scales for the measurement of mental states (the Krawiecka Scale; Krawiecka *et al*, 1977), problem behaviour (the Social Behaviour Schedule (SBS); Wykes & Sturt, 1986) are used along with assessments of living skills and interventions as a basis for measuring the process and outcome of care. The system keeps track of individual patients, charts progress and interventions, and prompts and helps unify service responses. It also highlights individuals requiring detailed needs assessment through the availability of wide-ranging automated reports, for example listing patients who have not been assessed for several months, those missing appointments or depot injections, those who are actively psychotic and refusing interventions, or those without key support staff in the community. In addition, SafetyNet collects administrative Korner data, other clinical data (aftercare management, past psychiatric history, admission and discharge data, physical information, medication, ICD–9/10 diagnoses), social data (benefits, social networks, accommodation), staff-contact information (key workers and current health service and non-health service contacts), legal-status information, and consumer feedback of the service on offer. Interventions recorded include medication, aftercare management, main intervention and up to five subsidiary interventions, and alert warnings. Despite the wide range of data collected, clinicians can access as much or as little of the SafetyNet system as they wish.

The SafetyNet dataset is summarised below:

Additional information
Accommodation and problems
Social networks
Daytime activities and skills
Benefits
Past psychiatric history
Health-service contacts
Aftercare plans/administration
Other service contacts
Admission/discharge information
Legal-status information
Medication (all drugs) and side effects
ICD–9/10 diagnoses (all codes)
Physical health/disabilities
Problems assessment (based on SBS)
Mental-state assessment (based on Manchester)
Mental state and problems reviews
Investigations
Consumer views on service
Rate on your own scales/questionnaires
(up to 98 additional scales added by end user)

Hardware & software

SafetyNet is available as an inexpensive system that will run on a standalone IBM-compatible personal computer (PC) with 1 MB RAM and a hard disk running MSDOS, on linked PCs where data is held on a central computer running on an MSDOS network or under a network running 386 SCO Xenix (or Unix compatible) operating systems. SafetyNet is fully compatible in its different guises so that users can start with a single-user PC version and upgrade later without loss of data.

Within SafetyNet is incorporated a system called ResearchBase whereby anyone (without programming expertise) can add in rating scales or questionnaires for time-series data collection. ResearchBase allows users to define questions which can be numeric ranges, dates, free text, or codes, each with an associated descriptor that will later appear in a window on screen for easy selection and automatic validation. The ResearchBase system allows users to add in up to 98 scales each with up to 999 questions (branching or non-branching). SafetyNet is written in the popular Dbase IV programming language which has become an international standard and has simple links to a variety of other packages for further graphical output, for example, spreadsheet, QuattroPro or statistical analysis, e.g. SPSS PC + . Services using SafetyNet who also purchased Dbase IV can interrogate the system in order to retrieve any combination of data and are not limited to the extensive range of reports that are provided with the system.

Building longitudinal records

Different mental health workers provide key clinical, personal and administrative information at each contact which will then be entered by the health worker concerned or a trained data-entry clerk to the central computer from peripheral IBM-compatible computers or terminals based in sites across the district and linked by a modem or lease line. Because each contact is time and date stamped and recorded (whether an individual attends or not) the system will alert all staff to individuals who have missed appointments, or who have refused depot medication. The system also draws up lists of people not seen for a specified time period, automatically prompting workers to arrange follow-up for these individuals, and keeps track of Mental Health Act information and Section 117 Aftercare provision. Before any patients are taken off the system, policy should dictate that attempts are made to assess them and to contact any relevant health workers to ensure that the patient is not in need of long-term support. The system provides problem-orientated automated reviews allowing the definition of management plans, a responsible key worker, and review data to be recorded. Automated frontsheet summaries of clinical or administrative data can be generated immediately, and listings of a workers caseload, or conversely of all mental health workers seeing an individual patient, can be provided on screen or as a printout.

The SafetyNet system actively archives all data so that an immediately accessible longitudinal record is built up which follows each individual's progress over the years. Health workers can choose to view records for a selected patient longitudinally on screen so that, for instance, problems can be viewed as they change over time. An extensive range of reports are available either in letter format to GPs on screen, to a file, or as printouts, the aims being to ensure that once data are entered into the system they are available to the end user and do not disappear into a 'Black Hole' from which they can never be retrieved.

Graphical charts can also be displayed showing the most recent problems or mental-state ratings. Alternatively, users may view and print out graphs showing the changes in ratings of a selected mental-state symptom or problem over time, or a time-series chart plotting management interventions or chlorpromazine equivalents against selected mental states, problems, or research ratings (Fig. 14.2). This allows the possibility of relating changes in outcome to interventions. Further developments currently underway include resource management and costing modules. All sensitive information

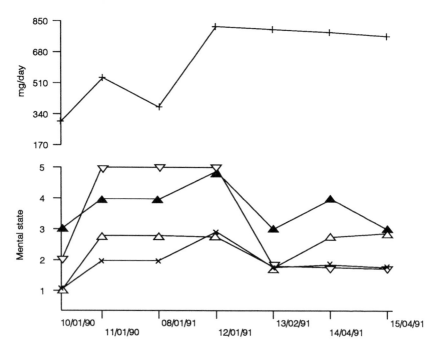

Fig. 14.2. Selected mental state signs: hallucinations (▽—▽), delusions (▲—▲), anxiety (△—△) and depression (×—×), and chlorpromazine equivalents (+—+)

(names and addresses) within SafetyNet is stored as encrypted code and the system has extensive security features to allow the user to set limited access by consultant, sector, or GP, or to limit access by individual mental health workers to selected screens or reports. SafetyNet also incorporates a full appointment-booking system, although users do not have to implement this if they choose to use existing systems.

Portable barcode-reading interface

A barcode-reading interface has been developed allowing community workers to collect key data on portable barcode readers which read standard code 39 barcodes (the readers are not connected to the machine but have RAM memory). Workers can download the information at the end of the day or every few days to the computer via a PC-linked device. This appears to be an effective means of collecting data from community sources. It is less expensive than data clerks and allows for immediate input of clinical data. The barcode system acts like a multiple-choice format questionnaire. The user reads a barcode which acts as a root identifier for each relevant data item (such as depression) and then reads a barcode rating (say between 1 and 5 for depression) from a single form with concatenating codes (ranging from 0 to 9). These barcode forms are cheap to produce, can be photocopied and laminated, and are easily portable in the community. Furthermore, if for any reason the barcode reader is misplaced, the data are more secure than if carried on a portable computer or on hand-filled forms. Floppy disk-based data entry options (Mini-net) are currently being programmed as separate modules (SafetyNet itself will run on a laptop or notebook computer with a hard disk).

East of data entry

Case-register systems are prone to failure because of the time taken to input relevant clinical data. Virtually every field item in SafetyNet can display a list of possible options for that data item and the user can pick one (or more) from that list by one key press (Fig. 14.3). The code for that item is then directly transferred and stored, and the selected code and its associated descriptor text (the rubric) is displayed on screen. Each data field has a maintenance option. Codes and descriptors can be customised by the system administrator without additional programming, thus allowing any user to collect data relevant to their local service.

CRISP

CRISP (Computer Recorded Information System for Psychiatry) was designed to be both a tool for clinicians and a source of 'bottom-up' data,

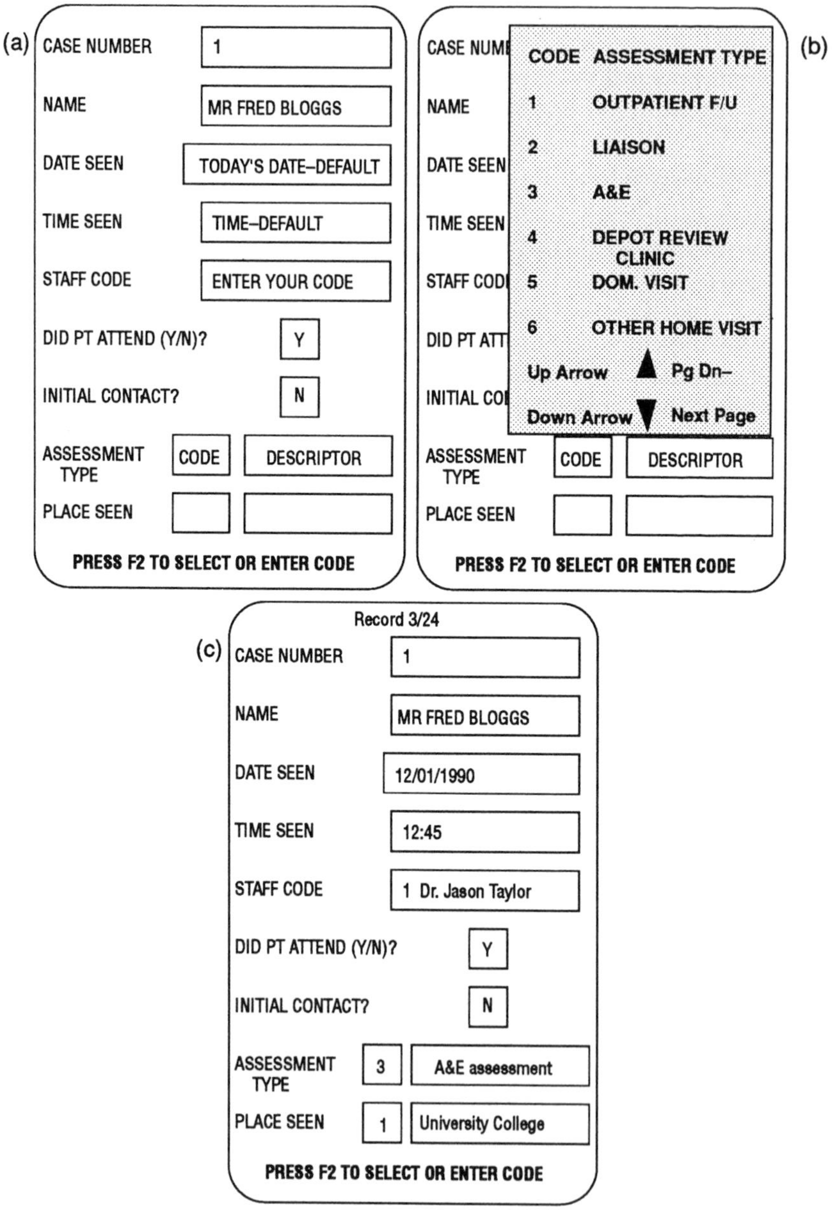

Fig. 14.3. Contact screens for data entry (a) and (b) (showing list of codes & descriptors on key F2 press) and for data view (c) (showing active archiving of contact records)

i.e. reliable clinical information which can be used for statistical and research purposes.

St Mary Abbots Hospital in Kensington, London W8, contains a District General Hospital Psychiatric Unit which was one of the first in London when it opened in 1966. It has continued to serve a very mixed area adjacent to the hospital, providing in-patient, day, out-patient, and community care. The CRISP system was developed in this setting.

A new psychiatric assessment procedure was introduced in 1983 involving emergencies being assessed on the day of referral by a multidisciplinary team, usually working in pairs. The needs of this assessment team, and indeed the needs of community care for psychiatric patients, highlighted the deficiency of the traditional medical records. These are paper records, with the bulk of entries being medical, but with provision for other disciplines to enter their contributions. These records work well enough for in-patients, but problems sometimes arise in an out-patient setting where the notes have to follow the patient. They become seriously inadequate when each discipline wishes to keep separate records and the patient or client may be seen at several different sites in the course of a week. Thus, the same patient may be sleeping in the hospital where he is technically an in-patient, attending a day hospital or a day centre under the local authority, visiting a psychologist for therapy and attending an out-patient appointment later in the week with a doctor.

In addition to the problem of the record being unable to be in more than one place at once, the needs of a multidisciplinary team may be for a more socially orientated record than the traditional medical history. There has been a gradual shift in the last 20 years towards recognition that help and care plans require more emphasis than they have previously had in psychiatric records which were often more preoccupied with diagnosing the problems than looking at the solutions.

One result of setting up the assessment procedure was the development of a data set and data-collection form. This was similar to a psychiatric summary and was intended to be computerised so that it could be available at more than one site and so that the data would be available for analysis. Out of these beginnings evolved the CRISP system. The data set contains all the clinical and administrative information that might normally be found in a psychiatric assessment or discharge summary, together with additional material. The system allows these data to be changed and updated any number of times and all the changes are archived. Thus a longitudinal record of changes within patients and populations is readily available. Because many professionals dislike using or will not use computers, all staff are offered the choice of direct entry into the computer or of completing a data-entry form on paper and handing it to the team secretary who will insert the material for them.

The data-entry form is completed the first time the patient is seen (in practice, completion of the form only takes about eight minutes for a practised clinician who has just assessed the patient). After data entry, the data set is printed out immediately as a current clinical summary (CCS). The CCS is then placed in the front of the notes, and whenever the patient is reviewed from then onwards, it is scanned briefly. If it is still correct, it is left alone – if there have been any changes, it is amended by the clinician, either by direct entry into the computer or by dictating the changes to the team secretary. A new CCS is then printed, and replaces the previous one in the notes. There is no need to save the previous CCS since the computer can reproduce a CCS for any past date. This cycle of revision can be repeated any number of times so as to reflect the actual changes that take place in the management of a patient. The more onerous task of completing the data-entry form is only required once in a patient or client's contact with the service. The main components of the dataset are given below:

basic demographic data
assets and coping resources
rating of involvement of relatives
details of family history and past history
a problems list with free text for amplification of detail
a brief mental state based on the Present State Examination (PSE;
    Wing *et al*, 1974)
help plans with free text for amplification
list of involved professionals and key workers who are concerned with
    patient care.

The dataset is largely self-explanatory, with the demographic data being approximately those found on a normal hospital frontsheet, but there are some additional items. Assets and coping resources are rated in an attempt to look at the positive side of the patient; the involvement of the family allows information concerning the patient's relationships. A list of problems, provided with space for free text, provides a reasonable compromise between a need for full information about the patient's present complaints and coding of problems to allow for searches.

A brief mental state consists of seven items produced by aggregation of Present State Examination (PSE) items. The ratings are similar to the PSE and it is designed so that the PSE glossary can be used as a guide for rating the mental state. Help plans (or care plans) allow site and nature of treatments planned, and, as with the problems, there is sufficient free text area for adequate description of the treatment planned. Each plan is tagged with the name of one professional who is primarily responsible and there may be any number of plans inserted. Lists of 'involved professionals' and key workers are also provided. The involved professionals are defined as those persons outside the service covered by the computer such as the GP, local authority social worker, and counsellor. Key workers are those who

TABLE 14.1
Basic input and output for CRISP system

Input	Output
Admissions	Clinic lists
Bookings	Lists of defaulters
Attendance registers	Standard letters
Changes of setting	Activity statistics
Other NHS computers	Korner statistics etc.
Midnight returns	Current clinical summary
Discharges etc.	Interagency referrals
Clinical review	Discharge letters
	Report for review MH act
	Review tribunals
	Nursing-process forms
	List and reminders
	Longitudinal data
	Research

are involved within the service and will generally include not just a key worker who is taking a special responsibility for the patient, but all those with a legitimate interest such as the 'Nursing Process' nurse for an in-patient, the social worker who may be attached to the team, the junior doctor and the consultant. The basic input and output of the system and the way in which it can be used by varying the output format are given in Table 14.1.

Separate modules provide for pharmacy and Mental Health Act administration. Once such a system is in regular use, the advantages for professionals are considerable. Clinical management is helped by immediate access to: individual records (CCS); lists of case load etc.; reminders and defaulters; and in-depth review, using Past CCS and Life Charts.

The 'scans' part of the output program can be used to interrogate the database for both clinical and research purposes. Using a suitable letter-writing package, the basic CCS data can be re-worked automatically by the machine to provide discharge summaries, summaries for the Mental Health Tribunal, etc. These then require only small amounts of typing for individual messages before they are sent out. The life chart and individual reporting facilities offer opportunities for longitudinal study of individual patients and surveys on the whole patient population.

The current version of the Mental Health Connection (MHC2) is written in the 'C' programming language and runs under the Unix operating system. This enables the software to be run on a variety of hardware from laptop PCs to mini computers. In addition to the CRISP element, it provides for the whole range of administrative and clinical functions required by a district psychiatric service. Data import and export are available to suit local requirements and the software is also available in modules to reduce the cost to users not requiring a district-wide system.

Results of the pilot project

The pilot project on the CRISP system commenced in April 1987 at St Mary Abbots Hospital and lasted for just over a year, using the CRISP concepts incorporated into the existing software developed for the Napsbury Hospital by Protechnic Computer Company of Cambridge (The Mental Health Connection). The main findings are described below.

The insertion of user-coded fields, debugging the software, and learning how to use the system, all took much longer than anticipated. Although there was much interest in the hospital, the lack of a key person who could master the intricacies of the system and devote enough time to this task was felt. A full time systems administrator was subsequently appointed and it was a conclusion of the pilot project that it is essential that there should be one key person who has the ability and the time to master the workings of the whole system and to teach clinical, secretarial and administrative staff how to make the best of it. The question of entry of user-coded fields is important. These are the items of information that the service wishes to collect. In spite of the fact that these had been largely worked out in advance, it still took a long time to insert them and get used to using them, and lack of firm control on entering new fields meant that some logical inconsistencies crept in.

By the latter half of the pilot project, just under 500 patients were on the system as names and registration numbers. Just under 400 patients had basic demographic data. By the end of the pilot project, 150 patients had full CCS and the majority of these had their CCS upgraded on a number of occasions. Towards the end of the pilot project it became apparent that these summary revisions were so frequent (because the system was being used) that a method of incorporating progress notes had to be added to the CCS and used as an alternative to revising the whole summary. Some 60 patients had summaries involving progress notes and this number was continuing to rise at the end of the project.

The pilot consultant team (PDR) was operating with the CCS as the primary record of clinical decision-taking by the team by the end of the pilot project. There was no deliberate intention to replace existing clinical notes, and it was always claimed that this was a summary rather than a full record. However, in areas such as day care where clinical notes tend to be quite scrappy and fragmented, the CCS appeared to be taking over as the definitive record. When there was a survey of follow-up information for purposes of Section 117 of the Mental Health Act, it was noted by an independent researcher that those patients with the CCS were the best documented of those attending day care. During the latter half of the project, the CCSs were providing a useful resource, and received favourable comments from Mental Health Review Tribunals, managers and GPs, as well as local staff.

The dataset proved acceptable to the clinical team and appeared to be a reasonable compromise between conflicting requirements. The CCS contains a mixture of data which are coded, and therefore easily analysable, and free text which puts flesh on the bones of the coded data. As implemented, the system allows a space for free text after all the major coded items such as family history, personal history, problem groups, help plans, etc. This was welcomed by staff members and was a major factor in making the printouts acceptable to users who were not interested in computers.

Guidance for the implementation of a computer system

It cannot be emphasised often enough that designing and implementing a computer system is very complicated, requires a great deal of work, and every aspect must be thought through. It certainly generally takes much longer and is much more difficult than anyone concerned visualises! In addition to decisions about the computer and its software, it is essential that decisions are taken about the non-computer aspects. Indeed, it can be argued that these are far more important than the computer-related topics. The first essential is a working group, consisting of key persons who are going to devote time and thought to the project. This must represent a compromise between the need for a group that is large enough to consider all potential users, but not so large that it cannot make decisions. Some successful systems have started in the mind of one individual. This may be very helpful and useful in developing the system, and indeed in seeing it as a coherent whole, but there then has to be a stage in which a working group is either persuaded to accept the overall model or has a say in making sure that the project is going to have something in it for all users. However, the difficulty about group decisions is the lack of a coherent group memory. There is a risk that the final product is flawed because there are conflicting elements that have not been reconciled.

Decisions to be made by the working group

(a) What is the system for and how widely available is it going to be within the service?

The group needs to consider the advantages and disadvantages of computer systems. It is likely that any system purporting to replace clinical notes is going to come up against insuperable resistance from at least some of the clinicians concerned. A system which summarises the situation along the lines that are indicated above has real appeal, however, particularly if the opportunity is made to provide the summaries and output at a number of different sites so that the computerised record is in fact of assistance in coordinating the care for the individual. This is particularly helpful in modern psychiatric services where much of the care may take place on different sites at different times, involving a number of professionals. If a system (whether this be an approach to audit or flagging up people whose mental health sections are due to expire) is not already operational in some form, then buying in computers and software without clear forethought, discussion and operational procedures may well have costs which outweigh the benefits.

(b) Can a dataset be agreed?

Mental health professionals have wide-ranging interests and target different patient groups. They may also have fundamentally different ideologies making common ground difficult beyond establishing a minimum administrative dataset. An alternative approach is to develop a system in modular fashion whereby the most fragmented services or those patient groups most in need of follow-up are given priority. Comprehensive clinical case-record systems will eventually incorporate datasets targeted at different populations but initially it may be difficult to please everyone.

(c) Who is going to operate the system?

It is essential to the running of the system that there is one individual who knows it well enough to operate all its aspects and can take responsibility for coordinating and training others. This may be the role of the innovator or even, if a professional has been involved in programming, the programmer. What is required is a coordinator who will have this as part of his/her job description with time set aside for it.

(d) Who is going to collect and enter the data?

The use of existing secretaries to put in clinical data has the advantage that they are used to typing and if the system is going to be generating letters and summaries, they have a vested interest in inserting data so as to reduce their own labour. There is no objection to clinicians entering data directly, but it is almost certainly unrealistic to imagine that all clinical staff will routinely enter data into a computer system. Some will be enthusiastic, others will be tolerant, but there will be a hard core who will resist any request to have hands-on experience with a computer. Peripheral data-entry devices such as bar codes, portable computers or optical-character reading of specially designed questionnaires may be used to minimise the task for professionals.

(e) Selecting a system

A general model of use, and an initial plan of the overall system and how it will operate, should arise out of these early decisions of the working group. Once this has been achieved, it may be worth considering software (computer programmes) to achieve this model of functioning. There are a number of choices here, of which the principal is whether to use an existing system which approximately matches, or can be modified to match, these requirements, or whether to develop a new system. It is essential to recognise that developing a computer system from nothing is time-consuming and that everybody underestimates the problems involved. Programmers have difficulty in grasping the functioning of a modern psychiatric service, and the professionals in that service have considerable difficulty in putting into words how they operate, even if they recognise it themselves! For the new system to survive it must be capable of proving itself attractive to unmotivated users who know very little of its origins. There is a grave risk of systems failing once the originators have left, or after the 'honeymoon' period, when users may feel that the ratio of work put in to benefit gained is unfavourable.

(f) Stationery and form-design considerations

Once a dataset and the software route have been decided, at least in outline, the clinical implementation should be considered again in more detail. Some fairly basic non-computer elements will be extremely important to the acceptance of the system, for example, what stationery will be required for data entry and for print-out? If possible the data-entry form, and indeed data-entry screens, should contain enough information so that a manual is unnecessary. Ideally, the data-entry forms should mimic the computer screens for ease of data transfer. The outputs need to be attractive and self-explanatory so that the information contained is easily digested and the outputs sell themselves to professionals.

(g) How many terminals and printers, and where?

There is a strong case for making generous provision in a networked system so that access is easy. This helps ensure that clinicians make use of the information on the system which, in turn, helps motivate them to keep it up to date.

(h) Who is going to be in charge of access, training and trouble-shooting?

This should be decided in some detail. It is desirable that all established professionals have access to a clinical computer system, even if only to selected parts. It is an advantage of a computerised record or summary that it can collect together the information gathered in different departments and make it available to all, thus harmonising the work of a multidisciplinary team. It is also possible that some individuals, such as say volunteers or staff concerned with administration, should have access to limited parts of the system only. It might be appropriate, for instance, to allow volunteers to know who the key workers involved with a particular patient are, but not the clinical information.

Training needs to be thought of at an early stage so that staff are aware that there is going to be a change in their working practices and they are given adequate explanation and preferably hands-on experience of the new system. There should be an emphasis on the rewards of the system. Training needs to be backed up by a clear trouble-shooting and support routine. It is recommended that the system coordinator or some identified person makes themselves available for requests for information and problems, particularly initially. There will always be new people arriving in a psychiatric service who will need training and there will also be those who forget quite elementary matters, such as how to turn on a printer.

It is important that persons who do not require it are not allowed access to parts of the computer programme that they might interfere with. Once more, this underlines the need for a named person or persons who should be contacted in the event of problems rather than allowing amateur computer experts to try and put things right. The staff required need to be identified in some detail and a timetable for training and implementation constructed by the working group.

(i) Who will have access?

The Data Protection Act (Office of the Data Protection Registrar, 1985) gives clear guidelines on access to data by subjects. Agreement must be reached about access to read and/or add data by different professional groups, and also whether access to information will be granted to patients/clients without their applying for this through more formal channels. Recent developments concerning the right of access to clinical notes have brought the situation for written notes into line with access to electronic data storage. It is good practice for all notes to be written with subject access in mind.

All systems must be secure. Password entry is used on most systems and data encryption (where any sensitive data are stored as meaningless code until the correct passwords are entered) on some. It would be desirable for systems to employ magnetic card readers (similar to those used by the banking dispensing machines). These card-entry systems, together with individual PIN numbers, can be arranged to set different access levels to the computer system. They are now available for IBM-compatible personal computers. This approach encourages an increased sense of personal responsibility for security.

(j) Coding requirements

Most clinical case-record systems store codes although some allow large quantities of free text to be typed in. Codes are less expensive in terms of computer disk storage and each code is often linked to a descriptor so that the code and descriptor can be displayed on the screen, for example, in ICD–9, 295.3 = paranoid schizophrenia. Codes speed up data input and can often be modified on any well designed computer system to meet the needs of different services. One of the greatest barriers to generalisation of models is that until very recently there were no widely adopted standards for coding of assessment, diagnoses and management in medicine.

Read codes[1], introduced by Dr James Read, have now been accepted as a national standard in general practice and increasingly in hospital practice as well. These codes cover all aspects of medicine and it is intended that they will expand into psychiatry with the cooperation of the Royal College of Psychiatrists. They are kept up-to-date with regular updates from the NHS Centre for Coding and Classification, which was founded after the Department of Health bought the copyright of the Read codes in 1990. Coding within psychiatry remains an area which is likely to require considerable clarification over the next few years. The diversity of approaches and ideologies within psychiatry may make the adoption of a standard set of codes difficult but there are many advantages to a nationally agreed coding system.

(k) Are links to existing systems needed?

Linking to existing systems is often problematic. There are a variety of patient administration systems (PAS) and if a community service covers a number of sites then linking to one or more of these may be desirable to prevent staff having to enter data twice. They may, however, run on completely different hardware with different computer-operating systems running different software. The situation may be further complicated by many units running Korner minimum data-set collection systems which may themselves not link to PAS or to any proposed clinical case-record system. If systems are linked, then attention needs to be given as to whether access is to be granted to users outside the mental health service, for example, general medicine, social services, etc.

Many PAS systems will use the hospital number as a unique patient identifier or create their own unique identifier from combining characters from the name and date-of-birth details. Some systems will not register community-based patients who have not attended out-patients or had admissions, for example, some GP referrals to the community psychiatric nursing service. A joint NHS/DoH working group set up in summer 1990 is dealing with the issues raised by the decision to use the NHS number for patient identification in data interchange by April 1993. Although the National Insurance number would perhaps be more useful, particularly for patients with long-term mental health problems (many of whom are not

---

1. Read codes are available from CAMS Computer Aided Medical Systems, Tannery Buildings, 58–60 Woodgate, Loughborough, Leicestershire LE11 2TQ

registered with GPs or have problems registering), few people know or carry them, and adoption of this as a standard raises ethical issues regarding the ease of identification of individuals.

(l) Hardware costs

These depend very largely on the size of the installation. If networking (linking several computers or terminals to a central machine), then the actual computer system is likely to be either a minicomputer or a microcomputer serving anything from two to 100 or so terminals and prices are therefore almost impossible to predict.

Computers, terminals, printers, cabling, and back-up, together with multiplexors and modems for communicating linkage and software support all need to be considered. It is important not to economise on the hardware, particularly on the terminals, printers, etc. because these are the public face of the computer system and their availability and quality will materially affect acceptability. There are additional hardware possibilities in terms of optical character reading, barcode readers, etc. which may make data entry a simpler task if carefully planned. Similarly, there is the possibility of hand-held computers being used for collecting data in the field which are then 'plugged in' to the main system. Recently there have been experiments with 'smart cards' whereby the patient carries around with them a credit card containing clinical information which can then be made available to various points where the individual contacts the service. It is the opinion of the authors, however, that these are not likely to prove satisfactory with psychiatric patients who tend to be somewhat unpredictable in their compliance with service requirements.

(m) Software costs

Once again, these vary widely between different systems and different development routes. Where the software is developed locally, with programming costs either being lost in a district budget or using the uncharged-for time of a professional, the cost is likely to be lowest. However, this may not be the best route. The questions that must be considered are whether the software is going to last, and how it will be supported and updated in future. A further consideration is that software and programmes written in an industry-standard language or database are much more likely to be acceptable in the long-run than some idiosyncratic or less well-known software, however sophisticated. Some software is more portable in the sense that it will run on a variety of different machines and operating systems. This does not tie the system to specific hardware and should allow the set-up to develop and expand in the future if it is successful without losing existing data. It is likely that in the life of a computer system of, say, ten years, the software will be revised extensively and the hardware might well be replaced at least once, hence the need for interchangeability.

(n) Staffing and support costs

It may be necessary to employ a new member of staff, particularly at the development stage. Failing that, adequate sessions must be made available for existing staff. It is likely that where secretaries are trained to use a computer system it will not save time (at least initially) although it may improve the quality of the service. Similarly, time must be set aside or money allocated both to train the initial staff group who are introducing the computer system and subsequently for a recurring programme of training for existing and new staff. Other support costs such as stationery and the costs of maintenance of both hardware and software need to be considered.

(o) Pitfalls

Systems which are badly thought out are likely to fail. It is common for inadequate attention to be paid to questions like the following. What is the system meant to do, and what outputs are expected from it? Who will collect, input, extract and, above all, update data? Staff need to be identified to carry out tasks of running and maintaining the system, with clear guidance about who they turn to if they cannot cope with a problem. Adequate decisions need to be taken by the clinical staff concerned as to how their practice is going to be modified to use and benefit from the computer system. The sheer hard work involved in preparing a system for use, devising local codes, descriptions, etc. needs to be considered and it is probable that the lack of agreed ways of coding is a handicap to generalisation of systems. The decision whether or not to employ Read codes is therefore of importance.

(p) The management of change

Once the working group has made the decisions above, the plans, the timetable and, above all, the advantages of the system should be widely publicised. Training sessions, with adequate 'hands on' experience should be arranged. All staff need to feel 'ownership' of 'their' system, so that loyalty and commitment are built up to sustain users through the inevitable teething troubles. Training needs to be planned on a continuing basis for new staff, with refresher courses available to existing users. Alternative modes of data entry may help minimise resistance from those reluctant to use a keyboard. Immediate support should be available to those having difficulties with either hardware or software. Feedback sessions should be arranged for users so that staff feel their views are being heard, and above all, users need to feel that they are getting rewards for their efforts.

The future

Computerised clinical case-record systems have developed from the older epidemiological case registers which generally ran on mainframe machines and provided little opportunity for interactive clinical case management. The rewards of a computerised record-keeping system are potentially enormous. If it is sufficiently flexible and easy to use, all the functions of a psychiatric service that require record keeping may be incorporated into the computer or details picked up from parallel systems such as PAS which may contain booking and admission data. The presence of a self-building psychiatric register across a service, with rapid access to both individual and statistical information, provides a major resource for clinicians, planners and researchers alike. It also enables the clinicians to review and audit their work in an unprecedented manner. It is likely to enhance coordination of patient care in a fragmented service through 'electronic shared care'.

The clinical task is made easier by appropriate output programmes, providing for preparation of summaries, letters, reminders, and lists, as well as statistics for both routine and special purposes. Extra modules may allow expert information to be available to clinicians, and questionnaires and datasets for special purposes to be grafted on to the standard dataset.

Decision-support systems which are linked to case registers, offering advice based on extensive data held in longitudinal case records, are likely to become increasingly prevalent over the next decade. An experimental system, APE (Anti-Psychotic medication Expert system) is currently under development, and can link to SafetyNet. APE aims to advise psychiatrists on the management of depot neuroleptic medication for individual patients. The system works through its knowledge of an individual patient's mental state, problems and admissions, as well as a knowledge of each individual's medication (converted to chlorpromazine equivalents) as it has changed over time. The system examines trends in specified symptoms or behaviour and explores this in relation to changes in medication and the patient's attitudes to their current treatment. Inbuilt rules allow the system to advise as to whether medication should be increased, decreased or remain unaltered, and offers suggestions as to appropriate medication. Needs-assessment programs, whereby programmed 'rules' could be applied to deduce needs from the database, have the merit of economy of clinical effort, and the advantage that the whole database could be scanned for those with unmet needs.

There remain major obstacles to employing such expert systems in routine clinical practice but the process of defining the rules by which we make clinical decisions is a potentially valuable task. Systems which feed back the rules by which a decision was reached may help towards a greater understanding of the complexities of clinical decision making.

Those clinical case-record systems which will sell themselves to potential users are those which work well, are used and liked by the practitioners, are well supported by hardware and software companies, and which perform the tasks required of them. Once the problems of clinical usage, regular updating, and reliability can be solved, the rewards are likely to be considerable.

References

ANDERSON, J. G., JAY, S. J., SCHWEER, H. M., *et al* (1986) Why doctors don't use computers: some empirical findings. *Journal of the Royal Society of Medicine*, **79**, 142–144.

CAMPBELL, P., TAYLOR, J., PANTELIS, C., *et al* (1990) Studies of schizophrenia in a large mental hospital proposed for closure and in two halves of an inner London borough served by the hospital. In *Proceedings of the International Conference on Schizophrenia: National Schizophrenia Fellowship* (ed. M. Weller). London: John Libby Publication.

HEDLUND, J. L. (1985*a*) *Computers in Mental Health: A Select Bibliography*. Missouri: Institute of Psychiatry.

—— (1985*b*) Mental Health in the 1980s. *Computers in Human Sciences*, **1**, 6–7.

HMSO (1989) *Working for Patients*. London: HMSO.

JAY, S. & ANDERSON, J. G. (1982) Computerised hospital information systems: their future role in medicine. *Journal of the Royal Society of Medicine*, **75**, 303–304.

KRAWIECKA, M., GOLDBERG, D. & VAUGHN, M. (1977) A standardised psychiatric assessment scale for rating chronic psychotic patients. *Acta Psychiatrica Scandinavica*, **55**, 299–308

OFFICE OF THE DATA PROTECTION REGISTRAR (1985) *The Data Protection Act 1984. An Introduction to the Act and Guide for Data Users and Computer Bureaux. Guideline No 1*. Wilmslow, Cheshire: Office of the Data Protection register.

TAYLOR, J., PANTELIS, C. & TAYLOR, C. (1988) Psychiatric case registers past, present and future. *British Journal of Clinical and Social Psychiatry*, **3**, 71–73.

—— & BHUMGARA, K. (1990) SafetyNet. *British Journal of Health Care Computing*, **7**, 33–34.

WYKES, T. & STURT, E. (1986) The measurement of social behaviour in psychiatric patients: an assessment of the reliablity and validity of the Social Behaviour Schedule, *British Journal of Psychiatry*, **148**, 1–12.

WING, J. K., COOPER, J. E. & SARTORIUS, N. (1974) *Description and Classification of Psychiatric Symptomatology: An Instruction Manual for PSE and CATEGO System*. Cambridge: Cambridge University Press.

—— (ed.) (1989) *Health Services Planning and Research. Contributions from Psychiatric Case Registers*. London: Gaskell Publications.

YOUNG, D. W. (1984) What makes doctors use computers? *Journal of the Royal Society of Medicine*, **77**, 663–667.

15 Computerised mental health assessments

GRAHAM THORNICROFT

The use of computers in clinical and research settings to aid in the assessment and treatment of patients with psychiatric disorders is now just past its infancy. During the last decade there has been an astonishing proliferation of computer applications in these areas (Selmi *et al*, 1990; Carr & Ghosh, 1983). This growth has recently differentiated into several distinct areas, of which the three most developed are computer-administered schedules (where patients use the computer directly themselves), computer-assisted interviews (in which the clinician or researcher uses the computer during the interview, for example for direct data entry), and case registers (Schwartz, 1990; Lieff, 1987; Baskin, 1990). This chapter will detail this rapidly growing field, comment on other areas which can be expected to become more important during the 1990s, such as expert systems, and consider with illustrations the advantages and limitations of computerisation for these purposes (Hedlund *et al*, 1981).

In addition to these direct methods of data collection about individual patients, other computerised systems have developed which aid both clinicians and researchers. For the researcher, computerised literature searches greatly simplify access to the scientific literature in a given area. Local databases have been developed which include information on attenders at lithium or depot clinics, and on patients detained under the terms of the Mental Health Act (and which may trigger reminder lists of patients whose period of detention is about to expire); these aspects are developed further in chapter 14.

The development of computer-administered assessments

The nature and extent of computer use for individual psychiatric assessments, and for aggregate service-use information, exactly parallels the technical progress of the available hardware and software. Applications were initially based on mainframe computers, moving to microcomputers, mainly using the CP/M operating system later in the 1970s, while during the 1980s systems have exploited the IBM personal computer (PC)/DOS standards to implement programmes that run on desktop computers. This sequence has meant that as computer systems able to run relevant psychiatric applications have decreased in size and cost, so the number of applications has vastly increased. This decentralisation of the tools needed to develop new programmes has allowed clinicians in particular to become actively involved, although their enthusiasm has often been offset by their relatively amateur programming skills.

During the 1960s several hospitals in the USA began to use mainframe computers to collect and analyse patient-specific data for management purposes. For example, in 1962 the Mayo Clinic in Minnesota began an early computer-based implementation of the Minnesota Multiphasic Personality Inventory (MMPI; Hathaway & McKinley, 1967). The early use of computers within mental health services was dominated by the computerisation of existing psychological tests. Other prototype computer interviews were conducted at the University of Minnesota in 1966, with questions appearing on a tiny cathode ray tube (Greist, 1990). More recently, Carr *et al* (1981) developed a computerised version of the Hamilton Rating Scale for Depression (HRSD; Hamilton, 1960) while the Eysenck Personality Inventory was converted for computer administration by Katz & Dalby (1981). At the same time Greist (1990) and his co-workers at the University of Wisconsin were developing a computer-scored version of the Hopkins Syndrome Checklist.

Many other questionnaires are now being published in computer-administered forms. In primary care, for example, a programme of research and development of computerised assessments has been carried out at the General Practice Research Unit at the Institute of Psychiatry in London. The Clinical Interview Schedule (CIS) has been implemented in a computer-administered form as PROQSY (Programmable Questionnaire System). The new version includes the 10 reported symptoms from the CIS, but excludes the 12 manifest abnormality items which were rated by the interviewer in the original version. The authors have reported reasonable levels of reliability, acceptability, accuracy, and ease of use (Lewis *et al*, 1988; Pelosi & Lewis, 1989; Wilkinson & Marcus, 1989).

Computer-assisted methods of assessment

In computer-assisted interviews, the patient or subject is questioned by the researcher or clinician and the data are entered directly into a computer, for example by a keyboard or barcode reader. While computer-administered methods are more suitable for self-administered questionnaires, computer-assisted techniques are used for interviews where trained staff are needed. Examples of standardised questionnaires which have been computerised to date include the Present State Examination (Wing *et al*, 1974) and the Composite International Diagnostic Instrument (Robins *et al*, 1985*a*). An illustration of this general approach is the C–DIS, or Computerised Diagnostic Interview Schedule. The Diagnostic Interview Schedule (Robins *et al*, 1985*b*), by virtue of its explicit operationalised diagnostic criteria and the algorithms controlling the generation of diagnoses, lends itself directly to computerisation (Comings, 1984). The DIS, designed to be administered by trained lay interviewers, is a highly structured interview that contains information necessary to make psychiatric diagnoses according to DSM–III criteria. Comparative testing of the computerised and manual versions of the DIS has shown the former to be no less reliable (Blouin *et al*, 1988; Greist, 1990).

Another example of the computer-assisted interview, the Geriatric Mental State (GMS), demonstrates the advantage of combining the data-collection step with the analysis programmes in a single session. The computerised GMS has been used as a case-finding instrument in a large (*n* = 1070) study of subjects aged over 65 in Liverpool. Using a split-half design, McWilliam *et al* (1988) demonstrated that the sensitivity, specificity and positive predictive values were no different between the two methods.

Computerised case registers

To establish and monitor locally-based mental health services, a clear, systematic and continuing method of collecting clinical, social-need, and service-usage data is required. The most comprehensive method of eliciting, coding and storing these data is the case register, which is defined as a local information system that records the contacts with designated social and medical services of patients or clients from a defined geographical area (Wing, 1989). The information is stored in a linked and cumulative file so that the care of any individual or group can be followed over time, no matter how complex the pattern of service attendance. Although such systems were formerly labour intensive, the recent availability of on-site microcomputers and minicomputers has made their more widespread use a practical option in many local areas.

The routine collection of clinical-contact data allows aggregate data to show patterns of service with respect to diagnoses (Der & Bebbington, 1987; Tansella & Williams, 1989), social class (Wiersma *et al*, 1983), and geographical mobility (Lesage & Tansella, 1989). Further, the use of standardised coding and diagnostic systems allows comparisons of service use within local areas (Giel *et al*, 1986), within regions (Torre *et al*, 1982), and between countries (ten Horn *et al*, 1986; Sytema *et al*, 1989). Such data can therefore indicate how variations in treated morbidity vary with local sociodemographic characteristics, with the nature and extent of local service provision, and with the service trends at the national level. Where one of the primary aims of developing local mental health services is to deliver services to identified priority groups of patients, then the detailed information produced by computerised case registers will be required to ensure that the outcome of implementation is consistent with the declared aims of the service. The increasingly widespread use of computerised clinical information by secretarial and administrative staff has recently opened up the possibility in many districts of developing meaningful case registers, so long as the key issues of data quality, reliability and completeness are properly addressed (see chapter 5).

Acceptability of computerised assessments

Although few studies have been carried out assessing the acceptability of computer-assisted interviews, reported results have been favourable. The Geriatric Mental State Schedule was used by Jones & McWilliam (1989) both on paper and with the use of a computer. In all, 22 subjects were interviewed using each method up to 14 days apart. Both methods produced similar results. The computer-assisted interview was seen to be advantageous for a number of reasons: the questions were presented on the screen and answered one at a time; certain aids were included to help with definition and the computer was programmed to accept responses within a certain range, reducing errors of input; questions which were not applicable could be skipped and the data was stored in a form suitable for further storage and analysis. Disadvantages noted included difficulties in training and interference with rapport, either by the structure of the interview or by the unease of the subject. The type of data that could be recorded was limited and data could easily be lost. The authors were also concerned about the acceptability of the computer to the interviewer.

The acceptability of computer-assisted interviews to patients and staff has also been assessed in studies in Baltimore and London using the Computer Acceptability Questionnaire (CAQ). This is a short seven-item computerised questionnaire, devised to compare the acceptability of paper-based and computerised interviews. The results of these studies, conducted with a wide range of staff and long-stay patients in both London and Baltimore, found no differences between any of the groups either by location or type of respondent. When asked if they had seen a computer before, there was a non-significant trend for the staff to be more likely to have had prior experience of computers. Both staff and patients showed a preference for our computer-assisted rather than paper-based version of the interview, with staff slightly but non-significantly more favourable. Approximately 75% of respondents found the computer very acceptable, with slightly more favourable responses by patients than staff. Conversely, more staff than patients were either neutral to the computer or found it unacceptable. Most respondents found that the computer did not distract them at all, the patients again scoring non-significantly higher on this rating than the staff. The majority of respondents did not report being disturbed either by a paper-based or by the computer-assisted interview. Most staff responded overwhelmingly in favour of being interviewed with the computer again, while a large but slightly lower proportion of the patient group felt that they would like to be interviewed again with the computer (O'Ryan *et al*, 1993). These results confirm previous findings from many studies that at least as many respondents prefer a computer to a human interview (Stein, 1987).

The items of the Computer Acceptability Questionnaire (CAQ) are outlined below.

(a) Have you had experience of computers before?
(b) How much does the computerised interview distract you?
(c) How much does the paper-based interview distract you?
(d) How much does the computerised interview disturb you?
(e) Do you prefer the paper-based or computerised interview?
(f) Overall, how acceptable to you is the computerised interview?
(g) Would you want to have a computerised interview again?

In child psychiatry, Sawyer *et al* (1990) collected information either using a computer-administered interview or a written questionnaire with parents, and compared this with an interview with the clinician. The study was primarily concerned with the parents' satisfaction with the methods of assessment. Before the interviews, their attitudes towards each method were recorded and the parents stated a preference for the interview with the clinician to the other forms of assessment, feeling it was more friendly and personal. Their preference for the computer-administered interview increased significantly after they had experienced it. In a recent study, Sarris & Sawyer (1990) stated that researchers should concentrate on trying to develop the potential of computerised interviews to support clinicians in the collection, storage, retrieval, and analysis of data.

Greist *et al* (1987) examined the acceptability of the computerised Diagnostic Interview Schedule (DIS) with 150 psychiatric patients. Greist (1990) also looked at the attitudes of the subjects to the computer-administered interview. He assessed the subjects' feelings about the computer on a five-point scale, and the subjects reported being significantly more comfortable with the computerised interview although it took longer. They concluded that a computer-administered interview was an acceptable way of collecting diagnostic information.

Mathisen *et al* (1987) conducted a similar study using the DIS on 135 in-patients and found that the diagnosis produced was accurate. They also examined the patients' attitudes to the computer, finding that 57% liked using the computer "quite a bit" or "extremely" and only 2% did not like using it at all. The majority of patients were able to express their ideas using the computer and 70% found it easy to use all the time. Indeed, 32% reported feeling more embarrassed giving information to the interviewer. Overall the participants were enthusiastic about the computer.

In London, Lewis *et al* (1988) conducted a computer-administered and an interviewer-administered interview on 45 subjects based on the CIS. Almost all of their subjects found the computer acceptable and no one refused to be interviewed because of the computer. Most found it easy to complete and only two reported it to be too superficial. Pelosi & Lewis (1989), however, did express concern about the validity of computer-administered interviews and feared the loss of communication, stating "the consultation is the beginning of therapy". Ancill *et al* (1985) compared computer-administered self-rating with interviewer-administered self-rating on 28 patients suffering from depression during a clinical drug trial, using the HRSD. Significant correlations were found between the two methods and they concluded that a computer-administered self-rating technique is worthwhile for both assessment and monitoring.

Computer-administered and computer-assisted interviews are becoming increasingly popular and the studies assessing these methods of data collection have given consistently favourable findings. The results from several studies are now convergent: the respondents, both staff and patients, found the computerised interview highly acceptable, they were already familiar with the technology, and they were neither distracted nor disturbed by it. These findings support the careful use of computers as useful tools for data collection in mental health evaluation.

Advantages of computerised assessment techniques

Why computerise psychiatric assessments? As has become clear from the discussion so far, the process of developing computer-based methods of data collection is expensive in terms of time, personnel, hardware, and in managing the process of change. The experience of most centres, however, is that when properly introduced, computer-based methods have many advantages. Decisions which follow explicit decision-trees are readily converted into computer programmes and this may reduce human error, for example, in the decision about whether needs are met or unmet in the MRC Needs for Care Schedule (see chapter 13). Procedures which are repetitive, such as eliciting basic sociodemographic data at patient registration can be computerised with considerable saving of clinical time.

For research purposes, computer applications have several potential advantages. Firstly, they eliminate observer bias generated by an interviewer responding to factors not directly related to the item being assessed. Secondly, both computer-assisted and computer-administered schedules avoid costly subsequent data entry into computer files, with the associated risk of transcription errors, and with a substantial time saving. Results which previously may have taken weeks or months to analyse may be incorporated into the main programme, so that a diagnostic result is available immediately after interviewing the patient. A further merit of this approach is that the programme can be designed so that no items are omitted from the interview, whereas paper-based interviews may be finished uncompleted, or may have followed branching options incorrectly. Where the schedules are self-administered, the interviewer is freed to undertake other tasks, or to arrange the assessment of several patients simultaneously.

A further area in which research has produced unexpectedly positive findings relates to the non-threatening nature of computer applications. In 1989, for example, Levine *et al* conducted a study of patients admitted to a general hospital after acts of self-harm. They compared computer- and psychiatrist-administered forms of the HRSD and a suicide-risk questionnaire. They found that patients disclosed more confidential and relevant information to the computer than to the clinician. In fact, they found that the computer was a better predictor of suicide risk than the doctor! Finally, a potential bonus for lengthy and complex instruments is that their ease of use improves with computerisation, and that patients and staff may report, as they did using the C–DIS (Blouin *et al*, 1988), that their expertise in using computers improves after the assessment.

Disadvantages of computerised assessments

A balanced appreciation of the use of computer-aided assessments in mental health must include consideration of the limitations of these developments. Many attempted computerised applications never reach an acceptable level of usability. Apart from issues of the reliability and validity of the assessment itself, the computer programme that can be widely and reliably used requires extensive testing across different hardware conditions, needs detailed and clear documentation to allow straightforward installation and use at remote sites, must have a satisfactory help facility within the programme, and needs an external support system for users who require assistance. Many of the programmes discussed in this chapter fail to fulfil several of these criteria.

Many potential users of computerised systems start with considerable reluctance to learn. This 'technophobia' means that successful applications require training programmes to teach the computer skills necessary. There may be important variations between staff groups in this respect. A study in Vancouver, for example, found that most reluctance to use computers came from psychiatrists and psychologists, while nursing, clerical and rehabilitation staff were most positive (Peters, 1990). Far more important, however, is that the staff who use these applications can see a direct benefit from the computer-based rather than the paper-based approach. Without such a sense of 'ownership', experience shows that the quality of the output results is severely limited by the poor calibre of input data. This is especially apparent in larger computer applications, such as wide-area case registers, in which coding decisions may be made by clerical staff with no direct contact with the patients described, and in this case both the completeness and the accuracy of some information, especially diagnosis, may fall to unacceptably low levels.

In terms of the psychometric properties of computerised assessments, it is possible that the presentation of items, usually with a display of one question on each screen, may affect reliability and validity. In paper-based versions, for example, respondents can read through the whole instrument quickly, answer in any order, gauge the length of the whole assessment at a glance, and readily check consistency between items. All of these may be more difficult when administered by computer, although the psychometric implications of this are unknown.

A further area of concern is how far data kept in computerised files are secure and confidential. The ease with which data files can be deleted or corrupted means that systematic, frequent, and continuing methods of copying, or backing up, files are required, with duplicates kept off-site and secure. In the absence of such systems, data are at risk of loss through carelessness, computer failure, or theft. Further, access to confidential data should be restricted to authorised users, and a potentially serious disadvantage of computerised recording systems is that, unless specifically limited, access to patient-specific data can be made enormously easier.

This raises a wider, related, issue: is it ethically acceptable to keep computerised records of individuals with current or past mental health problems? Sufficient concern has been expressed that some case registers, for example that in Mannheim, have closed under public pressure to limit the coordination of individual computerised data. This pressure needs firstly to be set against the practical requirements for clinicians to have rapid, complete and up-to-date information about patients, where a computerised record may allow such access. Secondly, during the next decade, computerisation may allow the introduction into clinical practice of standardised measures of patient outcome, which will facilitate the study of treatment efficacy (Department of Health, 1991; Thornicroft & Strathdee, 1991). Thirdly, computerised records of service use are now invaluable for epidemiological studies which seek to identify patterns in mental health contacts, and to seek explanations for those patterns which can inform future treatments.

Comprehensive computerised assessments for the long-term mentally ill

One potential use of computerised interviews is their combination to produce a comprehensive assessment of patient groups or cohorts. Field trials of such an approach have been undertaken recently in the COSTAR project in Baltimore (Thornicroft & Breakey, 1991), and at Friern and Claybury hospitals in North London (TAPS, 1990). At Friern Hospital, for example, until recently paper schedules were used for all interviews, each of which produced up to 24 pages with 502 items of information, all requiring filing and storage. The data were entered and verified for analysis up to 12 months after they were collected, at considerable financial cost. In February 1990, laptop computers were introduced for computer-assisted interviews. The IBM-compatible laptop computers chosen weighed around 4 kg, had a 20 Mb hard drive, and ran from mains or battery power. The programme used to computerise the questionnaires is called ENQUIRE and has been devised by Dr Gyles Glover (Glover, 1989).

The following 13 schedules have now been converted for computerised use using ENQUIRE:

Basic Everyday Living Skills Schedule
Brief Psychiatric Rating Scale
Environmental Index
Global Assessment of Functioning Scale
Living Unit Environmental Index
Mini-Mental State Examination
MRC Needs for Care Assessment
Patient Demographic and Psychiatric Past History Schedule
Patient Attitude Questionnaire
Physical Health Questionnaire
Present State Examination
Social Behaviour Schedule
Social Network Schedule.

They are administered by trained interviewers who enter data directly into the computer during the session with the respondent (patient or key informant). Most of the programmes have extensive on-line, context-sensitive help facilities to aid using the programmes, but also to make standard glossary definitions immediately accessible. Data output and storage is in character form in ASCII files. This allows easy use in a wide range of statistical programmes, but also makes the data recognisable to the eye. A single file for the raw results of each interview was generated using the patient's study number as the file name for ready identification.

The computer displays the questions on the screen one at a time allowing the interviewer to enter the respondents' answers directly. Each question and the possible responses are incorporated into one screen on the computer, with an optional help screen immediately available. A distinct advantage of this approach is that programmes to analyse the data can be run immediately after data collection. For example, the standardised assessment of the subjects' mental state used is the Present State Examination and the computerised version includes the CATEGO programme which converts the raw data into symptom and syndrome scores and an ICD diagnosis immediately after the interview. Standard output tables can be designed so that printed results can be incorporated, for example, in patients' clinical case notes.

These schedules produce a pattern of scores for each patient that form a rich descriptive array of information relevant to clinical and social needs. More specifically, the computerisation of the MRC Needs for Care Assessment greatly simplifies the interview procedure, and allows a direct method of quantifying the number of needs of each patient at each time period, and the proportion of needs that are met and unmet (see chapter 13). It also allows a meaningful measure of change in met and unmet need over time, both for individuals and for groups of patients (Tables 15.1 and 15.2).

TABLE 15.1

Example of output table from MRC Needs for Care Assessment Schedule computerised with ENQUIRE

Area	Problem status	Primary-need status
Clinical items		
Psychotic symptoms	current	met
Slowness/underactivity	current	met
Tardive dyskinesia	none	none
Neurotic symptoms	none	none
Dementia and delirium	current	no meetable need
Physical symptoms	none	none
Dangerous behaviour	recent	met
Embarrassing behaviour	current	unmet need for treatment
Distress	none	none
Social items		
Personal hygiene	none	none
Shopping	current: lack of performance	none
Get meals	current: lack of competence	met
Household chores	current: lack of performance	met
Use public transport	none	none
Use public amenities	none	none
Education	current: lack of performance	met
Occupation	none	none
Communication skills	none	none
Manage money	current: lack of competence	met
Manage own affairs	current: lack of competence	met

TABLE 15.2
Example of summary table from MRC Needs for Care Assessment Schedule computerised with ENQUIRE

Category	Number of items
Levels of functioning	
No problem	9
Recent problem	1
Current problem	10
Not known	0
Primary need status	
None	10
Met need	8
Unmet need for assessment	0
Unmet need for treatment	1
No meetable need	1
Secondary needs	
Future need	0
Overprovision	0
Possible need	0

Conclusions

A number of challenges lie between the present and the future realisation of the full potential of these tools. Firstly, it will be necessary to implement assessment techniques professionally, and this will require professional programming, marketing and support for assessment programmes, rather than the admirable but amateur attempts of clinical enthusiasts. Secondly, computer systems will need to operate efficiently across local and wide area networks as mental health services become progressively decentralised and interdependent (Aydin, 1989). Thirdly, it is likely that computers will be increasingly used for routine screening purposes – it has been demonstrated that computers are at least as effective in screening for alcohol dependence as are staff (Bernadt *et al*, 1989). For computerised assessment to become more clinically relevant, investment is required not just for hardware and software, but also for training staff both to input correct data, and to use the systems to enhance the quality of their clinical practice through the availability of better information.

Taking the potential contribution of data collection more widely, computers are now being increasingly used as clinical information systems. In Britain, for example, these predominantly use IBM-compatible PCs, running database applications in proprietary software (Table 15.3). It is striking how such systems have proliferated over the last five years, and it seems likely that an evolutionary cycle will rapidly identify those which do and do not deserve to survive and be disseminated.

Finally, one area seems set to become, although perhaps slowly, an important application in assessing mental health needs over the next decade: the expert system (Overby, 1987). In this context an expert system is a

TABLE 15.3
Summary of computerised clinical information systems in Britain in 1991

System	Site	Start	Hardware	Software	Scope	Comments
Bradford	Bradford	1988	IBM, ICL	UNIX, MSDOS	Community	Multi-user
Chipsy	Guy's	1990	IBM	Smartware	Child psychiatry	Stand-alone
CRAMS	Leeds, Derby, Leicester	1988	IBM	Psion Xchange	Comprehensive	Multi-user
CRISP	St Mary Abbots	1990	IBM		Comprehensive	Multi-user
CTMHE	Lewisham		IBM	Dbase III +, FOXPro	Psychogeriatric	Single-user
FPCD	Oxford	1989	IBM	MSDOS	Forensic	Stand-alone
GEPAS	Glasgow		IBM	Dbase III +	Lithium and depot	Stand-alone
MHITAS	Guy's		IBM	Smartware	Comprehensive	Multi-user
LFPDB	Leicester		IBM	Dbase IV	Forensic	Multi-user
Lothian	Edinburgh	1970	ICL		Comprehensive	Multi-user
M.H. Link	Hackney	1990	IBM	Clipper	Community	Single-user
P-Card	St George's		IBM	MSDOS	Child psychiatry	Multi-user
M.H. Connection	Napsbury, Bromley, Plymouth	1985	VAX	VMS, UNIX	Comprehensive	Multi-user
Bracken	Bexley	1990	IBM	Rbase	Forensic	Single-user
Concare	Lewisham, Canterbury, Tameside		IBM	Dbase III	Community	Single-user
St Bernards	Ealing		IBM	Smartware	Comprehensive	Multi-user
Marlborough	Camden		IBM	Smartware	Child and family	Stand-alone
Safety Net	Brighton, Edinburgh, NW Thames	1989	IBM	UNIX DOS 3.3	Community	Multi-user
Stylities	Southwark	1988	IBM	FOXPro	Community	Stand-alone
Monitor	York	1986	IBM	UNIX	Community	Stand-alone
Southampton	Southampton		IBM	Dbase III	Case register	Stand-alone

Based upon information collected by Wood S. & Sinclair M. (NHS Management Executive, 1992).

computer programme which aids in diagnosing and treating mental disorders. Five expert-system paradigms have been described: data-bank analysis, statistical-pattern recognition, Bayesian analysis, logical-flow charts, and knowledge-based systems (Morelli *et al*, 1987). A relatively simple illustration is the use of a computer database to indicate drug interactions (Schwartz, 1990), while such a system may also allow non-clinicians to make reasonable assessments of treatment needs, for example in remote sites (Hedlund *et al*, 1987).

Computer use in psychiatric assessment is set to become widespread over the next five years, and offers prospects for both a fragmentation of methods, and for a possible convergence of techniques and results. The rapidly diminishing cost of what was, until very recently, astonishing computer power will ensure that computers will soon be as widely used by clinical staff as they have become by secretarial staff in recent years.

Acknowledgements

I am pleased to acknowledge the major role played by Dr Gyles Glover in implementing assessment schedules for long-term psychiatric patients using the ENQUIRE programme. Drs Spitzer, Overall, and Folstein kindly gave permission for the Global Assessment of Functioning Scale, Brief Psychiatric Rating Scale and Mini-Mental State Examination respectively to be computerised using this system. I am grateful for the support of Dr W. Breakey in the Baltimore field trials of the laptop implementation of several of these instruments.

References

ANCILL, R., ROGERS, D. & CARR, A. (1985) Comparison of computerised self-rating scales for depression with conventional observer ratings. *American Journal of Psychiatry*, **71**, 315–317.

AYDIN, C. (1989) Occupational adaptation to computerised medical information systems. *Journal of Health and Social Behaviour*, **30**, 163–179.

BASKIN, D. (ed.) (1990) *Computer Applications in Psychiatry and Psychology.* New York: Brunner Mazel.

BERNADT, M., DANIELS, O., BLIZARD, R., *et al* (1989) Can a computer reliably elicit an alcohol history? *British Journal of Addiction*, **84**, 405–411.

BLOUIN, A., PEREZ, E. & BLOUIN, J. (1988) Computerized administration of the Diagnostic Interview Schedule. *Psychiatry Research*, **23**, 335–344.

CARR, A., GHOSH, A., ANCILL, R., *et al* (1981) Direct assessment of depression by microcomputer. *Acta Psychiatrica Scandinavica*, **64**, 415–422.

—— & —— (1983) Response of phobic patients to direct computer assessment. *British Journal of Psychiatry*, **142**, 60–65.

COMINGS, D. (1984) A computerised diagnostic interview schedule for psychiatric disorders. In *Using Computers in Clinical Practice* (ed. M. Schwartz), pp. 195–203. New York: The Haworth Press.

DEPARTMENT OF HEALTH (1991) *The Health of the Nation.* London: HMSO.

DER, G. & BEBBINGTON, P. (1987) Depression in inner London. A register study. *Social Psychiatry*, **22**, 73–84.

GIEL, R., HANNIBAL, J., HENDERSON, J., *et al* (1986) *Mental Health Services in Pilot Study Areas.* Copenhagen: World Health Organization.

GLOVER, G. (1989) *ENQUIRE Handbook.* London: Westminster Medical School.

GRIEST, J. (1990) Computers and psychiatric diagnosis. In *Computer Applications in Psychiatry and Psychology* (ed. D. Baskin). New York: Brunner Mazel.

———, LEWIN, M., ERDMAN, H., *et al* (1987) Comparison of computer- and interviewer-administered versions of the Diagnostic Interview Schedule. *Hospital and Community Psychiatry*, **38**, 1304–1311.

HAMILTON, M. (1960) A rating scale for depression. *Journal of Neurology, Neurosurgery and Psychiatry*, **23**, 56–62.

HATHAWAY, S. R. & MCKINLEY, J. C. (1967) *Minnesota Multiphasic Personality Inventory: Manual for Administration and Scoring.* New York: Psychological Corporation.

HEDLUND, J., VIEWEG, B., WOOD, J., *et al* (1981) *Computers in Mental Health: a Review and Annotated Bibliography.* Washington DC: NIMH.

TEN HORN, G., GIEL, R., GULBINAT, W., *et al* (eds) (1986) *Psychiatric Case Registers in Public Health.* Amsterdam: Elsevier.

JONES, J. & MCWILLIAM, C. (1989) The Geriatric Mental State Schedule administered with the aid of a microcomputer: a pilot study. *International Journal of Geriatric Psychiatry*, **4**, 215–219.

KATZ, L. & DALBY, T. (1981) Computer and manual administration of the Eysenck Personality Inventory. *Journal of Clinical Psychology*, **37**, 586–588.

LESAGE, A. & TANSELLA, M. (1989) Mobility of schizophrenic patients, non-psychotic patients and the general population in a case register area. *Social Psychiatry and Psychiatric Epidemiology*, **24**, 271–274.

LEWIS, G., PELOSI, A., GLOVER, E., *et al* (1988) The development of a computerised assessment for minor psychiatric disorder. *Psychological Medicine*, **18**, 737–745.

LEVINE, S., ANCILL, R. & ROBERTS, A. (1989) Assessment of suicide risk by computer-delivered self-rating questionnaire: preliminary findings. *Acta Psychiatrica Scandinavica*, **80**, 216–220.

LIEFF, J. (1987) *Computer Applications in Psychiatry.* Washington DC: American Psychiatric Association Press.

MATHISEN, K., EVANS, F. & MYERS, K. (1987) Evaluation of a computerised version of the Diagnostic Interview Schedule. *Hospital and Community Psychiatry*, **38**, 1311–1315.

MCWILLIAM, C., COPELAND, D., DEWEY, M., *et al* (1988) The Geriatric Mental State Examination as a case finding instrument in the community. *British Journal of Psychiatry*, **153**, 205–208.

MORELLI, R., BRONZINO, J. & GOETHE, J. (1987) Expert systems in psychiatry: a review. *Journal of Medical Systems*, **11**, 157–168.

O'RYAN, D., BAXTER, L., THORNICROFT, G., *et al* (1992) The TAPS Project (14). Computer-assisted evaluation of long-term psychiatric patients: acceptability to patients and staff. *International Journal of Methods in Psychiatric Research* (in press).

OVERBY, M. (1987) Psyxpert: an expert system prototype for aiding psychiatrists in the diagnosis of psychotic disorders. *Computer and Biological Medicine*, **17**, 393–395.

PELOSI, A. & LEWIS, G. (1989) The computer will see you now. *British Medical Journal*, **299**, 138–139.

PETERS, R. (1990) Attitudes of community mental-health staff toward computers. *Canadian Journal of Community Mental Health*, **1**, 155–162.

———, HELZER, J. E., ORVASCHEL, H., *et al* (1985*b*) The Diagnostic Interview Schedule. In *Epidemiologic Field Methods in Psychiatry: The NIMH Epidemiologic Catchment Area Program* (eds W. W. Eaton & L. G. Kessler). Orlando, Florida: Academic Press.

SAWYER, M., SARRIS, A., QUIGLEY, R., *et al* (1990) The attitude of parents to the use of computer-assisted interviewing in a child psychiatry service. *British Journal of Psychiatry*, **157**, 675–678.

SARRIS, A. & SAWYER, M. (1990) Automated information systems in mental health services. *International Journal of Mental Health*, **18**, 18–30.

SCHWARTZ, M. (1990) Clinical applications of computers: an overview. In *Computer Applications in Psychiatry and Psychology* (ed. D. Baskin). New York: Brunner Mazel.

SELMI, P., KLEIN, M., GRIEST, J., *et al* (1990) Computer-administered cognitive–behavioural therapy for depression. *American Journal of Psychiatry*, **147**, 51–56.

STEIN, S. (1987) Computer-assisted diagnoses for children and adolescents. In *Computerised Psychological Assessments* (ed. J. Butcher), pp. 145–158. New York: Basic Books.

SYTEMA, S., BALESTRIERI, M., GIEL, R., *et al* (1989) Use of mental health services in South-Verona and Groningen. *Acta Psychiatrica Scandinavica*, **79**, 153–162.

TANSELLA, M. & WILLIAMS, P. (1989) The spectrum of psychiatric morbidity in a defined geographical area. *Psychological Medicine*, **19**, 765–770.

TAPS (TEAM FOR THE ASSESSMENT OF PSYCHIATRIC SERVICES) (1990) *Better Out than In?* London: North East Thames Regional Health Authority.

THORNICROFT, G. & BREAKEY, W. (1991) The COSTAR programme 1: improving social networks of the chronic mentally ill through outreach case management services in E. Baltimore. *British Journal of Psychiatry*, **159**, 245–249.

—— & STRATHDEE, G. (1991) The Health of the Nation: Mental Health. *British Medical Journal*, **303**, 410–412.

TORRE, E., MARINONI, A., ALLEGRI, G., *et al* (1982) Trends in admission before and after an act abolishing mental hospitals: a survey of three areas in Northern Italy. *Comprehensive Psychiatry*, **23**, 227–232.

WIERSMA, D., GIEL, R., DE JONG, A., *et al* (1983) Social class and schizophrenia in a Dutch cohort. *Psychological Medicine*, **13**, 141–150.

WILKINSON, G. & MARCUS, A. (1989) PROQSY: a computerised technique for psychiatric case identification in general practice. *British Journal of Psychiatry*, **154**, 378–382.

WING, J. (ed.) (1989) *Health Services Planning and Research. Contributions from Psychiatric Case Registers*. London: Gaskell.

——, COOPER, J. E. & SARTORIUS, N. (1974) *The Measurement and Classification of Psychiatric Symptoms*. Cambridge: Cambridge University Press.

16 Services for the homeless mentally ill

WILLIAM R. BREAKEY, EZRA SUSSER and PHILIP TIMMS

Homelessness is not a new phenomenon in Western societies and it is probable that even decades ago a certain proportion of homeless people in British and American cities were mentally ill. More than 20 years ago, research on both sides of the Atlantic demonstrated the high prevalence of mental illness in homeless men (Whiteley, 1955; Bogue, 1963; Edwards *et al*, 1968; Spitzer *et al*, 1969). In the past decade, providers and policy makers of mental health services have been particularly concerned, partly because the high prevalence of mental disorder in the 'new homeless' has been linked to the phasing out of mental hospitals as the primary locus of care for the severely mentally ill. Whether or not this link is as clearly established as critics of deinstitutionalisation claim, the high prevalence of mental disorders in homeless people and their presumed need for mental health services is readily apparent. A new target population for mental health services has been identified.

The homeless mentally ill are only a subgroup within the much larger population of homeless people. In many respects their problems and needs are similar to those of other homeless people. Above all, they need a place to live which will offer safety, shelter, privacy, and a degree of permanence. They need dignity, acceptance, and friendship. They need financial support, which is more available currently in Britian than in America, and access to primary care, which is difficult for homeless people in both countries (Reid, 1989).

In addition to the needs they share with homeless people in general, the homeless mentally ill have particular needs for treatment, rehabilitation and support. This is a new area of specialisation for mental health services, with as yet no consensus about the effectiveness of different approaches. For example, it is still not clear whether it is preferable to have special service programmes for homeless people or to integrate them into the mainstream mental health service (Brent-Smith & Dean, 1990; Susser *et al*, 1992). There is, as yet, only a limited literature on the issues of service provision and only a few demonstration projects have been subjected to systematic evaluation. This chapter, therefore, describes briefly what has been learned in the past several years in North America and in the British Isles about the characteristics of the homeless mentally ill and their needs for services, and discusses some of the issues relevant to meeting those needs.

Studies of homeless mentally ill people show that, while many have had little contact with mental health services, significant numbers have been in treatment (Marshall, 1989). Thus, a problem for many is lack of access to services, while the problem for others is that whatever services have been rendered have clearly not enabled them to be resettled in permanent and adequate housing.

In assessing the service needs of homeless mentally ill people, a number of issues must be considered. First, there is the problem of defining the target population (Bachrach, 1984; Fischer & Breakey, 1986). Different subgroups of homeless people have different characteristics, and comprise a spectrum which extends from those who sleep under bridges or in abandoned buildings to those who are placed in motels or bed-and-breakfast, or doubled up in the homes of relatives. Definitions and sampling strategies used in epidemiological research have usually focused on those persons residing in shelters, hostels, or reception centres (e.g. Tidmarsh & Wood, 1972; Bassuk *et al*, 1984; Fischer *et al*, 1986; Susser *et al*, 1989; Scott, 1991). There are obvious dangers in generalising from these data to homeless people as a whole. Some investigators have reported findings on special subpopulations of homeless people, such as homeless families (e.g. Bassuk *et al*, 1986). Other studies of the homeless mentally ill have been based on clinical samples, in hospital or other treatment programmes, or individuals who have been selected because they were identified as mentally disabled. This introduces additional sources of bias, if the purpose is to get a measure of the needs of homeless people as a whole (e.g. Fernandez, 1984; Herzberg, 1987; Wright & Weber, 1987; Marshall, 1989). Because of the heterogeneity of the homeless population, findings from one setting can only be applied in another with caution. For this reason several surveys have attempted to obtain more widely representative samples by drawing subjects from a range of settings (e.g. Roth & Bean, 1986; Koegel *et al*, 1988; Vernez *et al*, 1988; Breakey *et al*, 1989).

A second issue concerns the concept of need. A traditional clinical perspective measures need in terms of those people who seek or are referred for services. The public health perspective, on the other hand, views need in terms of the population of all those who have specific health problems, including those who do not seek services. Homeless people do not give high priority to mental health needs (Ball & Havassy, 1984; Mulkern, 1985) and in many cases will not seek out care. Some, in fact, will actively avoid engagement with mental health services. A public-health perspective is essential in community mental health services generally, but especially in considering the needs of homeless people in view of their isolation, and in many cases their alienation, from the service system (Susser *et al*, 1992).

Another issue in considering need relates to clinical priorities and the definition of mental illness. Should programmes be solely concerned with the severely disabled, who are the focus of community care and support programmes, the so-called victims of deinstitutionalisation, or should they also aim to serve the less severely disturbed and disabled, including families and children? There is no doubt that virtually all homeless people have problems which would benefit from counselling and support, and different groups and agencies will respond differently to the question of priority for services. In this chapter, however, we focus on the needs of those persons with major mental illnesses, such as schizophrenia, bipolar affective disorders, major depressive illnesses, and related disorders.

A further consideration in attempting to assess needs is that a concept of service need is to some extent dependent upon an understanding of service effectiveness. At present there is little objective data on the effectiveness of specific interventions with homeless mentally ill people, so that stating a need for a particular intervention is necessarily based more on informed opinion than on established norms of practice.

At the end of the chapter we briefly review some of the current approaches to providing services for homeless people with major mental illnesses.

Estimating the need for clinical services

Keeping in mind the need for a broad range of basic human services to solve the problems shared by homeless and rootless people in general, there are two approaches to obtaining a measure specifically of the mental health service needs of homeless people. One is to obtain an estimate of the extent of morbidity in the population, and from that to estimate the numbers of people who need services. However, because the needs of individuals vary greatly, depending upon their particular circumstances and problems, the use of morbidity data provides very inexact estimates. More specific measures of the types of services or interventions needed require individual assessments of representative samples. We shall consider both approaches.

Morbidity

The service needs of homeless people can, to some extent, be predicted from the prevalence of psychiatric disorders, the degree of disability experienced by these individuals and the patterns of comorbidity, including co-occurring substance-use disorders and physical diseases. The literature on morbidity in homeless people has grown rapidly in recent years, but caution needs to be exercised in interpreting data drawn from different settings under different sampling conditions. The simplest method to get a rough measure of the extent of psychiatric morbidity is to obtain self-reports of their psychiatric histories. Surveys conducted in a variety of settings have found that as many as one-third to a half of homeless people report having been admitted at some time to a hospital for treatment of a psychiatric disorder; higher rates are reported in samples drawn from treatment settings (Fernandez, 1984; Herzberg, 1987; Brent-Smith & Dean, 1990). However, self-reporting histories of hospital admission may not be accurate (Susser & Struening, 1990) and this measure is neither sensitive nor specific as an index of the presence of mental illness or an indicator of need.

Another approach is to use a questionnaire, such as the Center for Epidemiological Studies–Depression Inventory (CES–D; Radloff, 1977), the Brief Symptom Inventory (BSI; Derogatis & Spencer, 1984), or the General Health Questionnaire (GHQ; Goldberg, 1972). Instruments such as these generally identify between one-third and a half of homeless people to be suffering from significant degrees of emotional distress, depression, or demoralisation, sufficient to warrant psychiatric attention (Fischer *et al*, 1986; Susser *et al*, 1989; Stark *et al*, 1989; Scott, 1991). Translating this information into a statement of need, however, is difficult because of its lack of specificity. Some of the persons so identified may need extensive professional interventions; others may need support from an empathic friend or counsellor; for others, the emotional distress will be relieved when steps are taken to solve the problems of poverty and lack of adequate housing.

Planning psychiatric services requires more specific information on the nature and severity of specific mental disorders. Recent research, using a variety of standardised diagnostic methods, indicates that the range includes the major mental illnesses, personality disorders, substance-use disorders, and a wide variety of others. Data from representative US studies which employed standardised diagnostic methods, drawing representative samples of subjects from non-treatment settings, are shown in Table 16.1. In spite of differences in sampling and diagnostic methods, there is a considerable degree of agreement in their findings. The prevalence rates for psychiatric disorders are compared with rates obtained in the NIMH Epidemiological Catchment Area study in five American cities (Regier *et al*, 1988).

Prevalence data from two British studies conducted before 1980, and two recent studies conducted in non-treatment settings are shown in Table 16.2. In general, prevalence rates of schizophrenia were higher than in the American studies, and rates of substance-use disorders were lower, although in at least some cases, the observed prevalence of substance abuse may be low because abusers were excluded from hostels which served as sampling sites.

Mental illness

UK and US studies demonstrate a remarkable degree of consistency in their

TABLE 16.1
Percentage lifetime prevalence of selected DSM–III mental disorders in homeless populations compared with the ECA Combined Five-Site Household Survey Population

Reference	Male: %	Schizo-phrenia	Affective disorder	Demen-tia	Substance-use disorders
Los Angeles Koegel *et al* (1988) (n = 328)	95.0	13.1	29.5	3.4	69.2
California Vernez *et al* (1988) (n = 315)	71.0	11.0	22.0	NR	69.0
Baltimore Breakey *et al* (1989) (n = 125M, 78W)	0 / 100.0	17.1 / 12.1	23.7 / 18.6	0 / 3.3	38.2 / 75.4
New York Susser *et al* (1989) (n = 177)	100.0	11.0	NR	NR	NR
USA: ECA (5 cities) Regier *et al* (1988) (n = 18 571)	41.0	1.3	8.3	1.3	16.4

TABLE 16.2
Percentage prevalence rates of selected psychiatric disorders in hostels, lodging houses and resettlement units in England and Scotland

		n	Schizo-phrenia	Affective disorders	Addiction
Hostels (Lodge Patch, 1970) (men)		123	14.6	8.1	21.1
Common lodging houses (Priest, 1976) (men)[1]		77	32.5	5.2	18.2
Resettlement units (Scott, 1991) (women)	Age < 31	24	8.3	20.8	20.8
	Age > 30	25	28.0	36.0	48.0
Direct access hostel (Timms & Fry, 1989) (men)	New arrivals	65	24.6	6.2	15.3
	Residents	58	38.0	0	1.7

1. 'Definite' and 'probable' cases combined.

overall finding that between one-third and a half of homeless people may be diagnosed with a major mental illness. In US studies, schizophrenia is diagnosed in 10–15% and major affective illnesses, unipolar or bipolar, in 20–30%. Scott's (1991) data on women in resettlement units in England are very similar, but in general, British studies provide higher estimates of the prevalence of schizophrenia, 15–30%, and lower estimates of the prevalence of affective disorders, 5–10%. It is quite possible that the lower rates of affective disorder reported in British studies relate to differences in definitions of disorders. The American studies quoted here reported lifetime prevalence rates, whereas British studies used diagnostic methods which focused on current disorders. What is more, the DSM–III criteria for major depression (American Psychiatric Association, 1980) used in American studies may have included some cases which would not have been classified as major affective disorders by British psychiatrists.

Substance-use disorders

Very high prevalence rates of substance-use disorders are reported in homeless populations, although there is great variability, possibly related to differences in sampling strategies, differences in methods of diagnosis, including confusion between lifetime and point-prevalence rates, or real differences between homeless populations in different places (Fischer, 1991). In Baltimore in the mid-1980s, alcohol abuse and dependence were found to be much more prevalent among homeless people than abuse of and dependence on other substances (Breakey *et al*, 1989), while in the same period, in New York, drug abuse was remarkably widespread among homeless men in the shelter system with cocaine being the most commonly used drug (Susser *et al*, 1989). Overall, in American studies, median rates for alcoholism of 47% in homeless men and 17% in homeless women can be estimated by compiling data from the many studies published in recent years; equivalent median rates for drug-use disorders are 23% in men and 26% in women (Fischer, 1991). In the UK, there is also great variation between studies. Stark *et al* (1989) reported that 42% of the long-stay male residents of reception centres in England had a definite drinking problem; Timms & Fry (1989) reported a rate of 2% in residents of a Salvation Army hostel in London. Substance abuse in one form or another has traditionally been perceived as the major problem of homeless people, and this stereotype still has considerable strength.

Mental illness–substance abuse comorbidity

The conspicuousness of substance-use disorders in homeless populations has at times obscured the importance of mental illness. Recently, in the United States, the level of public concern about mental illness in homeless people has tended to diminish the role of substance abuse. However, the importance of 'dual diagnosis' in the homeless – the co-occurrence of major mental illnesses and substance-use disorders – is increasingly apparent (Drake *et al*, 1991). Substance abuse occurs as frequently in the homeless mentally ill as in homeless people in general, and more frequently in the most disabled of the mentally ill. In Baltimore, 80% of severely mentally ill men also had a substance-abuse diagnosis, and in severely mentally ill women, the rate was close to 40%. The co-occurrence of mental illness and substance abuse increases the likelihood that a mentally ill person will become homeless (Drake *et al*, 1989; Belcher, 1989; Susser *et al*, 1991*b*) and poses considerable problems for service providers (Ridgely *et al*, 1986; Drake & Wallach, 1989). The treatment of the mental illness and rehabilitation of the mentally ill person are compromised by the effects of the substance use. Conversely, participation in treatment programmes for substance abuse which cater to the general population of substance abusers is difficult for persons with mental illness.

Other psychiatric disorders

A wide variety of other psychiatric conditions are found in addition to the major groups of the mental illnesses and substance-use disorders. Depressed mood and demoralisation are, understandably, common, even in those people whose disorder does not meet criteria for affective illness. Suicide attempts are quite frequently reported (Susser *et al*, 1989). Anxiety disorders, including disorders in the phobic and obsessive–compulsive categories, are also common, often occurring in association with substance abuse. Personality disorders are widespread, reported in 40% of homeless men and women in Baltimore (Breakey *et al*, 1989) and in 70% of young homeless mothers in Massachussetts (Bassuk *et al*, 1986). The most common personality disorders in the Baltimore sample were those which interfere with a person's capacity to establish helpful and supportive relationships, the schizoid, antisocial, and avoidant types.

Disability

The presence of a mental illness *per se* is not the most critical factor in determining a person's capacity to survive in the community. Many mentally ill individuals cope reasonably well with the demands of everyday life in the community. It is, rather, the level of functional impairment that determines the level of service that a given individual may require, and some investigators have focused their attention on estimation of functional capacity rather than diagnostic evaluation. The assessment of functional capacity in homeless people, however, is problematic for several reasons. Firstly, making such a determination generally requires a reliable observer and a period of observation in which the person's performance can be assessed. This may be costly, but also may not be feasible in a mobile population. Secondly, most standard instruments for assessing functional capacity are designed for in-patients or persons in residential settings. They rely upon the ratings of skills which a homeless person may have no opportunity to perform, such as food preparation, performing one's own laundry, or managing money.

Notwithstanding these difficulties, several research teams have attempted to assess functional capacity. Barrow *et al* (1989) devised an instrument specifically for use in homeless people; Marshall (1989) used the REHAB scale (Baker & Hall, 1988), first developed for hospital patients. Both groups concluded that many homeless mentally ill persons are quite severely impaired, and may be judged to need an extensive array of rehabilitation and supportive services.

Individual clinical-needs assessment

While prevalence data permit broad generalisations about service needs, a clearer picture can be obtained by defining the specific needs of individuals in a representative sample. This requires a careful evaluation of persons by clinicians who can develop individual profiles of need. Using this method, psychiatrists in Baltimore estimated that 50% of severely mentally ill homeless men would benefit from short-term hospital admission for stabilisation of their condition, but that only 14% of the severely mentally ill men (2% of the total sample of homeless men) would need long-term hospital care. The advantage of this method is that a series of recommendations can be produced which are very consonant with normal practice. The disadvantage is that the recommendations may be idiosyncratic to a particular clinician or group of clinicians, reflecting their particular outlook and experience, with consequent limitations in generalisability. However, standardised instruments for measuring the need for services of homeless people have not been developed, and instruments developed for use with domiciled individuals may not be appropriate.

Characteristics of the population affecting service provision

Most large cities in the USA now have one or more programmes to supply the needs of the homeless mentally ill, as do many health districts in the UK (Roderick *et al*, 1991). A body of specialised clinical experience is accumulating (Thomison & Cook, 1987; Blackwell *et al*, 1990; Brent-Smith & Dean, 1990; Susser *et al*, 1990; Breakey, 1992). Experience shows that the service needs of homeless mentally ill people are determined by their psychopathology and functional capacity, as described, but strategies for meeting those needs must take into consideration a number of special characteristics. These include the distrust that many homeless mentally ill people have of the mental health service, their relative lack of the supports upon which patients and therapists in other situations can usually rely, and their poverty.

Distrust

Programmes for helping homeless people frequently face the dilemma that those whose needs seem greatest may be the most reluctant to accept help. The distrust of homeless people for helpers and helping agencies probably has several roots. Paranoid symptoms noted by psychiatrists may to some extent be understandable responses to the dangerous environment in which homeless people exist and the distrust of mentally ill persons may arise from earlier bad experiences of mental health care. They may be fearful of being 'put away'. Some lack insight into the reality of their illness, or may have made a conscious decision to avoid psychotropic drugs because of their unpleasant side-effects. Service programmes for homeless people must be prepared to encounter this mistrust and adjust their expectations and approaches accordingly. They should not expect that all who need services will seek them, and they should not expect that proffered help will in all cases be gratefully accepted.

Many outreach workers employ strategies first developed in New York City (Cohen, 1990; Barrow *et al*, 1991) to gain the trust of homeless street people. In many cases street-dwelling men and women are so fearful of those who try to help them that months may be required to establish even a minimally trusting relationship. Workers at first may be able to do nothing more than to give a person a sandwich. Susser has described the reluctance of women in a shelter to trust a psychiatrist. One of the strategies he used to gain their trust was to conduct a weekly bingo game in the shelter (Susser, 1992). The Simon Community in England has adopted a philosophy of unconditional acceptance, 'no questions asked', and a minimum of rules in their shelters, as a way of minimising the barriers to the acceptance of help (Leach, 1979).

Lack of supports

Research has repeatedly demonstrated the relative isolation of homeless people (Roth *et al*, 1985), including those who are severely mentally ill (Farr *et al*, 1986). They are rarely in an active marital relationship; in many more cases than expected, they have never been married; they report few friends, few confiding relationships, and tend to describe themselves as loners. They do not have the relationships found in a normal workplace or neighbourhood. More often than expected, they have childhood histories of disruptive family relationships, for instance have been placed in foster care (Susser *et al*, 1991*a*). Providing services for a population such as this is very different from providing them for a typical domiciled population, where a treatment provider can assume that the person is supported by a certain array of relationships. What is more, for the homeless, other supportive factors are lacking, such as a permanent place to sleep and live, personal safety, a reasonable diet, a degree of financial security. Their extremely precarious circumstances should be reflected in treatment and rehabilitation approaches.

Poverty

The homeless are the poorest of the poor. Even where relatively good social security systems are in place, their resources are clearly inadequate to meet their basic needs. Mentally ill persons in general often have difficulty in obtaining entitlements (Allen, 1989). This is certainly the case for mentally ill homeless people, in part because of their inability to tolerate the cumbersome procedures for obtaining these resources. The amount of public assistance is generally based upon poverty indices and provides minimally adequate resources for survival. An intelligent, healthy and well-organised person may be able to sustain a minimal standard of living with supports of this sort, but for a mentally ill person, the challenge may be too great.

Homeless women

In most places where homeless people congregate, men predominate. Shelters, missions, reception centres, and hostels have in the past catered mostly to the needs of men. Until quite recently, homelessness among women was considered rare, and an indication of severe social disorder (Caplow *et al*, 1968). Research, therefore, has focused more on homeless men than on women. In the past several years, however, homelessness among women has risen dramatically in the US, especially among single mothers (Bassuk, 1991). Families with children are reported to account for more than 40% of the homeless population in many major cities, including New York, Los Angeles and Philadelphia (US Conference of Mayors, 1990). A number of studies of homeless women have been reported (Bassuk & Rosenberg, 1988; Weitzman *et al*, 1992). Only a few permit comparisons between men and women (Fernandez, 1984; Herzberg, 1987; Breakey *et al*, 1989; Scott, 1991).

Several studies have suggested that women are generally less socially isolated than men, for example, they maintain closer contacts with their families. They are also somewhat more successful than men in obtaining financial entitlements. There is an impression among many investigators that the prevalence of psychiatric disorders and level of disability in women on their own in the shelter system is higher than in men, but this has not been clearly supported by empirical research.

Two distinct groups of homeless women, with somewhat different characteristics, have been described. One is the group of mothers of homeless families. These are generally younger women, with prevalence rates of mental illness and substance-use disorders that are little different from the general population, but who may have higher rates of personality disorder. The other is composed of women who are generally older, are not accompanied by children and are to be found in places frequented by single homeless people. In this group the prevalence of substance use and mental illness is considerably higher than in the general population. However, their rates of substance-use disorders are generally lower than those in homeless men.

Service strategies

Meeting the mental health service needs of homeless mentally ill persons may be tackled through the establishment of a special programme, or by making existing programmes more responsive to their special needs (Brent-Smith & Dean, 1990). Whichever approach is taken, there are certain basic requirements for a responsive service. A high level of clinical expertise is required, in view of the complexity of the clinical problems presented. Some form of outreach is needed, because many patients will not readily seek treatment, and close integration with social services is essential to help persons deal with their many social-service needs. Providing adequate treatment to a person who is 'on the street' is extremely difficult. It is thus vital to get people housed, and for this purpose to have access to a variety of housing options. Close collaboration with substance-abuse services is essential, as with primary health-care services. Finally, close linkages with other parts of the mental health-care network are needed, so that as soon as possible people may move on into the mainstream.

Service models

Special clinics for the homeless

Because of the reluctance of many homeless people to make use of regular health-care facilities, and the reluctance of some health-care providers to accept homeless people for treatment, special clinics have been set up in many places, where access for homeless people will be easier. Often such clinics are designed to provide primary health care, but they also serve the needs of the mentally ill (Wright & Weber, 1987; Thomison & Cook, 1987; Joseph, 1990; Brickner *et al*, 1990).

Shelter-based interventions

An alternative approach has been to move the mental health (or primary care) service providers into shelters or other places where homeless people are served. This approach has been employed, for example, in the very large shelters in New York City (Caton *et al*, 1990; Gounis & Susser, 1990).

Street outreach programmes

To examine more vigorously the problem of prospective patients' reluctance to seek treatment, most programmes have found it essential to have outreach workers whose job it is to seek out people who need treatment. Some individuals accept offers of help relatively easily, but others may be extremely resistant, so that repeated contacts may be needed before the person can be persuaded to accept help (Cohen *et al*, 1984; Cohen, 1990; Wobido *et al*, 1990). The outreach team may conclude that a person is in clear danger through self-neglect, or failure to protect herself or himself. In this situation, workers may have to use involuntary admission procedures to get a person to treatment, a process which may bring the team into conflict with advocacy or libertarian groups (Cournos, 1989).

Mobile assertive-treatment programmes

An extension of the outreach principle is the development of mobile treatment teams. The treatment model may be based on the Training in Community Living model developed by the Program for Assertive Community Treatment (PACT; Stein & Test, 1985), adapted for a mobile population. In this model, rather than the outreach worker bringing the patient in to the centre, the treatment team goes out to the patient wherever their intervention is needed. What is more, instead of this being thought of as a temporary expedient to improve access to treatment, it is a long-term commitment to the patient, for as long as the treatment programme is needed.

Case-management programmes

Case management has emerged in recent years as an important component in many mental health programmes. The variety of services that are needed to meet individuals' needs, and the complexity of the processes required to obtain services and entitlements need both expertise and a level of organisation beyond the capacities of many mentally ill people. Case management for homeless people requires special knowledge of the situations they face and of the various systems to bring together services for income maintenance, housing, treatment, and rehabilitation. There is some evidence that case management may have a specific effect in helping a person to develop networks of supportive relationships (Thornicroft & Breakey, 1991; Goering *et al*, 1992) and may thus have a particularly valuable role with homeless people.

Evaluating services for homeless people

Evaluation of service programmes involves an estimation of the extent to which they attain their declared objectives. Programmes for supplying the mental health needs of homeless people are likely to have objectives which are different from those of service programmes which are designed to meet the needs of more conventional populations. Whereas another programme may define its objectives as reducing in-patient hospital use, reducing levels of symptoms, or increasing employability in its patients, the objectives for a programme for the homeless mentally ill may be more basic. A fundamental objective for any programme will be to enable its clients or patients to escape from homelessness. However, there may be many other objectives, some parallel to that, and some which could be considered as intermediate goals on a path to attaining the ultimate objective. For example, some homeless mentally ill people are reluctant to have anything to do with treatment providers, and simply reaching the point where a person will talk with a worker may be a legitimate initial goal. Another intermediate goal towards the eventual objective of improved psychosocial functioning may be to link a patient successfully into the mental health service (Mowbray *et al*, 1991). The concept of a hierarchy of needs (Maslow, 1954), which holds that it is not possible to address higher order needs, such as medical treatment, until basic needs, such as those for food and clothing, have been met, is basic to service provision for homeless people and is echoed in the opinions of homeless people themselves (Ball & Havassy, 1984; Mulkern *et al*, 1985).

With homeless individuals, their social situation may need changing more than their psychopathology. Changes, as usually defined in evaluation studies, seem particularly irrelevant unless the client's circumstances improve. Symptom scales or target behaviours may therefore be of limited relevance. Social indices such as type of accommodation, access to benefits, work, etc., are likely to be more meaningful. An evaluator must recognise that the attainment of these objectives is strongly dependent on factors outside the control of the psychiatric service provider, such as the vagaries of the housing supply and social service policy decisions.

A hierarchy of objectives can be constructed, from the most basic to the most sophisticated as shown below:

Accepts sandwich from outreach worker
Maintains eye contact with outreach worker
Accepts clean clothing
Accepts housing/shelter assistance
Permits interview with clinician
Accepts medication
Spontaneously attends to personal hygiene
If dangerous, is brought to emergency facility
Attends clinic regularly
Manifests reduction in symptoms
Improvement in self-care ability
Adjusts satisfactorily to sheltered living programme

Participates in social activities
Maintains mutually satisfactory relationship
Transfers from homeless programme to generic programme
Participates in vocational rehabilitation programme
Able to live independently
Sustains competitive employment.

Programmes will vary in the degree to which they focus on particular segments of the hierarchy. A programme which reaches out to the most alienated of street people will have basic objectives. A programme which provides clinical services to persons in hostels or transitional living programmes will have different objectives that are higher on the hierarchy.

Standardised measures of psychopathology, functional capacity, quality of life, etc. are thus likely to have limited application in evaluating programmes for the homeless unless they are used to assess a focused objective, such as alcohol abuse, or can be adapted to examine particular issues of concern. Obtaining appropriate housing is an outcome of central importance where standard instruments are not available. A method of ranking housing options is needed, from the most basic to the most supportive, differentiating those that provide conjugate living arrangements from those that provide independent living arrangements, those where food is provided and those where the person must provide his/her own food, and so forth. An evaluator will then be concerned not simply with whether a person has a residence, but the extent to which the type of residence obtained matches the needs of the individual. Another example of an outcome where special evaluation tools would be needed is in measuring a client's degree of success in gaining access to benefit programmes to which he or she is entitled.

Prevention

Service programmes for the homeless mentally ill are essential, but in essence are merely palliative and do not solve the basic causes of the problem. It should be accepted that part of the role of the generic mental health service system in the era of community care is to provide a system of services which prevent mentally ill people from becoming homeless. Effective mental health service strategies are needed to prevent individuals from falling through the cracks and mental health services should be evaluated as to the extent to which they actively implement preventive strategies.

It should be emphasised once again that, in many respects, the problems of the homeless mentally ill are little different from those of homeless people in general. The prevention of homelessness for them, as for other homeless people, begins with a consideration of the causes of poverty, the shortage of low-income housing, changes in the employment market, deficiencies of the educational systems and other broad societal issues that are beyond the scope of mental health agencies.

Considering the particular problems of the seriously mentally ill, however, the critical factors which cause a particular person to become homeless are still not clearly established. A first stage in developing rational preventive strategies is the identification of risk factors. Childhood placement in foster care is a risk factor for homelessness later in life (Susser *et al*, 1987, 1991*a*), as is substance abuse co-occurring with mental illness (Belcher, 1989; Drake *et al*, 1989). If risk profiles can be established, a basis for identifying people at risk can be established, and special preventive interventions can be developed in mental health programmes.

The usefulness of computerised case registers should be investigated to assist service systems in providing continuity of care. Most importantly, however, a range of housing options, with varying degrees of supervision to meet the varied needs of disabled persons is essential to a well-developed mental health service system, and basic to preventing homelessness. Mentally ill people, as others, have preferences about the setting in which they live. If their preferences are ignored, one response is to leave, even to become homeless, rather than to stay in an unsatisfactory situation. The provision of a variety of good housing options would be calculated to decrease the likelihood of a mentally ill person becoming homeless. District or catchment-area service systems can be evaluated on the extent to which they provide appropriate housing for mentally ill people in the service area, and the frequency with which individuals drop out of the system or become homeless.

Summary and conclusion

The homeless mentally ill constitute a substantial subgroup of the burgeoning homeless populations of the USA and UK. Their needs for mental health services can be estimated from the high prevalence of major mental illnesses, the extent of comorbidity with substance-use disorders, their high levels of functional impairment, their lack of social supports, and their poverty. Individual assessments indicate that only a small number would be considered, by contemporary criteria, to require long-term hospital care, but many need a complex and well coordinated system of community-based care.

Experience with mental health services for the homeless indicate that special clinics orientated to their needs may be more effective than trying to integrate homeless people straight away into the mainstream mental health service system. Outreach to shelters and street locations is essential and close integration with primary care is advantageous, in view of the high prevalence of somatic illness in the homeless population. Case management may have a particularly valuable role in advocacy, coordinating needed services and assisting homeless clients to develop supportive relationships.

References

ALLEN, D. S. (1989) The uptake of social security benefits among psychiatric day hospital patients. *Psychiatric Bulletin*, **13**, 626–627.

AMERICAN PSYCHIATRIC ASSOCIATION (1980) *Diagnostic and Statistical Manual of Mental Disorders (3rd edn) (DSM–III)*. Washington, DC: APA.

BACHRACH, L. L. (1984) Interpreting research on the homeless mentally ill: some caveats. *Hospital and Community Psychiatry*, **35**, 914–916.

BAKER, R. & HALL, J. N. (1988) REHAB: a new assessment instrument for chronic psychiatric patients. *Schizophrenia Bulletin*, **14**, 97–111.

BALL, F. L. J. & HAVASSY, B. E. (1984) A survey of the problems and needs of homeless consumers of acute psychiatric services. *Hospital and Community Psychiatry*, **35**, 917–921.

BARROW, S. M., HELLMAN, F., LOVELL, A. M., *et al* (1989) *Effectiveness of Programs for the Mentally Ill Homeless. Final Report, Community Support Systems Evaluation Program*. New York: New York Psychiatric Institute.

——, ——, ——, *et al* (1991) Evaluating outreach services: lessons from a study of five programs. In *Psychiatric Outreach to the Mentally Ill* (ed. N. L. Cohen). San Francisco: Jossey Bass.

BASSUK, E. L. (1991) Homeless families. *Scientific American*, **265**, 66–74.

——, RUBIN, L. & LAURIAT, A. S. (1984) Is homelessness a mental health problem? *American Journal of Psychiatry*, **141**, 1546–1550.

——, ——, —— (1986) Characteristics of sheltered homeless families. *American Journal of Public Health*, **76**, 1097–1101.

—— & ROSENBERG, L. (1988) Why does family homelessness occur? A case control study. *American Journal of Public Health*, **78**, 783–788.

BELCHER, J. R. (1989) On becoming homeless: a study of chronically mentally ill persons. *Journal of Community Psychology*, **17**, 173–185.

BLACKWELL, B., BREAKEY, W. R., HAMMERSLEY, D., *et al* (1990) Psychiatric and mental health services. In *Under the Safety Net* (eds P. W. Brickner, L. K. Scharer, B. A. Conanan, *et al*), pp. 184–203. New York: Norton.

BOGUE, D. J. (1963) *Skid Row in American Cities*. Chicago: University of Chicago Press.

BREAKEY, W. R. (1992) Mental health services for homeless people. In *Homelessness: a National Perspective* (eds M. Robertson & M. Greenblatt), pp. 101–108. New York: Plenum Publishing.

——, FISCHER, P. J., KRAMER, M., *et al* (1989) Health and mental health problems of homeless men and women in Baltimore. *Journal of the American Medical Association*, **262**, 1352–1357.

BRENT-SMITH, H. & DEAN, R. (1990) *Plugging the Gaps: Providing a Service for Mentally Ill People*. London: Lewisham and North Southwark Health Authority.

BRICKNER, P. W., SCHARER, L. K., CONANAN, B. A., *et al* (eds) (1990) *Under the Safety Net*. New York: Norton.

CAPLOW, T., BAHR, H. M. & STERNBERG, D. (1968) Homelessness. *International Encyclopedia of the Social Sciences*, **6**, 494–499.

CATON, C., WYATT, J. W., GRUNBERG, J., *et al* (1990) An evaluation of a mental health program for homeless men. *American Journal of Psychiatry*, **147**, 286–289.

COHEN, N. L. (1990) *Psychiatry Takes to the Streets*. New York: Guilford.

——, PUTNAM, J. F. & SULLIVAN, A. (1984) The mentally ill homeless: isolation and adaptation. *Hospital and Community Psychiatry*, **35**, 922–924.

COURNOS, F. (1989) Involuntary medication and the case of Joyce Brown. *Hospital and Community Psychiatry*, **40**, 736–740.

DEROGATIS, L. R. & SPENCER, P. M. (1984) *Administration and Procedures: BSI Manual–I*. Baltimore: Johns Hopkins University.

DRAKE, R. E. & WALLACH, M. A. (1989) Substance abuse among the chronic mentally ill. *Hospital and Community Psychiatry*, **40**, 1041–1046.

——, —— & HOFFMAN, J. S. (1989) Housing instability and homelessness among aftercare patients of an urban state hospital. *Hospital and Community Psychiatry*, **40**, 46–51.

——, OSHER, F. C. & WALLACH, M. A. (1991) Homelessness and dual diagnosis. *American Psychologist*, **46**, 1149–1160.

EDWARDS, G., WILLIAMSON, V., HAWKER, A., *et al* (1968) Census of a reception centre. *British Journal of Psychiatry*, **114**, 1031–1039.

FARR, R., KOEGEL, P. & BURNHAM, A. (1986) *A Study of Homelessness and Mental Illness in the Skid Row Area of Los Angeles*. Los Angeles: LA Department of Mental Health.

FERNANDEZ, J. (1984) "In Dublin's Fair City": the mentally ill of no fixed abode. *Bulletin of the Royal College of Psychiatrists*, **8**, 187–190.

FISCHER, P. J. (1991) *Alcohol, Drug Abuse and Mental Health Problems among Homeless Persons: a Review of the Literature, 1980–1990*. Washington, DC: US Department of Health and Human Services, ADAMHA.

—— & BREAKEY, W. R. (1986) Homelessness and mental health: an overview. *International Journal of Mental Health*, **14**, 6–41.

——, SHAPIRO, S., BREAKEY, W. R., *et al* (1986) Mental health and social characteristics of the homeless: a survey of Baltimore shelter users. *American Journal of Public Health*, **76**, 519–524.

GOERING, P., WASYLENKI, D., ST. ONGE, M., *et al* (1992) Gender differences among clients of a case management program for the homeless. *Hospital and Community Psychiatry*, **43**, 160–165.

GOLDBERG, D. P. (1972) *The Detection of Mental Illness by Questionnaire*. London: Oxford University Press.

GOUNIS, K. & SUSSER, E. (1990) Shelterization and its implications for mental health services. In *Psychiatry Takes to the Streets* (ed. N. Cohen). New York: Guilford Press.

HERZBERG, J. L. (1987) No fixed abode: a comparison of men and women admitted to an East London psychiatric hospital. *British Journal of Psychiatry*, **150**, 621–627.

JOSEPH, P. L. A. (1990) A psychiatric clinic for the single homeless in a primary care setting in Inner London. *Psychiatric Bulletin*, **14**, 270–271.

KOEGEL, P., BURNAM, A. & FARR, R. K. (1988) The prevalence of specific psychiatric disorders among homeless individuals in the inner city of Los Angeles. *Archives of General Psychiatry*, **45**, 1085–1092.

LEACH, J. (1979) Providing for the destitute. In *Community Care for the Mentally Disabled* (eds J. K. Wing & R. Olson). Oxford: Oxford University Press.

LODGE PATCH, I. (1970) Homeless men in a London survey. *Proceedings of the Royal Society of Medicine*, **63**, 437–441.

MARSHALL, M. (1989) Collected and neglected: are Oxford hostels for the homeless filling up with disabled psychiatric patients? *British Medical Journal*, **299**, 706–709.

MASLOW, A. H. (1954) *Motivation and Personality*. New York: Harper and Row.

MOWBRAY, C. T., COHEN, E. & BYBEE, D. (1991) Services to individuals who are mentally ill: implementation evaluation. In *Evaluating Programs for the Homeless* (ed. D. Rog). San Francisco: Jossey Bass.

MULKERN, V., BRADLEY, V. J., SPENCE, R., *et al* (1985) *Homelessness Needs Assessment Study: Findings and Recommendations for the Massachussets Department of Mental Health*. Boston: Massachussets Department of Mental Health.

PRIEST, R. G. (1976) The homeless person and the psychiatric services: an Edinburgh survey. *British Journal of Psychiatry*, **128**, 128–136.

RADLOFF, L. S. (1977) The CESD Sale: A self-report depression scale for research in the general population. *Applied Psychological Measurements*, **1**, 174–181.

REGIER, D. A., BOYD, J. H., BURKE, J. D., *et al* (1988) One month prevalence of mental disorders in the United States. *Archives of General Psychiatry*, **45**, 977–986.

REID, J. (1989) The homeless and the changing British National Health Service. *American Journal of Public Health*, **79**, 965–966.

RIDGELY, M. S., GOLDMAN, H. H. & TALBOTT, J. A. (1986) *Chronically Mentally Ill Young Adults with Substance Abuse Problems: A Review of Relevant Literature and Creation of a Research Agenda*. Baltimore: University of Maryland School of Medicine.

RODERICK, P., VICTOR, C. & CONNELLY, J. (1991) Is housing a public health issue? A survey of directors of public health. *British Medical Journal*, **302**, 157–160.

ROTH, D., BEAN, J., LUST, N., *et al* (1985) *Homelessness in Ohio: a Study of People in Need*. Ohio: Department of Mental Health.

—— & —— (1986) The Ohio study: a comprehensive look at homelessness. *Psychosocial Rehabilitation Journal*, **9**, 31–38.

SCOTT, J. (1991) *A Survey of Female Users of Resettlement Units*. Newcastle-upon-Tyne: University of Newcastle-upon-Tyne, Department of Psychiatry.

SPITZER, R. L., COHEN, G., MILLER, J. D., *et al* (1969) The psychiatric status of 100 men on skid row. *International Journal of Social Psychiatry*, **15**, 230–234.

STARK, C., SCOTT, J., HILL, M., *et al* (1989) *A Survey of the "Long-Stay" Users of DSS Resettlement Units*. Newcastle-upon-Tyne: University of Newcastle-upon-Tyne, Department of Social Policy.

STEIN, L. & TEST, M. A. (1985) *The Training in Community Living Model: A Decade of Experience*. San Francisco: Jossey Bass.

SUSSER, E. (1992) Working with people who are mentally ill and homeless: the role of a psychiatrist. In *Homelessness and its Prevention* (ed. R. Jahiel), pp. 207–217. Baltimore Md.: Johns Hopkins University Press. (In press).

——, STRUENING, E. L. & CONOVER, S. (1987) Childhood experiences of homeless men. *American Journal of Psychiatry*, **144**, 1599–1601.

——, —— & —— (1989) Psychiatric problems in homeless men. *Archives of General Psychiatry*, **46**, 845–850.

—— & —— (1990) Diagnosis and screening for psychotic disorders in a study of the homeless. *Schizophrenia Bulletin*, **16**, 133–145.

——, GOLDFINGER, S. M. & WHITE, A. (1990) Some clinical approaches to the homeless mentally ill. *Community Mental Health Journal*, **26**, 463–480.

——, LIN, S., CONOVER, S., *et al* (1991*a*) Childhood antecedents of homelessness in psychiatric patients. *American Journal of Psychiatry*, **148**, 1026–1030.

——, —— & —— (1991*b*) Risk factors for homelessness in patients admitted to a state mental hospital. *American Journal of Psychiatry*, **148**, 1659–1664.

——, VALENCIA, E. & GOLDFINGER, S. (1992) Clinical care of homeless mentally ill individuals: strategies and adaptations. In *Treating the Homeless Mentally Ill* (eds H. R. Lamb, L. L. Bachrach & F. Kass). Washington, DC: American Psychiatric Press.

THOMISON, A. R. & COOK, D. A. G. (1987) Rootlessness and mental disorder. *British Journal of Clinical and Social Psychiatry*, **5**, 5–8.

THORNICROFT, G. & BREAKEY, W. R. (1991) The COSTAR programme. 1: Improving social networks of the long-term mentally ill. *British Journal of Psychiatry*, **159**, 245–249.

TIDMARSH, D. & WOOD, S. (1972) Psychiatric aspects of destitution. In *Evaluating a Community Psychiatry Service: The Camberwell Register 1964–71* (eds J. K. Wing & A. M. Hailey), pp. 327–340. London: Oxford University Press.

TIMMS, P. W. & FRY, A. H. (1989) Homelessness and mental illness. *Health Trends*, **21**, 70–71.

US CONFERENCE OF MAYORS (1990) *A Status Report on Hunger and Homelessness in America's Cities*. Washington, DC: The US Conference of Mayors.

VERNEZ, G., BURNAM, M. A., MCGLYNN, E. A., *et al* (1988) *Review of California's Program for the Homeless Mentally Disabled*. Santa Monica, CA: RAND Corporation.

WEITZMAN, B. C., KNICKMANN, J. R. & SHINN, M. (1992) Predictors of shelter use among low-income families: psychiatric history, substance abuse and victimization. *American Journal of Public Health*, **82**, 1547–1550.

WHITELEY, J. S. (1955) Down and out in London: mental illness in the lower social groups. *Lancet*, **ii**, 608–610.

WOBIDO, S. L., FRANK, T., MERRITT, B., *et al* (1990) Outreach. In *Under the Safety Net* (eds P. W. Brickner, L. K., Scharer, B. A. Conanan, *et al*), pp. 328–339. New York: Norton.

WRIGHT, J. D. & WEBER, E. (1987) *Homelessness and Health*. Washington, DC: McGraw-Hill.

17 Needs of relatives of long-term psychiatric patients

LIZ KUIPERS

Relatives of the psychiatrically ill are not given a choice. It happens that someone they live with and have a relationship with has psychiatric problems. Thus for this group – the relatives of those with schizophrenia or depression – the needs are not so much about their own functioning, or lack of it, as about the demands placed on them by their acceptance of the caring role. In the literature, the needs of relatives are not even considered unless they are also carers. Thus, the impact of a severe mental illness on those who relinquish a caring role or who do not take it up is not taken into account. 'Peripheral' relatives such as grandparents or siblings, who do not take on caring as a primary role, also tend to be ignored. At this stage, relatives' needs have been documented only for the main carers of the psychiatrically ill – often elderly parents, spouses (especially if the patients' diagnosis is depression) and a few siblings and adult children. Carers of the psychiatrically ill are likely to be female if they are parents, but, unlike other groups, a substantial number of the spouses, siblings and adult children will be male.

Needs for care, as defined elsewhere in this volume, do not apply to relatives: they do not initially have 'an illness or disability for which there is an acceptable and effective treatment or cure'. However, in the process of remaining involved as a patient becomes mentally ill they do develop problems associated with this caring role. These problems can be defined as relatives' needs. Unfortunately these problems have often not been recognised; the idea that relatives have needs for care on their own behalf has taken a remarkably long time to be accepted, let alone acted upon. In the past, relatives have been blamed, ignored, or just left to cope, by professionals concerned only with 'the patient'.

This situation has begun to change. Partly because of the impact of self-help groups such as The National Schizophrenia Fellowship (NSF) and The Manic–Depressive Fellowship, relatives' views are beginning to be taken seriously. However, few relatives belong to self-help groups and, as a group, relatives remain poor advocates on their own behalf.

Relatives as carers are now becoming even more essential. Mental hospitals continue to close and admission time in the remaining hospital beds continues to reduce. Alternative provision such as hostel accommodation or group homes remains unevenly distributed around the country and increasingly dependent on local and charitable initiatives. Figures on those with major mental illnesses who return home to live with relatives vary, but are about 60% for first admission (MacMillan *et al*, 1986) and 50% if first and subsequent admissions are included (Gibbons *et al*, 1984). Even in the case of long-term patients, between 40 and 50% either live with or are in close contact with relatives, or have other patients in their network who take on this caring role (Creer *et al*, 1982). The central role of families in providing long-term care is not in dispute (Gibbons *et al*, 1984). Without relatives it seems likely that professional services would be overwhelmed by the needs of patients trying to live in the community. However, in order both to maximise the care that such patients receive and to ensure it is not delivered at the cost of another vulnerable group in society – the unpaid carers (Lefley, 1987) – it is necessary to consider in detail the effects of providing care for the mentally ill.

Since the 1950s, when patients first began to return to live in the community after the introduction of the phenothiazines, there has been interest in, and studies of, the effect that this had on relatives. However, the sobering fact emerges that a great deal of what was documented then is still being documented in the 1990s. This seems to reflect a basic difficulty professionals have in accepting that relatives might have needs and, that if they do, these should have implications for service provision. There has been, and remains, a tendency for professionals to think that relatives are 'someone else's job'. It is only in the last decade that opportunities for working in partnership with relatives have developed. Only now are there some signs that relatives are being seen as a resource rather than as a nuisance (Kuipers & Bebbington, 1985, 1990; Mintz *et al*, 1987) and that they are being offered support and help, so that those who want to can continue in a caring role without being exploited or made to feel guilty if they refuse.

The measurement of family burden

To explore the problems that families may experience as a consequence of their caring role, the concept of family burden has been developed. Platt (1985) in a review of the issues involved in measuring burden defines it as "the presence of problems, difficulties or adverse events which affect the life (lives) of the psychiatric patients' significant others (e.g. members of the household and/or the family)" (p. 385). There are other definitions but in Platt's view they share a common underlying frame of reference "the effect of the patient upon the family" (Goldberg & Huxley, 1980, p. 127);

"the impact of living with a [psychiatric] patient on the way of life, or health of family members" (Brown, 1967, p. 53); "the difficulties felt by the family of a psychiatric patient" (Pai & Kapur, 1981, p. 334).

Hoenig & Hamilton (1966) were the first to make a clear attempt to distinguish between two dimensions of burden; the 'objective' and 'subjective' burden of caring. Objective burden is any disruption of family life which is potentially verifiable and observable such as financial problems, social isolation, or having to cope with violent behaviour. Subjective burden refers to the personal feelings that relatives attribute to the caring role such as distress or upset. In the better studies these are now assessed independently (e.g. Fadden *et al*, 1987*b*).

More recently, there has been some attempt to distinguish between an event and its perceived cause; what has been called patient relatedness (e.g. Platt *et al*, 1983). This enables independent analysis of an event and its specificity to the problems of living with a psychiatric patient. Families may have financial problems, which may or may not be attributable to a patient living in the household.

Measures of burden vary in what they ask about, how well they separate objective and subjective burden, and which informants they use. However, what they attempt to examine is the basic loss of reciprocity in relationships that can be caused by severe mental illness, which breaks down the usual mechanisms that maintain an equable and supportive relationship. It seems to be this imbalance which may prevent the relationship from being intrinsically reinforcing and lead carers to feel that they need external support in order to maintain the caring role. The degree of burden that relatives of patients with severe psychiatric disorders report has been reviewed (Fadden *et al*, 1987*a*; MacCarthy, 1988). As MacCarthy (1988) discusses, the evidence of burden has varied depending on the criteria used and on the fact that relatives, as a group, are remarkably uncomplaining. Nevertheless, it is clear that burden exists and is usually extensive.

Mandelbrote & Folkard (1961*a,b*) estimated the degree to which families were restricted or disturbed by the presence of schizophrenic patients in the home. Despite a rather crude method of assessment, they found that over half of the families were disturbed in some way, although only 2% reported severe stress. Mills (1962) studied psychiatric patients without selecting for diagnosis and found that most were a source of some anxiety to their relatives. More than half were described as difficult at home, and only a small minority caused no practical problems. In Grad & Sainsbury's study (1963*a,b*) almost two-thirds of the families had been experiencing hardship because the patient was living at home and in one-fifth the burden was severe. Two years later, 20% of their initial sample remained heavily burdened.

Wing *et al* (1964) followed 113 schizophrenic patients for a year after discharge. When patients returned to live with their families, social relations were strained in nearly two-thirds of cases. Waters & Northover (1965) similarly reported that many schizophrenic men occasioned moderate to severe hardship to their relatives in terms of social embarrassment, inconvenience, and behaviour which frightened them or caused tension in the family. Hoenig & Hamilton (1966, 1969) found that three-quarters of their patients had some kind of adverse effect on the household.

Creer *et al* (1982) interviewed 52 relatives of long-term patients and found that up to 60% of households had to contend with at least moderate levels of disturbed behaviour. Gibbons *et al* (1984), in a sample of 141 patients, found a similar proportion suffered hardship, often severe. In their study, only 10% of the sample gave no evidence of family hardship. Carers were coping with high levels of disability; 65% of patients showed disturbed behaviour and 78% had restricted social performance. In these last two studies, as MacCarthy (1988) points out, supportive relatives were included even if they did not always live with the patient; as even a short break from continuous care ('respite') seems to reduce subjective burden, these high levels of hardship may still underestimate the problems faced by full-time carers.

The problems that severe mental illness can cause to relationships are reflected in high rates of divorce and separation in marriages where one member is mentally ill. Brown *et al* (1966) noted that in many cases the patient's illness had been instrumental in bringing about divorce and separation, and in their study the rates for patients were three times the national average for women and four times for men. Clinically it appears that if a carer is a spouse, they will always have considered separation or divorce. However the guilt engendered by a decision to leave when a partner is in obvious difficulties will mitigate against it; several studies note this. An early study of spouses (Yarrow *et al*, 1955a) found that even those contemplating separation or divorce had elected to give the relationship another try. Fadden *et al* (1987b) in a study of the spouses of long-term depressive patients found a similar adherence to the marriage despite considerable difficulties.

Effects on social and leisure activities

An obvious consequence of living with a relative with persistent mental illness is the damaging effect on social and leisure activities. This is often considerably worse for women, who are more likely to be the main carers (Fadden *et al*, 1987b). Yarrow *et al* (1955b) noted that wives (carers) consistently believed that mental illness was stigmatised by others and expressed fears of social discrimination. As a consequence, one-third of them adopted a pattern of 'aggressive concealment', making drastic changes in order to avoid former friends; some even moved house. Another third had told only members of the family, or close friends who either understood the problem or had been in a similar situation themselves.

A number of other studies have documented the restriction of social activities experienced by those who live with and care for patients with schizophrenia (e.g. Mandelbrote & Folkard, 1961*a,b*; Wing *et al*, 1964; Waters & Northover, 1965). This can be especially marked when the relative is elderly (Leff *et al*, 1982). Similar observations have also been made for spouses of severely depressed patients (Fadden *et al*, 1987*b*). These relatives spent over 60 hours per week in face-to-face contact with the patient and were correspondingly socially isolated. In MacCarthy *et al*'s (1989*b*) study, relatives averaged 49 hours per week contact with long-term patients. Anderson *et al* (1984) found a decrease in the social networks of some relatives who lived with schizophrenic patients. MacCarthy (1988) notes that relatives of those attending long-term day care have very few social contacts other than the patient, few are employed, and many remain isolated in their own homes. She also points out that social isolation is a "pervasive problem, which impairs the relationship between patient and supporter and reduces coping resources more fundamentally than material hardship". It is clear that isolation and stigma, while not new problems, still exist in the community and remain as difficulties to be faced by relatives in the caring role (Kuipers *et al*, 1989).

Financial and employment difficulties

These have been emphasised in a number of studies (Yarrow *et al*, 1955*b*; Mandelbrote & Folkard, 1961*a,b*; Mills, 1962; Hoenig & Hamilton, 1966, 1969; Stevens, 1972; Fadden *et al*, 1987*b*). They are likely to be greatest when the carer is a spouse, as caring may interfere quite substantially with the opportunity to stay in work and the spouse may not be able to take on the role of financial provider. Because severe psychiatric disorders may interfere with long-term earning capacity, higher levels of burden occur when patients who were formerly earning are affected than when the illness begins early in life. In the latter case, expectations and financial commitments may not yet have developed. Many patients in long-term care never become financially independent, and relatives, such as parents, who have always supported them may find this a less difficult transition. Nevertheless, the loss of potential earnings, whether of a previous main earner or of a person who might have been expected to be economically viable, is likely to have effects on caring relatives and to lead at the very least to a more impoverished family setting than otherwise. Because the psychiatric illness is often long-term these effects are likely to be underestimated.

How do relatives adjust to these illnesses?

Viewing disturbed or unusual behaviour as symptomatic of illness or relapse is what professionals are trained to do. Carers are not, however, and they may make various attributions in an attempt to understand and deal with the day-to-day issues. They may decide an individual is being 'difficult' or 'lazy' and blame them for their behaviour. This is typical of relatives rated as critical or hostile according to the Expressed Emotion (EE) measure (Leff & Vaughn, 1985; Brewin *et al*, 1991). Alternatively, they may deny, or fail to see, any behaviour as problematic (Jackson *et al*, 1990).

Relatives are likely to feel high levels of anxiety, exacerbated by the fact that often there is a crisis before any professional help can be obtained. It is also likely that guilt, anger and feelings of rejection will surface. These reactions were noted by Clausen *et al* (1955a) and Yarrow *et al* (1955a). Most of the relatives described by Creer & Wing (1974) had at times expressed anger at the way their lives had been spoiled, and grief when they recalled what the patient had been like before the illness. Fadden *et al* (1987b) found that many of the spouses of the depressed patients expressed not only anger and guilt, but a sense of loss as if they had been physically bereft of the person they married. This grief has been likened to a bereavement process both in terms of impact and the length of time it can take to accept the patient as they are now (Lefley, 1987; Kuipers *et al*, 1989).

Things may not become easier over time. Objective hardships are likely to increase (Grad & Sainsbury, 1968; Hoenig & Hamilton, 1969; Lefley, 1987). However, resignation, which is associated with less objective stress, is also more common (Gibbons *et al*, 1984; MacCarthy *et al*, 1989b).

Relatives' own mental health

It is only relatively recently that it has become routine to investigate the psychological impact of caring while assessing the severity of burden. Effects were documented initially for those living with depressed or neurotic partners (Kreitman, 1964; Kreitman *et al*, 1970; Ovenstone, 1973a) and for those living with schizophrenic patients (Brown *et al*, 1966; Hoenig & Hamilton, 1966, 1969; Stevens, 1972; Creer & Wing, 1974). More recently, relatives have been assessed using standardised measures such as the General Health Questionnaire (GHQ; Goldberg & Hillier, 1979) and the Present State Examination (PSE; Wing *et al*, 1974). The consistent finding then emerges that around one-third of relatives are likely to have raised levels of anxiety and depression connected to the caring role (Creer *et al*, 1982; Fadden *et al*, 1987b). MacCarthy *et al* (1989b) found that 77% of the sample of 45 carers of long-term patients described at least one symptom of distress and 14 (33%) reported experiencing three or more such symptoms – considerably higher levels of disorder than would be expected in the general population. As MacCarthy (1988) had earlier pointed out, "calculating the costs of maintaining a patient in need of continual care in the community should include that of providing psychiatric treatment for up to one third of the main dispensers of this care" (p. 216).

Burdensome symptoms

Behaviour problems in patients are the best predictors of complaints from carers and are major correlates of burden (Lefley, 1987). In practice these seem to fall into two categories – socially disruptive behaviour and social withdrawal.

In Mills' (1962) study, carers were commonly concerned that patients might be a danger to themselves or to others. Problems frequently arose with neighbours as a result of patients' behaviour. Many relatives complained of disturbed nights. In Grad & Sainsbury's (1963*a,b*) study, psychotic patients were more problematic than those with neurotic problems. Severe burden was related to aggression, delusions, hallucinations, confusion, and poor self-care. However, problems that were complained of most often were the frustrating, depressive, and hypochondriacal preoccupations of patients. Brown *et al* (1966) found the number of problems and the distress experienced by relatives were related to the degree of disturbed behaviour shown by patients with schizophrenia who lived with them. Hoenig & Hamilton (1966,1969) confirmed that most frequently relatives reported both aggressive behaviour and extreme seclusion and withdrawal as problematic.

Creer & Wing (1974), in a study of 80 long-term carers, 50 of whom were members of the NSF, found that negative symptoms of social withdrawal, lack of conversation, underactivity, slowness, and having few leisure interests were rated most often as problems. Socially embarrassing behaviour and obviously disturbed behaviour were also difficult. Gibbons *et al* (1984) reported that disruptive behaviour caused the most distress to relatives. Even though they were minority behaviours, offensive behaviour, rudeness, and violence were found by almost all carers to be upsetting if they had to cope with them. According to another study (Fadden *et al*, 1987*b*), sleeplessness was the main problem for carers of depressed patients, followed by misery, worry, guilt, and the inactivity of patients.

MacCarthy *et al* (1989*b*) found patients' lack of independent self-help skills and disruptive antisocial behaviour, followed by negative symptoms and difficulties in relating to the patient, as the main problems named by carers.

The burden of depressive symptoms

The specific burdens of depressive illnesses on carers are not often separated in the literature, and the relatively limited information available is mainly concerned with the effects on spouses – the main carers (Kuipers, 1987; Fadden *et al*, 1987*a*). In these marriages there is frequently conflict (Hinchcliffe *et al*, 1978), particularly over role functions (Ovenstone, 1973*b*), and a high level of dependence (Birtchnell & Kennard, 1983). With increasing pathology on the part of the husband, fewer joint decisions are made (Collins *et al*, 1971), and the wives of depressed patients may have significantly less independent social activity than controls (Nelson *et al*, 1970). Partners may find it difficult to take over roles in the marriage; spouses not only find that they have increased responsibilities but that they have lost their own support and intimate confidant in the marriage (Fadden *et al*, 1987*b*). Adolescent children living with chronically depressed parents have increased levels of psychiatric morbidity (Hammen *et al*, 1987). These disturbances may be more marked when life events have to be coped with (Hirsch *et al*, 1985).

Behaviour of professionals towards relatives

Not many studies have looked at this specifically. The Clausen study (Clausen *et al*, 1955*b*) investigated how attitudes held by both patients' wives and their psychiatrists affected the services provided (Deasy & Quinn, 1955). Wives mainly made requests for information regarding aetiology, diagnosis, and prognosis, and advice on how to deal with the patient when he returned home. In nearly two-thirds of cases, however, wives expressed dissatisfaction because they did not receive this information or the professionals were inaccessible. Deasy & Quinn reported that the psychiatrists frequently felt that they had to protect patients from their wives as they believed that factors in the relationship had caused the illness.

General dissatisfaction with services, mental health professionals and service-delivery systems continues to be expressed by carers (Lefley, 1987). That carers are rarely involved in decision making, that services need to be available continuously and not just in a crisis, and that carers of the long-term mentally ill may have to deal with the complexities not only of the mental health services but also of legal and criminal systems is still being documented.

The only study so far to look specifically at how adequately a service provides for the needs of relatives of those attending long-term day care was by MacCarthy *et al* (1989*b*). This study was one of a series of surveys of high-contact users of psychiatric services, in which the MRC Needs for Care Assessment was used to measure both functioning and whether interventions had been attempted; this led to judgements of whether needs had been met or not (Brewin *et al*, 1987, 1988). MacCarthy *et al*'s study (1989*b*) was unique in adapting these standardised measures of need to look at the problems relatives might have, thereby allowing definitive comment on whether adequate services were being provided. Subjects were 145 patients attending day care locally. Of these, 61 (42%) were living with at least one other relative. Patient functioning was assessed by interviewing the relatives with a modified version of the MRC Social Behaviour Schedule (Wykes & Sturt, 1986). Questions were asked about difficulties with finances, employment, children and their own physical and mental health in order to assess objective burden. Relatives were also asked how much any particular problem could be attributed to the patient. Finally they were asked about contact with services and their satisfaction with these.

MacCarthy *et al* found that relatives had problems most frequently in the areas of information and advice, emotional support, and respite care. These three areas were also the ones with most unmet need. They found that practical needs, such as for housing, child care, and help with benefits were most often met. However, information and advice had only been offered successfully to about half of the relatives. Support for emotional burdens had the highest rate of underprovision. Some relatives were being offered help, but one-fifth of the sample needed help that had not yet been offered. Respite care had been rarely identified as a problem and had only been met for one family out of 61. This study confirmed again that relatives tolerated their demanding role, had difficulty articulating what other help they would like, and were not likely to complain.

Implications for service provision

It is clear from the literature reviewed that relatives of the long-term mentally ill have a demanding and often unsupported role, and may be extensively burdened by it, both objectively and in terms of the emotional impact of these disorders. The degree of burden may be severe and can affect the carers' own mental well-being, particularly as caring is likely to last for a lifetime (Lefley, 1987) without respite (MacCarthy *et al*, 1989*b*). Services seem more likely and able to respond to crises than to the continuous, changing requirements of families as they go through the life cycle. Patients' stability may vary and interact with these changes. Services do provide practical help but even now, 40 years after the problem was first documented, they have difficulty in providing information and advice, and particularly in providing effective emotional support.

Relatives have needs both for their own mental health and quality of life, and to enable them to provide an adequate, stimulating and yet not over-stressful environment for the patient. Some relatives do manage this, but it cannot be assumed. There is also some evidence that the resignation that can characterise long-term caring relationships may be detrimental to patients' functioning and well-being (MacCarthy *et al*, 1989*a*).

There is hardly any mention in the literature of benefits that might occur in the caring role. Lefley (1987) notes that positive aspects have not been adequately assessed. It seems instead that the role is often accepted because of a lack of community alternatives. This lack runs right through the literature; there is limited support offered, and no choices for carers to decide how to take up the caring role. Caring appears at present to involve total care, with all the social and personal costs involved; the alternative is to reject the role altogether.

Specific needs for services

The needs outlined above seem to suggest a rather pessimistic view of whether anything will ever change. There is a danger of professionals and the services available becoming as overwhelmed and even as burdened by the families' problems as the carers themselves. There is sometimes a sense that whatever is offered, it will not be enough. However, a careful look at the specific services that might be provided, together with evidence from some current studies on effectiveness, does suggest pointers for the future.

(a) The need for collaborative rather than adversarial relationships between professionals and carers

Over the last decade there has been evidence of some change from professionals 'blaming' families for problems, to being willing instead to work with them in partnership to use the resources both sides have available to help improve and maintain patients' recovery from serious mental illnesses. The change has been most noticeable in the literature on the successful family interventions using social and pharmacological treatment in schizophrenia (reviewed by Kuipers & Bebbington, 1988, 1990). This, of course, is based on the earlier work on EE (Leff & Vaughn, 1985) which suggests that family attitudes, while not being the cause of schizophrenia, have an effect on its course. Despite some contrary views (Hatfield *et al*, 1987), this theory has led to the development of techniques whereby the family can be helped to cope more effectively (Leff *et al*, 1985; Falloon *et al*, 1985; Tarrier *et al*, 1988). There is also some evidence that EE and burden are linked (Jackson *et al*, 1990).

Another requirement of a collaborative stance by professionals is that they are prepared to take the carers' viewpoint seriously, to act if asked rather than wait for the crisis, and to work on prevention of relapse rather than just treating symptoms once a relapse has occurred. Even a 24-hour crisis team can fail to provide adequate long-term support and rehabilitation (Reynolds *et al*, 1990). Some recent work suggests that carers are well able to assess early signs of relapse in patients who live with them and that this information can be used with clinicians to prevent more serious symptoms from developing (Birchwood *et al*, 1989).

Another strand of research which may reduce the distance between professional staff and carers is the recently replicated finding that not only do staff and carers have to cope with many of the same behaviour problems in patients (Creer *et al*, 1982), but that they also share a range of EE ratings (Watts, 1988). Typically, around 40% of staff in long-term care will be rated as high EE towards one or more key patients (Moore *et al*, 1992). This finding has implications for the importance of staff training and for allowing carers access to specialised help for patients' behaviour that staff also have problems in coping with.

(b) A need to understand

It must now be obvious that informing carers is a necessary first step in any interaction between carers and professionals. Information helps carers to understand the condition they are dealing with and its implications, both in terms of long-term care and emotional impact. Telling carers the name of a condition such as schizophrenia or depression helps alleviate some of the confusion and misattribution that is likely to arise otherwise. Giving information to carers is by no means straightforward. Because of high levels of anxiety that carers might have when in first contact with professionals, there may be considerable difficulties in understanding and accepting what is said. At best, education provides a diagnosis and some optimism and is the basis for engaging relatives in further intervention (Smith & Birchwood, 1987; Berkowitz *et al*, 1990). Staff must be prepared to continually answer questions, to admit when answers are uncertain or unknown, and to discuss implications for the individual family over many months. Changes in the situation, a cyclical illness or other unpredictability, will often mean the whole process starting again.

(c) Help in problem solving

Difficult behaviour is a correlate of burden in carers. Thus, helping carers to cope with it successfully is an important issue and one that is very frustrating for carers if avoided or handled superficially. Giving advice does not mean that staff tell carers what to do – this is perceived as arrogant, and lacks credibility because staff are seen as not having to cope continuously with these problems. Family members need to be encouraged to try out new and constructive behaviour patterns, one problem at a time, broken into manageable steps, with possible solutions negotiated rather than imposed on all involved, including the patient. There is now much literature available on the techniques that can be successfully applied (Falloon *et al*, 1984; Anderson *et al*, 1986; Kuipers & Bebbington, 1990; Kuipers *et al*, 1992).

(d) Need for emotional support

The emotional impact of illness, particularly severe mental illness, continues to be underestimated. Families are likely to have a wide range of emotional responses. Shock and denial characterise first contacts with professional services. Later, guilt, grief, loss, anger, and rejection are likely, as is worry about the future and the patient's vulnerability, given perceived and actual deficits in role performance. Isolation, stigma, and poor understanding from friends and family are common. Hopelessness and finally resignation – nothing ever changes – may set in. It is not surprising that professionals may feel daunted and not attempt to offer help. However, there is evidence that help can be given successfully. Most of the intervention studies with a positive outcome offered support either implicitly or explicitly (Leff *et al*, 1982, 1989; Falloon *et al*, 1982; Hogarty *et al*, 1986; Tarrier *et al*, 1988). MacCarthy *et al* (1989*a*) were able to improve attitudes and coping, although not burden, using education and support groups for relatives giving long-term care. Brooker and colleagues showed that CPNs were rated by carers as successful in offering both information and emotional support to families coping with schizophrenia (Brooker *et al*, 1992).

(e) Needs for care to continue

One of the worst aspects of professional services that carers discuss is high staff turnover. Busy hospitals, particularly teaching hospitals, are not ideal places for staff to form long-term relationships as advocates for families (MacCarthy *et al*, 1989*a*). As staff move on, carers have to start again with new professionals. However, in the same way that continuity of care is a reasonable aim for long-term patients (Watts & Bennett, 1983), so it can be for long-term carers. The self-help groups have taken on this role over the last ten years, offering support groups and helplines. Professional services can, via a keyworker system, ensure that even if staff change, information is handed on effectively and monitoring and intervention strategies are not lost. However, it does need a positive commitment, probably from senior staff members in a multidisciplinary team, that carers merit this level of input.

(f) Need to look after themselves

The damage to a carer's own health from the caring role, including the personal and social costs (Noh & Turner, 1987), is now well documented. Carers risk increased psychological problems, isolation, family impoverishment, and a likelihood that the family will become enmeshed and overdependent (Lefley, 1987). Nevertheless, carers often want to offer help to their relatives, and see what they do as a positive contribution – one that can enhance patient recovery and social functioning. The issue seems to be the lack of choice. Feeling forced into a difficult and often unrewarding role will not make it work to either carers' or patients' advantage. Carers can offer a valuable resource, a possible lifetime commitment to a patient and a 'normal' setting in the community. They provide contact with a social network for patients whose own networks are likely to be restricted (Hamilton *et al*, 1989). If carers feel exploited and left to cope unaided, this resource will not necessarily continue to be available.

In order to look after themselves, carers may need staff to allow them time off, to ask for respite, and to develop their own independent interests. It is difficult to accept that it can be caring to leave a patient to cope alone some of the time. These interventions have been shown to be effective, both in changing overprotective relationships and in allowing relatives to enjoy themselves without experiencing guilt (Leff *et al*, 1982, 1989).

If there were more alternatives available in the community, both in the range of accommodation, the flexibility of support, and the importance attributed to the caring role, it is possible that burden would diminish. A report of the facilities available in Germany suggests that this can indeed be done (Hoffman & Hubschmid, 1989).

(g) Need for respite care

The specific use of respite care for psychiatric patients and their families is not established. It is accepted that elderly patients can be admitted to relieve carers but it is often not seen as justified for patients, who may be well, to be given a hospital bed 'just' for social reasons.

The need for respite care for relatives has been identified (MacCarthy *et al*, 1989*b*). What services can offer is planned respite care. This entails deciding beforehand with the family that a patient can be admitted for a short stay each month, for example, over a weekend. The offer does not have to be taken up. This procedure acknowledges that there is a problem and that respite is a legitimate request. A preventative offer of respite may well avert a crisis, as it is a certainty of relief that can often only be guaranteed otherwise by waiting for, or escalating, a crisis.

Another model is not to rely on hospital beds – an increasingly scarce and expensive resource – but to offer other accommodation in the community specifically for this use. The NSF have pioneered the use of houses in local areas for this purpose.

(h) The needs of 'peripheral' relatives

Relatives who are not the main carer, but who are often still involved with the patients' concerns, are hardly ever considered by services. In recent years there have been some local attempts to form support groups which will consider these needs; so far these are groups for siblings of patients and for children of patients.

Siblings have particular problems which include feelings of anger and resentment at the attention the patient is receiving in the family and fear that they themselves will have mental illness problems as well. Later on, siblings report feeling guilt at the anger and fear, and also guilt at their own achievements which may highlight the continuing difficulties and lack of progress of a brother or sister. There is often also misunderstanding of the problems, followed by avoidance and leaving home early to make sure the burden of care is not passed on to them. Ambivalent feelings may remain in the relationship between an ill and a well sibling.

Children share some of these feelings, and often also have a very confused relationship with the ill parent who may not be able to offer consistent care. Children will often blame themselves for this, and later feel anger and resentment if care is lacking or sporadic. It seems likely that at least one capable parent or carer is necessary to a child's development, and children from settings where this has not been possible because of mental illness may have specific problems.

Services need to be aware that 'peripheral' relatives exist, but may be neither as vocal, nor as easy to contact as the main carer. They are likely to have similar needs to the main carer; for basic information, advice, for help to cope with specific problems, for reassurance, and for emotional support.

Conclusions

At present, the needs of relatives of the long-term mentally ill living in the community are extensive and unlikely to be met in full. We have known about the needs for 40 years, and they have not changed substantially. There is now awareness of the problems, but still a 'scatter shot' approach (Kreisman & Joy, 1974) to the implementation of solutions. There is evidence suggesting that the existing needs do not have to be overwhelming for services. Provision of support for carers will enable them to make informed decisions about their commitment, level of involvement, and how they take up the role. Meeting needs now is also likely to be cost effective as it can prevent aspects of future morbidity in both carers and patients who live with them.

Relatives have little choice over the position they find themselves in and its impact on them. Their needs are intrinsic to the role and are likely to develop over time, as they continue a valuable and difficult job. In the 1990s, it is time to stop simply cataloguing the problems and to start providing services that are geared to these needs.

References

ANDERSON, C. M., HOGARTY, B., BAYER, T., *et al* (1984) EE and social networks in parents of schizophrenic patients. *British Journal of Psychiatry*, **144**, 247–255.
——, REISS, D. J. & HOGARTY, C. E. (1986) *Schizophrenia in the Family: a Practitioner's Guide to Psycho-education and Management.* New York: Guilford Press.
BERKOWITZ, R., SHAVIT, N. & LEFF, J. P. (1990) Educating relatives of schizophrenic patients. *Social Psychiatry and Psychiatric Epidemiology*, **25**, 216–220.

BIRCHWOOD, M., SMITH, J., MACMILLAN, F., *et al* (1989) Predicting relapse in schizophrenia: the development and implementation of an early signs monitoring system using patients and families as observers, a preliminary investigation. *Psychological Medicine*, **19**, 649–656.

BIRTCHNELL, J. & KENNARD, J. (1983) Does marital maladjustment lead to mental illness? *Social Psychiatry*, **18**, 79–88.

BREWIN, C. R., WING, J. K., MANGEN, S. P., *et al* (1987) Principles and practice of measuring needs in the long-term mentally ill: the MRC Needs for Care Assessment. *Psychological Medicine*, **17**, 971–981.

———, ———, ———, *et al* (1988) Needs for care among the long-term mentally ill: a report from the Camberwell High Contact Survey. *Psychological Medicine*, **18**, 457–468

———, MACCARTHY, B., DUDA, K., *et al* (1991) Attribution and expressed emotion in the relatives of patients with schizophrenia. *Journal of Abnormal Psychology*, **100**, 546–554.

BROOKER, C., TARRIER, N., BARROWCLOUGH, C., *et al* (1992) Training community psychiatric nurses for psychosocial intervention: report of a pilot study. *British Journal of Psychiatry*, **160**, 836–844.

BROWN, G.W. (1967) The family of the schizophrenic patient. In *Recent Developments in Schizophrenia* (eds A. J. Coppen & A. Walk), pp. 43–59. London: Royal Medico-Psychological Association.

———, BONE, M., DALISON, B., *et al* (1966) *Schizophrenia and Social Care*. Oxford: Oxford University Press.

CLAUSEN, J. A. & YARROW, M. R. (1955a) The impact of mental illness on the family. *Journal of Social Issues*, **11**, 3–64.

———, ———, DEASY, L. C., *et al* (1955b) The impact of mental illness: research formulation. *Journal of Social Issues*, **11**, 6–11.

COLLINS, J., KREITMAN, N., NELSON, B., *et al* (1971) Neurosis and marital interaction: III. Family roles and functions. *British Journal of Psychiatry*, **119**, 233–242.

CREER, C. & WING, J.K. (1974) *Schizophrenia at Home*. Surbiton: National Schizophrenia Fellowship.

———, STURT, E. & WYKES, T. (1982) The role of relatives. In *Long-Term Community Care: Experience in a London Borough* (ed. Wing J. K.), pp. 29–39. *Psychological Medicine*, Monograph Supplement No. 2.

DEASY, L. C. & QUINN, O. W. (1955) The wife of the mental patient and the hospital psychiatrist. *Journal of Social Issues*, **11**, 49–60.

FADDEN, G. B., BEBBINGTON, P. E. & KUIPERS, L. (1987a) The burden of care: the impact of functional psychiatric illness on the patient's family. *British Journal of Psychiatry*, **150**, 285–292.

———, KUIPERS, L. & BEBBINGTON, P. E. (1987b) Caring and its burdens: a study of the relatives of depressed patients. *British Journal of Psychiatry*, **151**, 660–667.

FALLOON, I. R. H., BOYD, J. L., MCGILL, C. W., *et al* (1982) Family management in the prevention of exacerbations of schizophrenia. A controlled study. *New England Journal of Medicine*, **306**, 1437–1440.

———, ——— & ——— (1984) *Family Care of Schizophrenia*. New York: Guilford Press.

———, ———, ———, *et al* (1985) Family management in the prevention of morbidity of schizophrenia. Clinical outcome of a two year longitudinal study. *Archives of General Psychiatry*, **42**, 887–896.

GIBBONS, J. S., HORN, S. H., POWELL, J. M., *et al* (1984) Schizophrenic patients and their families. A survey in a psychiatric service based on a district general hospital. *British Journal of Psychiatry*, **144**, 70–77.

GOLDBERG, D. & HUXLEY, P. (1980) *Mental Illness in The Community*. London: Tavistock.

GRAD, J. & SAINSBURY, P. (1963a) Evaluating a community care service. In *Trends in Mental Health Services* (eds J. Farndale & H. Freeman), pp. 303-317. New York: MacMillan.

——— & ——— (1963b) Mental illness and the family. *Lancet*, **i**, 544–547

——— & ——— (1968) The effects that patients have on their families in a community care and a control psychiatric service: a two year follow-up. *British Journal of Psychiatry*, **114**, 265–278.

GOLDBERG, D. P. & HILLIER, V. G. (1979) A scaled version of the GHQ. *Psychological Medicine*, **9**, 139–146.

HAMILTON, N. G., PONZOHA, C. A., CUTLER, P. L., *et al* (1989) Social networks and negative versus positive symptoms of schizophrenia. *Schizophrenia Bulletin*, **15**, 625–633.

HAMMEN, C., ADRIAN, C., GORDON, D., *et al* (1987) Children of depressed mothers: maternal strain & symptoms as predictors of dysfunction. *Journal of Abnormal Psychology*, **96**, 190–198.

HATFIELD, A., SPANIOL, L. & ZIPPLE, A. M. (1987) Expressed emotion: a family perspective. *Schizophrenia Bulletin*, **13**, 221–226.

HINCHCLIFF, M. K., HOOPER, D., & ROBERTS, F. J. (1978) *The Melancholy Marriage*. Chichester: John Wiley.

HIRSCH, B. J., MOOR, R. H. & REISCHL, T. L. (1985) Psychological adjustment of adolescent children of a depressed, arthritic or normal parent. *Journal of Abnormal Psychology*, **94**, 154–164.

HOENIG, J. & HAMILTON, M. W. (1966) The schizophrenic patient in the community and his effect on the household. *International Journal of Social Psychiatry*, **12**, 165–176.

—— & —— (1969) *The Desegregation of the Mentally Ill*. London: Routledge and Kegan Paul.

HOFFMAN, H. & HUBSCHMID, T. (1989) The social dependence of the long-term patient: a study in social psychiatric ambulatory care. *Psychiatrie Praxis*, **16**, 1–7.

HOGARTY, E. G., ANDERSON, C. M., REISS, D. J., *et al* (1986) Family psychoeducation, social skills training and maintenance of chemotherapy in the aftercare of schizophrenia. *Archives of General Psychiatry*, **43**, 633–642.

JACKSON, H. T., SMITH, N. & McGORRY, P. (1990) Relationship between EE and family burden in psychotic disorders: an exploratory study. *Acta Psychiatrica Scandinavica*, **82**, 243–249.

KREISMAN, D. E. & JOY, V. D. (1974) Family response to the mental illness of a relative: a review of the literature. *Schizophrenia Bulletin*, **10**, 34–57.

KREITMAN, N. (1964) The patient's spouse. *British Journal of Psychiatry*, **110**, 159–173.

——, COLLINS, J., NELSON, B., *et al* (1970) Neurosis and marital interaction: I.Personality and symptoms. *British Journal of Psychiatry*, **117**, 33–46.

KUIPERS, L. (1987) Depression and the family. In *Coping with Disorder in the Family* (ed. J. Orford). London: Croom Helm.

—— & BEBBINGTON, P. (1985) Relatives as a resource in the management of functional illness. *British Journal of Psychiatry*, **147**, 465–470.

—— & —— (1987) *Living with Mental Illness*. London: Souvenir Press.

—— & —— (1988) Expressed emotion research in schizophrenia: theoretical and clinical implications. *Psychological Medicine*, **18**, 893–909.

—— & —— (1990) *Working in Partnership: Clinicians and Carers in the Management of Long-standing Mental Illness*. Oxford: Heinemann Press.

——, MacCARTHY, B., HURRY, J., *et al* (1989) Counselling the relatives of the long-term adult mentally ill: (ii) a low cost supportive model. *British Journal of Psychiatry*, **154**, 775–782.

——, LEFF, J. & LAM, D. (1992) *Family Work for Schizophrenia: A Practical Guide*. London: Gaskell.

LEFF, J., KUIPERS, L., BERKOWITZ, R., *et al* (1982) A controlled trial of social intervention in the families of schizophrenic patients. *British Journal of Psychiatry*, **141**, 121–134.

——, ——, ——, *et al* (1985) A controlled trial of social intervention in the families of schizophrenic patients. Two year follow up. *British Journal of Psychiatry*, **146**, 594–600.

—— & VAUGHN, C. (1985) *Expressed Emotion in Families*. London: Guilford Press.

——, BERKOWITZ, R., SHAVIT, N., *et al* (1989) A trial of family therapy versus a relatives' group for schizophrenics. *British Journal of Psychiatry*, **154**, 58–66.

LEFLEY, H. P. (1987) Ageing parents as care givers of mentally ill adult children: an emerging social problem. *Hospital and Community Psychiatry*, **38**, 1063–1070.

MacCARTHY, B. (1988) The role of relatives. In *Community Care in Practice* (eds A. Lavender & F. Holloway). Chichester: John Wiley.

——, KUIPERS, L., HURRY, J., *et al* (1989a) Counselling the relatives of the long-term adult mentally ill: evaluation of the impact on relatives and patients. *British Journal of Psychiatry*, **154**, 768–775.

——, LESAGE, A., BREWIN, C. R., *et al* (1989b) Needs for care among the relatives of long-term users of day-care. *Psychological Medicine*, **19**, 725–736.

McMILLAN, J. F., GOLD, A., CROW, T. J., *et al* (1986) The Northwick Park Study of first episodes of schizophrenia: IV. Expressed emotion and relapse. *British Journal of Psychiatry*, **148**, 133–143.

MANDELBROTE, B. M. & FOLKARD, S. (1961a) Some problems and needs of schizophrenics in relation to a developing psychiatric community service. *Comprehensive Psychiatry*, **2**, 317–328.

—— & —— (1961b) Some factors related to outcome and social adjustment in schizophrenia. *Acta Psychiatrica Scandinavica*, **37**, 223–235.

MILLS, E. (1962) *Living with Mental Illness: A Study in East London*. London: Routledge and Kegan Paul.

MINTZ, L. I., LIBERMAN, R. P., MIKLOWITZ, D. J., et al (1987) Expressed emotion: a call for partnership among relatives, patients and professionals. *Schizophrenia Bulletin*, **13**, 227–235.

MOORE, E., BALL, R. & KUIPERS, L. (1991) Expressed emotion in staff working with the long-term adult mentally ill. *British Journal of Psychiatry* (in press).

NELSON, B., COLLINS J., KREITMAN, N., et al (1970) Neurosis and marital interaction: II. Time-sharing and social activity. *British Journal of Psychiatry*, **117**, 47–58.

NOH, S. & TURNER, R. J. (1987) Living with psychiatric patients: implications for the mental health of family members. *Social Science and Medicine*, **25**, 263–272.

OVENSTONE, I. M. K. (1973a) The development of neurosis in the wives of neurotic men. Part I: Symptomatology and personality. *British Journal of Psychiatry*, **122**, 33–43.

—— (1973b) The development of neurosis in the wives of neurotic men. Part 2: Marital role functions and marital tension. *British Journal of Psychiatry*, **122**, 711–717.

PAI, S. & KAPUR, R. L. (1981) The burden on the family of a psychiatric patient: development of an interview schedule. *British Journal of Psychiatry*, **138**, 332–335.

PLATT, S. (1985) Measuring the burden of psychiatric illness in the family: an evaluation of some rating scales. *Psychological Medicine*, **15**, 383–393.

——, WEYMAN, A. & HIRSCH, S. (1983) *Social Behaviour Assessment Schedule (SBA)* (3rd edn). Windsor, Berks: NFER, Nelson.

REYNOLDS, I., JONES, J. E., BERRY, D. W., et al (1990) A crisis team for the mentally ill: the effect on patients, relatives and admissions. *Medical Journal of Australia*, **152**, 646–652.

SMITH, J. & BIRCHWOOD, M. J. (1987) Specific and non-specific effects of educational intervention with families living with a schizophrenic relative. *British Journal of Psychiatry*, **150**, 645–652.

STEVENS, B. (1972) Dependence of schizophrenic patients on elderly relatives. *Psychological Medicine*, **2**, 17–32.

TARRIER, N., BARROWCLOUGH, C., BAMRAH, J. S., et al (1988) The community management of schizophrenia: a controlled trial of behavioural intervention with families to reduce relapse. *British Journal of Psychiatry*, **153**, 532–542.

WATERS, M. A. & NORTHOVER, J. (1965) Rehabilitated long-stay schizophrenics in the community. *British Journal of Psychiatry*, **111**, 258–267.

WATTS, F. N. & BENNETT, D. H. (1983) *Theory and Practice of Psychiatric Rehabilitation*. Chichester: John Wiley.

WATTS, S. (1988) *A Descriptive Investigation of the Incidence of High EE in Staff Working with Schizophrenic Patients in a Hospital Setting*. Unpublished dissertation for Diploma in Clinical Psychology. Leicester: British Psychological Society.

WING, J. K., MONCK, E., BROWN, G. W., et al (1964) Morbidity in the community of schizophrenic patients discharged from London mental hospitals in 1959. *British Journal of Psychiatry*, **110**, 10–21.

——, COOPER, J. E. & SARTORIUS, N. (1974) *Measurement and Classification of Psychiatric Symptoms*. Cambridge: Cambridge University Press.

WYKES, T. & STURT, E. (1986) The measurement of social behaviour in psychiatric patients: an assessment of the reliability and validity of the SBS schedule. *British Journal of Psychiatry*, **148**, 1–11.

YARROW, M., CLAUSEN, J. & ROBBINS, P. (1955a) The social meaning of mental illness. *Journal of Social Issues*, **11**, 33–48.

——, SCHWARTZ, C. G., MURPHY, H. S., et al (1955b) The psychological meaning of mental illness in the family. *Journal of Social Issues*, **11**, 12–24.

18 Measuring and meeting mental health needs

JOHN WING, GRAHAM THORNICROFT and CHRIS R. BREWIN

This book is about methods of ensuring that clinical and administrative attempts to meet mental health needs are better informed and therefore potentially more rational and useful. Measurement in mental health depends upon achieving conceptual clarity, but the complexities are such that it is impossible to avoid controversy. This makes public discussion and debate essential. The clearer the definitions are, the more precise the measurements will be, and therefore the more sharply focused the debate.

It is fair to say that all the contributors to the book are dissatisfied with the statistical information currently available, whether for clinical or managerial purposes. The dissatisfaction would have been even more marked if the net had been spread more widely, to include primary care and social services. Several authors (Chapters 2, 3, 7 and 8) have emphasised that the focus of care has been shifting rapidly from a specialist context towards a community approach in which the present administrative boundaries of social services and primary care have become obstacles to progress. There have always been opportunities to cross them, exploited by forward-looking collaborators from the different camps, but this depended on individual initiatives and chance groupings. Now the impetus is such that a degree of integration between information systems is becoming inevitable.

We have limited the scope of the book to information and audit systems serving specialist mental health services because this is where most current expertise and pioneering work is located. However, the principles involved are no different for general practice, local authorities, or other organisations involved in mental health care. The Salford Case Register (Chapter 5) has long collected data from health services and social services alike. Experience with the Read codes in general practice has led to their modification for use in specialist settings (Chapter 14).

The overlap of services necessitated when specialist carers operate from Community Mental Health Centres is already leading to shared local registers.

Because of their wide distribution, their broad spectrum of type and severity, and their effects on social functioning, mental disorders are characteristic of conditions that require common information systems to meet community health needs. Because laboratory investigations have not, up to now, been as helpful as in other areas of medicine, greater expertise has had to be acquired in the accurate delineation and measurement of mental symptoms, behavioural problems, diagnostic criteria, social disablement and disadvantage, and quality of the social environment. This experience is highly relevant for other disciplines in medicine, even those most technologically based, as well as for the caring professions beyond medicine. We suggest therefore that the content of the book can be applied with suitable modifications to most other situations where good quality data are necessary to determine care. To give only one example, the MRC Needs for Care Assessment has been adapted to measure the needs of patients with diabetes (Brewin *et al*, 1991).

The definitions of need in Chapters 1 and 13 are clinical, while that in Chapter 3 expresses the purchaser's view, but they are largely identical. Clinicians, in their role as providers, are interested in measuring and meeting the needs of each individual receiving their service (individually-based need); the purchaser is concerned with measuring and meeting the aggregated needs of the population (epidemiologically-based need). Much of this book is concerned with the relationship between the two dimensions of need. It seems axiomatic that the more accurate and reliable the observations at the clinical level, the better will be the planning decisions for the community at large, and the more useful will be the local, regional, and national statistics.

At the level of individual care there is considerable scope for adopting more systematic and comprehensive treatment plans. At present, care is largely determined by the beliefs and preferences of individual clinicians and by the constraints of local provision. This is perfectly adequate when patients respond to the treatment offered, but may not be either efficient or effective for patients who respond only partially or not at all. In a survey of the long-term mentally ill in Camberwell (Brewin *et al*, 1988), there were many examples both of impoverished ideas about the possible range of treatment strategies and of persistence with ineffective treatments, in other words, overprovision. Similarly, Brugha *et al* (1992) have found that standard treatment of depression by psychiatrists is frequently marred by inadequate doses of antidepressant medication.

Without a treatment protocol there is a risk that in many cases some viable treatment options will not be considered systematically, and that, in the absence of alternatives, ineffective treatments will be continued for too long. A treatment protocol can ensure that a minimum set of treatment options are routinely considered and, where possible, implemented. The MRC Needs for Care Assessment described in Chapter 13, which embodies a simplified model of care for the long-term mentally ill, spelling out specific treatment options and implementation rules, represents a first step towards such a protocol. Similar protocols could be of benefit in many other areas of mental health, particularly in the acute services.

Alongside the development of more formal care plans, meeting needs depends on close monitoring of service effectiveness. Parry (1992) outlines how psychotherapy services could be improved by incorporating principles of audit and evaluation routinely. Following Maxwell (1984), she proposes six criteria on which to judge the success of a service: is it relevant and appropriate, is it equitable, is it available, is it acceptable, is it effective, and is it efficient? The latter two criteria should be fulfilled by the existence of care plans and protocols, and by routine monitoring of outcome. The first four criteria are useful for assessing whether there is a match between the needs (both self-defined and professionally defined) of a local target population and the type of care offered. Even if the service offers effective and efficient treatments, the population needs may still remain unmet if the problems are of a different kind, if some users are unfairly excluded on grounds such as race or class, if there are geographical or administrative blocks impeding access to the service, or if the care offered is unacceptable to users.

Evidence accumulated over more than two decades has shown that service use varies with local indices such as household composition, social isolation, poverty, and ethnicity, as well as age and sex. Marital status was usefully incorporated into the old Resources Allocation Working Party (RAWP) formula for psychiatric services on the basis of this evidence. Regrettably, the mechanism most recently proposed reverts to the Standardised Mortality Rate (SMR), which is not an effective measure of morbidity. Chapter 4 reviews the use of a range of indices and concludes that marital status would still be an appropriate index to use. The Jarman score also has some merit because of the weight of empirical evidence brought forward (Thornicroft *et al*, 1992). Local targets would thus be set for local needs rather than on the basis of average national 'norms'. Although the Jarman score has been incorporated in part into the funding formula for primary-care practitioners, the mechanism that is proposed for weighted capitation allowances to hospital services is based upon the SMR, as detailed in Chapter 4. It seems probable that this will underestimate the extent to which areas of greater material poverty make greater use of mental health services. The result is likely to be a relative diversion of funding away from inner-city services, with a commensurately greater difficulty in meeting needs at the service level (Kings Fund Commission of London, 1992).

Related to this, it is difficult to foresee that the proportion of meetable needs can be increased even for the most seriously disabled target groups unless an effective mechanism is introduced rapidly to protect (or 'ring-fence') mental health expenditure from predation from other health and social-service demands.

The new arrangements may forge alliances between statutory and voluntary agencies that have hitherto been moribund. This may occur, for example, between psychiatric services and housing departments through joint-assessment procedures or through effectively purchased 'packages' of care for the seriously mentally ill. In the near future, many localities will install small individual databases or local-area networks to provide the information infrastructure to support purchasing and service-provision decisions, and by the end of the decade these may have effectively crossed the boundaries between health-service, social-service and voluntary agencies to allow fuller data integration, with all the resulting ethical implications (see Chapter 14). It is clear that putting local and needs-led services in place will require a balance between establishing enduring systems of collaborative care, and responding pragmatically to opportunities that arise in practice, often at short notice.

The content and structure of mental health information systems (MHIS)

Earlier sections of this book (Chapters 5 and 14) deal with systems for the routine collection of mental health information. They recommend adopting the structure of the psychiatric case register, in which dated contacts with specified agencies or agents are recorded and relevant clinical data entered (ten Horn, 1986; Wing, 1989). There is an enormous variety of computerised MHIS, each with its own profile and advantages. A national lead is necessary to provide a minimum specification that would be common to all. A representative group from the Royal College of Psychiatrists has drafted recommendations on minimum technical and data speci-fications. National standards – 'The Data Manual' and the 'Clinical Terms Project' – are also in preparation. These will help determine the common content of the systems, which should be able to accommodate local variations in information requirements.

National direction is needed on how local services should develop information systems to support clinical work, and the idea of a 'virtual case register' that rests within a computerised clinical information-support system has much to recommend it (see Chapter 5). In this case, detailed central leadership, for example from the Royal College of Psychiatrists, is needed on minimum technical and data specifications, so that local modifications can be added to this common core. It may then be helpful for purchasing consortia, or regions, to establish information support units to oversee local and wide-area network commissioning, installation, maintenance and development, along with data quality assurance procedures. A minimum clinical data set can be collected for local use in all districts, also guaranteeing a minimum set of local, regional, and national statistics. This dataset should, however, act as the top level of a more complex structure, each item leading to options for a more detailed description of problems, interventions, outcomes and costs.

This broader context within which assessment of mental health needs must be discussed raises complex ethical issues that require separate discussion. There is an ethical duty to provide the most effective service possible and therefore to base all decisions, from individual face-to-face assessment and care to the planning and monitoring of effective service delivery, on good quality information. At the same time there is an ethical duty to preserve confidentiality and to protect from adventitious harm (ten Horn *et al*, 1986). Informing patients or clients of their rights to access such MHIS under the Data Protection Act is also essential. Further problems will be met when proposals are made to merge registers across professional boundaries. However, the main difficulty is likely to be getting agreement on shared access to identifiable data, under strict local security. If that can be reached, there should be no difficulty in maintaining confidentiality.

Far-reaching policy changes embodied in the *NHS and Community Care Act* (House of Commons, 1990) ensure that the way in which local mental health services will be developed for the remainder of the 1990s will be substantially different from the past. The division between the service purchasing and provision roles of health authorities has already seen an amalgamation of many adjacent districts for purchasing purposes, and it now seems likely that these consortia will formally merge with Family Health Service Authorities (FHSAs) by 1995, although details are still unclear. This will serve to integrate primary and secondary levels of health care even further, but at the same time may partially or fully erase the significance of previous district health authority boundaries, with mixed economies of social and health providers within each larger consortium area (Audit Commission, 1992). Secondly, fund-holding primary-care practices will play an increasingly forceful role in this modified market place, and will be able to negotiate service criteria that meet their agenda for service needs more fully. Against this, the newly established remit of public-health departments, on the purchasing side (see Chapter 3), will aim to estimate at the population level, and later to measure, a 'local-needs profile' as the starting point for service contracting. The resultant of all these newly established vectors is, in 1992, difficult to predict, but we can expect that the respect traditionally accorded to established patterns of service provision will rapidly become a mark of nostalgia rather than practice.

Many opportunities now exist that allow more rational planning of services for a local community – such as a health district or sector – if both the will to achieve change and the information on which to continuously monitor and adjust it are available together. Much can be achieved by either alone, but the combination would be unstoppable. In this new arena, what changes are required for clinicians to make the transition from service-led to needs-led provision? As the roles of the districts and the regions become more indistinct, we propose that this transition needs to be considered at two levels: the local and the national.

At the local level, positive changes in the following areas will facilitate services that may more closely correspond to needs. The development of local consortia of stakeholders (see Chapter 7) will broaden the base of those claiming to define service needs. In particular, users of services and their informal carers have not yet been adequately involved in designing services which are meant to meet their needs. Further, jointly purchased, and later jointly commissioned, provision will tend to attenuate what many practitioners, at least from the health-service perspective, see as a divisive and destructive definitional split between 'health' and 'social' care. Carefully considered, locally developed and locally evaluated models of care management, which can draw the purchaser/provider dividing line at different levels within social service departments (SSDs) and also examine outcomes, will help to establish how to put into practice the still notional 'lead' role of SSDs in community care (Social Service Inspectorate 1991*a*, *b*). This will be especially true where local conditions point to specific service gaps, for example for the homeless mentally ill (see Chapter 16).

At the national level, detailed guidance is required on definitions, information, mechanisms, and targets. First, as was mentioned earlier in relation to 'serious mental illness', much planning and implementation of mental health services occurs in a definitional vacuum. Most key terms are not operationally defined. To take a number of examples, no agreement has been established on what respite care, new long-stay, dual-diagnosis, sector, or sheltered work mean. Until and unless there is such a centrally coordinated dissemination of terminology, comparisons between local areas will remain schematic and the results of coordinated needs-led planning will not be comparable between areas.

To move beyond this reliance on scraps of out-of-date information (in recent public-health reports, for example, relying upon data from case registers recorded up to 30 years ago, upon surveys conducted 20 years ago, upon information gathered in North America 15 years ago, or upon census data now 11 years out of date), we require two kinds of tool. Firstly, we need brief, standardised outcome assessments of social and clinical functioning in important areas of ability and disability (see

Chapters 1 and 2) that can be easily learned and reliably used in a wide range of settings. There are plenty of well-investigated but lengthy instruments to use for 'validation' purposes. Secondly, we require coordination by and for public-health doctors on the most important measures of local morbidity that can be routinely collected in every area, and which can be assembled at national level. The replacement of the Mental Health Enquiry data by Körner and Health Service Indicator data in the 1980s was in this respect in many ways regressive.

A national lead is also required now to refine and disseminate needs-assessment mechanisms. This book shows that a wide variety of approaches can portray the needs of patients or clients as individuals or as groups. It remains true, however, that these, even in combination, contribute only a partial understanding of the total needs in each local area, and that many of the sources identified here are missing or incomplete in most localities. We therefore find ourselves in the situation of archaeologists uncovering fragments of information from different periods of the past, and attempting to assemble these shards into a mosaic that is meaningful.

Planning needs-led services for the future

For long-term planning of service developments, we suggest that the discipline of setting targets will be invaluable. Indeed, Prince Charles put forward such a view to the Annual Meeting of the Royal College of Psychiatrists at Brighton in 1991:

> "The time for debate about whether locally based forms of care should supplant traditional institutions is over . . . we should now formulate and co-ordinate clear mental health targets and strategies at each level to achieve their implementation over the next decade."

Setting service targets is a means to direct services along agreed paths, for example towards being more fully needs-led, and to set benchmarks of achievement against which actual progress can be measured. The recent White Paper *The Health of the Nation* (Department of Health, 1992), creates an opportunity to initiate target-setting for mental health services. It may, for example, supplement the work of advisory and inspectorate agencies (see Chapter 10) in establishing minimum levels of services in each local area, since we know that districts vary enormously in their levels and ranges of provisions, and that whole categories of services may be entirely absent (Thornicroft, 1988; Wing, 1992). We therefore propose that local service needs should not be estimated by national norms, of the type set out in *Better Services for the Mentally Ill* (Department of Health and Social Security, 1975). Rather, having established basic minima, it may be better to set target ranges, acknowledging that areas differ considerably, that we should focus on the number of 'places' needed rather than on 'beds', and that provisions within service categories are highly interdependent, as indicated in Chapter 8.

While attempting in this book to set out clearly the state of the art of needs assessment for mental health, we must also place this rational approach within the wider context of changes in the British National Health Service – for we work among dangers and opportunities. The dangers offered by the progressive division between purchasers/commissioners and providers of services is that the former will aggregate to the supradistrict level (sometimes coterminous with old Area Health Authorities) to optimise purchasing power and to attract sufficient public health expertise, while the providers reduce in size to service units. In both cases the geographical identity with, and responsibility for, the health district (usually about a quarter of a million population) is lost. In particular, service providers will increasingly be bound and driven by the service contracts which will specify costs, volume, and quality criteria, but which have no necessary link with the measured or estimated needs of the whole local population. Equally, at the purchaser level, as Farrow (1991) has shown in a survey of District Public Reports, there is in most districts insufficient interest or expertise in assessment of mental health needs even to warrant mention. This split therefore invites the fragmentation palpable in many parts of the mental health system in the United States.

At the same time, there is within SSDs a real danger that the 1990 *NHS and Community Care Act* will be enacted only in the statutory requirements (making client needs assessments) rather than in the discretionary elements (delivering the consequent care). This is especially likely if the Social Services Inspectorate guidance is adopted: that a 'brokerage' model be used in which case managers have no direct care responsibilities. This would offer an intriguing comparison to the working of the parallel purchaser/provider split: at the authority level for health services, and at the team level in social services.

In parallel with these dangers, the current multiple initiatives affecting how health and social-care agencies provide services offer exceptional opportunities. The requirement to prepare joint community-care plans provides a vehicle in which local agencies may share a common direction. The availability of the Mental Illness Specific Grant does go some way to prime new locally-based services, the requirements of the Care Programme Approach do furnish a mechanism to plan hospital discharge and to coordinate care, and the assumption of the planning remit by purchasing authorities does set a framework within which the definition of needs can be attempted, and substitution of service-led by needs-led priorities may be required.

All these centripetal and centrifugal forces are powerfully active within the mental health services in Britain in the early 1990s. We hope this book will focus attention on the possibility that intentions to introduce needs-led services will be frustrated by an uncontrolled entrepreneurial diversity, leading to widely different standards of care. The way to avoid such a danger is to ensure that top-down epidemiologically-based commissioning and quality control interact at all levels with bottom-up clinical information about how far population and individual needs are being met.

References

AUDIT COMMISSION (1992) *Community Care: Managing the Cascade of Change*. London: HMSO.
BREWIN, C. R., WING, J. K., MANGEN, S. P., *et al* (1988) Needs for care among the long-term mentally ill: a report from the Camberwell High Contact Survey. *Psychological Medicine*, **18**, 457–468.
——— , BRADLEY, C. & HOME, P. (1991) Measuring needs in patients with diabetes. In *The Technology of Diabetes Care: Converging Medical and Psychosocial Perspectives* (eds C. Bradley, P. Home & M. Christie). Reading: Harwood.
BRUGHA, T. S., BEBBINGTON, P. E., MACCARTHY, B., *et al* (1992) Antidepressant may not assist recovery in practice: a naturalistic prospective survey. *Acta Psychiatrica Scandinavica*, **86**, 5–11.
DEPARTMENT OF HEALTH AND SOCIAL SECURITY (1975) *Better Services for the Mentally Ill*, Cmnd 6233. London: HMSO.
DEPARTMENT OF HEALTH (1991) *The Health of the Nation*. London: HMSO.
FARROW, S. (1991) Introduction to annual reports of public health. In *Indicators for Mental Health in the Population* (eds R. Jenkins & S. Griffiths). London: HMSO.
HOUSE OF COMMONS (1990) *National Health Service and Community Care Act*. London: HMSO.
KINGS FUND COMMISSION ON LONDON (1992) *London Health Care 2010: Changing the Future of Health Services in the Capital*. London: Kings Fund.
MAXWELL, R. J. (1984) Quality assessment in health. *British Medical Journal*, **288**, 1470–1472.
PARRY, G. (1992) Improving psychotherapy services: applications of research, audit and evaluation. *British Journal of Clinical Psychology*, **31**, 3–19.
SOCIAL SERVICES INSPECTORATE (1991*a*) *Care Management and Assessment. Practitioners' Guide*. London: HMSO.
——— (1991*b*) *Care Management and Assessment. Managers' Guide*. London: HMSO.
TEN HORN, G., GIEL, R., GULBINAT, W., *et al* (1986) *Case Registers in Public Health: a Worldwide Inventory*. Amsterdam: Elsevier.
THORNICROFT, G. (1988) Progress towards DHSS targets for community care. *British Journal of Psychiatry*, **153**, 257–258.
——— , MARGOLIUS, O. & JONES, D. (1992) The TAPS project 6. New-long stay psychiatric patients and social deprivation. *British Journal of Psychiatry*, **161**, 621–624.
WING, J. (ed.) (1989) *Health Services Planning and Research. Contributions from Psychiatric Case Registers*. London: Gaskell.
——— (1992) *Epidemiologically-Based Mental Health Needs Assessment*. London: Department of Health.

Index

Compiled by Stanley Thorley